CORPVS MEDICORVM GRAECORVM

EDIDIT

ACADEMIA BEROLINENSIS ET BRANDENBVRGENSIS
CVM ACADEMIIS HAVNIENSI ATQVE LIPSIENSI

V 3,2

GALENI

DE PROPRIIS PLACITIS

EDIDIT, IN LINGVAM ANGLICAM VERTIT,
COMMENTATVS EST

VIVIAN NUTTON

IN AEDIBVS ACADEMIAE SCIENTIARVM

GALEN

ON MY OWN OPINIONS

EDITION, TRANSLATION AND COMMENTARY
BY
VIVIAN NUTTON

AKADEMIE VERLAG

Dieser Band wurde durch die Bund-Länder-Kommission für Bildungsplanung
und Forschungsförderung im Akademienprogramm mit Mitteln des Bundes (Bundesministerium
für Bildung, Wissenschaft, Forschung und Technologie) und des Landes Berlin
(Senatsverwaltung für Wissenschaft, Forschung und Kultur) gefördert.

Die Deutsche Bibliothek - CIP-Einheitsaufnahme

Galenus :
On my own opinions / Galen. Ed., transl. and commentary
by Vivian Nutton. - Berlin : Akad. Verl., 1999
(Corpus medicorum Graecorum ; 5,3,2)
Einheitssacht.: De propriis placitis
Parallelsacht.: Galeni De propriis placitis
ISBN 3-05-003340-1

ISSN 0070-0347

Der Akademie Verlag ist ein Unternehmen der R. Oldenbourg-Gruppe.

Das eingesetzte Papier ist alterungsbeständig nach DIN/ISO 9706.

Druck und Bindung: Druckhaus „Thomas Müntzer“, Bad Langensalza

Printed in the Federal Republic of Germany

TABLE OF CONTENTS

Bibliography 7
Introduction 14
A. The sources for the text 14
I. The Greek manuscripts 14
a) Parisinus gr. 2332 14
b) Vindobonensis med. gr. 15 15
c) Parisinus suppl. gr. 634 15
d) Neapolitanus III.D.15 (229) 16
e) Yalensis 234 16
f) Parisinus gr. 2147 16
g) Ambrosianus gr. 659 17
h) Laurentianus gr. 74,5 18
i) Marcianus gr. 281 18
j) Parisinus suppl. gr. 35 19
k) Codex Adelphi 19
II. The relationship between the Greek manuscripts 21
III. The Arabo-Latin translation 22
a) Parisinus lat. 6865 23
b) Malatestianus S.V 4 23
c) Dresdensis Db 92 24
d) Parisinus Academicus 51 25
e) Biturigensis 299 (247) 25
f) The lost Paris manuscript 25
IV. The relationship between the Latin manuscripts 27
V. Date and authorship of the Arabo-Latin translation 29
VI. The Arabo-Latin translation and the Greek original 30
VII. The excerpt in Hebrew translation 31
VIII. The Graeco-Latin translation of chapters 14–15 (= De substantia) 33
a) Parisinus lat. 6865 33
b) Malatestianus S.V 4 33
c) Malatestianus S.XXVI 4 34
d) Matritensis lat. 1978 34
e) Monacensis lat. 490 34
f) Neapolitanus VIII D 38 34
g) Wellcomensis 286 34
IX. The relationship between the Latin manuscripts of De substantia 35
X. Authorship of the Graeco-Latin translation 36
XI. The Graeco-Latin translation and the Greek manuscripts 36
B. The textual history of De propriis placitis 37
C. Editorial principles 45
D. De propriis placitis and Greek autobiography 45
Text and translation 51
Commentary 126

Indices 219
A. Index nominum Graecorum 219
B. Index verborum Graecorum 219
C. Index nominum Latinorum 228
D. Index verborum Latinorum 230
E. Index nominum Hebraicorum 246
F. Index verborum Hebraicorum 246
G. Voces Arabicae Latinis litteris scriptae 247

BIBLIOGRAPHY[1]

Alcinoos, Enseignement des doctrines de Platon, ed. and comm. J. Whittaker, transl. P. Louis, Paris, 1990 (Collection des Universités de France)

Alexandri Aphrodisiensis praeter commentaria scripta minora: De anima liber cum Mantissa, ed. I. Bruns, Berlin, 1887 (Supplementum Aristotelicum II 1)

– In Aristotelis Topicorum libros octo commentaria, ed. M. Wallies, CAG II 2, Berlin, 1891

– praeter commentaria scripta minora: Quaestiones, De fato, De mixtione, ed. I. Bruns, Berlin, 1892 (Supplementum Aristotelicum II 2)

The refutation by Alexander of Aphrodisias of Galen's treatise on the theory of motion, ed., transl., and comm. N. Rescher and M. E. Marmura, Islamabad, 1965

B. Alexanderson, Galenos, Περὶ κρίσεων. Überlieferung und Text, Gothenburg, 1967 (Studia Graeca et Latina Gothoburgensia XXIII)

M. Th. d'Alverny, review of Iohannis Alexandrini Commentaria in librum De sectis Galeni, ed. C. D. Pritchet, Leiden, 1982, in: Scriptorium 38, 1984, pp. 361–366

Anonymi Londinensis ex Aristotelis iatricis Menoniis et aliis medicis eclogae, ed. H. Diels, Berlin, 1893 (Supplementum Aristotelicum III 1)

ANRW = Aufstieg und Niedergang der Römischen Welt, ed. W. Haase and H. Temporini

Apulei Platonici Madaurensis Opera quae supersunt, vol. III: De philosophia libri, ed. C. Moreschini, Stuttgart and Leipzig, 1991

Archimedis Opera omnia cum commentariis Eutocii, ed. J. L. Heiberg, vol. II, Leipzig, 1913 (repr. Stuttgart, 1972)

Aristarchus see Heath

Aristotelis Opera cum Averrois commentariis, vol. V, Frankfurt a. M., 1962 (repr. of the Juntine edition, Venice, 1562)

– qui ferebatur liber De pomo, versio Latina Manfredi, ed. M. Plezia, Warsaw, 1960 (Auctorum Graecorum et Latinorum opuscula selecta II)

Aristoteles – Werk und Wirkung, P. Moraux gewidmet, ed. J. Wiesner, 2: Kommentierung, Überlieferung, Nachleben, Berlin and New York, 1987

Artemidori Daldiani Onirocriticon libri V, ed. R. A. Pack, Leipzig, 1963

P. Athanassiadi, Philosophers and oracles: shifts of authority in late paganism, Byzantion 62, 1992, pp. 45–62

C. Atherton, The Stoics on ambiguity, Cambridge, 1993

J. Barnes, Galen and the utility of logic, in: Galen und das hellenistische Erbe, pp. 33–52

G. Bergsträßer, Neue Materialien zu Ḥunain ibn Isḥāq's Galen-Bibliographie, Leipzig, 1932 (Abh. f. d. Kunde d. Morgenlandes 19,2)

H. H. Biesterfeldt see Galens Traktat

J. Ch. Bürgel, Averroes „contra Galenum". Das Kapitel von der Atmung im Colliget des Averroes als ein Zeugnis mittelalterlich-islamischer Kritik an Galen, Nachrichten d. Akademie d. Wiss. in Göttingen, philol.-hist. Kl. 1967,9, pp. 276–290

CAG = Commentaria in Aristotelem Graeca

Timaeus a Calcidio translatus commentarioque instructus, ed. J. H. Waszink, London and Leiden, 1962 (Corpus Platonicum Medii Aevi, Plato Latinus IV)

[1] Works cited once are described in full in the appropriate place.

Censorini De die natali liber ad Q. Caerellium, ed. K. Sallmann, Leipzig, 1983
CMG = Corpus Medicorum Graecorum
K. Deichgräber, Die griechische Empirikerschule. Sammlung der Fragmente und Darstellung der Lehre, um Zusätze vermehrter anastatischer Neudruck der Ausgabe von 1930, Berlin and Zurich, 1965
Ph. De Lacy, The third part of the soul, in: Le opere psicologiche, pp. 43–63
– see Galeni De semine
H. Diels, Doxographi Graeci, 2nd ed., Berlin and Leipzig, 1929
– see Galeni In Hippocratis Prorrheticum I comm. III
H. Diels and W. Kranz, Die Fragmente der Vorsokratiker, 3 vols., 7th ed., Berlin, 1954 (= D.-K.)
J. Dillon, The Middle Platonists. A study of Platonism 80 B.C. to A.D. 220, London, 1977
Diogenes of Oinoanda, The Epicurean inscription. Edition with introduction, translation, and notes by M. F. Smith, Naples, 1993 (La scuola di Epicuro, Suppl. 1)
Pedanii Dioscuridis Anazarbei De materia medica libri quinque, ed. M. Wellmann, 3 vols., 2nd ed., Berlin, 1958
D. M. Dunlop, The Muntakhab Ṣiwān al-ḥikmah of Abū Sulaimān as-Sijistānī. Arabic text, introduction and indices, The Hague, Paris, New York 1979 (Near and Middle East Monographs IV)
B. Einarson, A note on the Latin translation of Galen De propriis placitis, Classical Philology 54, 1959, pp. 258–259
Epicuro, Opere. Introduzione, testo critico, traduzione e note di G. Arrighetti, nuova edizione riveduta e ampliata, Turin, 1973 (Biblioteca di cultura filosofica 41)
Erasistrati Fragmenta, ed. I. Garofalo, Pisa, 1988
Eusebius, Werke, Zweiter Band: Die Kirchengeschichte, ed. E. Schwartz; die lateinische Übersetzung des Rufinus, ed. Th. Mommsen, erste Hälfte, Leipzig, 1903 (Die griechischen christlichen Schriftsteller der ersten drei Jahrhunderte 9,1)
D. Frioli, Catalogo di manoscritti filosofici nelle biblioteche italiane, vol. IV, Florence, 1982
Claudii Galeni Opera omnia, ed. C. G. Kühn, 20 vols., Leipzig, 1821–1833 (= K.)
Claudii Galeni Pergameni Scripta minora, ed. J. Marquardt, I. Müller, G. Helmreich, 3 vols., Leipzig, 1884–1893 (repr. Amsterdam, 1967)
Galeni Institutio logica, ed. K. Kalbfleisch, Leipzig, 1896
Galeni De temperamentis libri III, ed. G. Helmreich, Leipzig, 1904 (repr. Stuttgart, 1969)
Galeni De usu partium libri XVII, ed. G. Helmreich, 2 vols., Leipzig, 1907/1909
Galeni De optimo docendi genere, Exhortatio ad medicinam (Protrepticus), ed. and transl. A. Barigazzi, CMG V 1,1, Berlin, 1991
Galeni De elementis ex Hippocratis sententia, ed., transl., and comm. Ph. De Lacy, CMG V 1,2, Berlin, 1996
Galeni De constitutione artis medicae ad Patrophilum, ed. and transl. St. Fortuna, CMG V 1,3, Berlin, 1997
Galeni De semine, ed., transl., and comm. Ph. De Lacy, CMG V 3,1, Berlin, 1992
Galeni De propriorum animi cuiuslibet affectuum dignotione et curatione, De animi cuiuslibet peccatorum dignotione et curatione, De atra bile, ed. W. de Boer, CMG V 4,1,1, Leipzig and Berlin, 1937
Galeni De placitis Hippocratis et Platonis, ed., transl., and comm. Ph. De Lacy, 3 vols., CMG V 4,1,2, Berlin, 1978–1984
Galeni De sanitate tuenda libri VI, ed. K. Koch; De alimentorum facultatibus libri III, ed. G. Helmreich, in: CMG V 4,2, Leipzig and Berlin, 1923
Galeni De praecognitione, ed., transl., and comm. V. Nutton, CMG V 8,1, Berlin, 1979
Galeni In Hippocratis De natura hominis comm. III, ed. J. Mewaldt, in: CMG V 9,1, Leipzig and Berlin, 1914
Galeni In Hippocratis Prorrheticum I comm. III, ed. H. Diels; In Hippocratis Prognosticum comm. III, ed. J. Heeg, in: CMG V 9,2, Leipzig and Berlin, 1915

Galeni In Hippocratis Epidemiarum libr. I comm. III, ed. E. Wenkebach; In Hippocratis Epidemiarum libr. II comm. V, transl. F. Pfaff, CMG V 10,1, Leipzig and Berlin, 1934
– In Hippocratis Epidemiarum libr. III comm. III, ed. E. Wenkebach, CMG V 10,2,1, Leipzig and Berlin, 1936
– In Hippocratis Epidemiarum libr. VI comm. I–VI, ed. E. Wenkebach; comm. VI–VIII, transl. F. Pfaff, CMG V 10,2,2, 2nd ed., Berlin, 1956
Galeni Adversus Lycum et Adversus Iulianum libelli, ed. E. Wenkebach, CMG V 10,3, Berlin, 1951
Galeni In Platonis Timaeum comm. fragmenta, ed. and comm. H. O. Schröder, CMG Suppl. I, Leipzig and Berlin, 1934
Galeni De consuetudinibus, ed. J. M. Schmutte, CMG Suppl. III, Leipzig and Berlin, 1941
Galeni De instrumento odoratus, ed., transl., and comm. J. Kollesch, CMG Suppl. V, Berlin, 1964
Galeni De partibus artis medicativae, De causis contentivis, De diaeta in morbis acutis secundum Hippocratem libellorum versiones Arabicae, ed. and transl. M. Lyons; De partibus artis medicativae, De causis contentivis libellorum editiones alterius ab Hermanno Schoene, alterius a Carolo Kalbfleisch curatae, new ed. by J. Kollesch, D. Nickel, G. Strohmaier, CMG Suppl. Or. II, Berlin, 1969
Galeni De optimo medico cognoscendo libelli versio Arabica, ed., transl., and comm. A. Z. Iskandar, CMG Suppl. Or. IV, Berlin, 1988
Galen, Über die medizinischen Namen, ed. and transl. M. Meyerhof and J. Schacht, Abh. d. Preuß. Akademie d. Wiss. 1931, phil.-hist. Kl. 3, Berlin, 1931
Kitāb al-aḫlāq li-Ǧālīnūs, ed. P. Kraus, Bulletin of the Faculty of Arts of the Egyptian University 5, 1939, pp. 1–51
Galen, On medical experience, ed. and transl. R. Walzer, London, New York, Toronto, 1944
Galeni Compendium Timaei Platonis aliorumque dialogorum synopsis quae extant fragmenta, ed. P. Kraus and R. Walzer, London, 1951 (Corpus Platonicum Medii Aevi, Plato Arabus I)
Galens Traktat ‚Daß die Kräfte der Seele den Mischungen des Körpers folgen' in arabischer Übersetzung, ed. H. H. Biesterfeldt, Wiesbaden, 1973 (Abh. f. d. Kunde d. Morgenlandes 40,4)
Galen's commentary on the Hippocratic treatise Airs, Waters, Places in the Hebrew translation of Solomon ha-Me'ati, ed., transl., and comm. A. Wasserstein, Jerusalem, 1982 (The Israel Academy of Sciences and Humanities, Proceedings VI 3)
Galen on respiration and the arteries. An edition with English translation and commentary of De usu respirationis, An in arteriis natura sanguis contineatur, De usu pulsuum, and De causis respirationis, by D. J. Furley and J. S. Wilkie, Princeton, 1984
Galenus, Anatomicarum administrationum libri qui supersunt novem. Earundem interpretatio arabica Hunaino Isaaci filio ascripta, ed. I. Garofalo, vol. I: libri I–IV, Naples, 1986
Galens Kommentar zu Platons Timaios, ed. C. J. Larrain, Stuttgart, 1992 (Beiträge zur Altertumskunde 29)
Galeni De crisibus see Alexanderson
Galen, De septimestri partu see Walzer, Galens Schrift
Galeni Subfiguratio empirica see Deichgräber, Empirikerschule
[Galen], Ad Gaurum quomodo animetur fetus see Kalbfleisch, Die neuplatonische ... Schrift
Galen und das hellenistische Erbe. Verhandlungen des IV. Internationalen Galen-Symposiums, veranstaltet vom Institut für Geschichte der Medizin am Bereich Medizin (Charité) der Humboldt-Universität zu Berlin, 18. – 20. September 1989, ed. J. Kollesch and D. Nickel, Stuttgart, 1993 (Sudhoffs Archiv, Beih. 32)
Galeno: obra, pensamiento e influencia (Coloquio internacional celebrado en Madrid, 22 – 25 de Marzo de 1988), ed. J. A. López Férez, Madrid, 1991

Galen's Method of healing. Proceedings of the 1982 Galen Symposium, ed. F. Kudlien and R. J. Durling, Leiden et al., 1991 (Studies in Ancient Medicine 1)

L. García Ballester, Soul and body, disease of the soul and disease of the body in Galen's medical thought, in: Le opere psicologiche, pp. 117–152

P. Gas see Pagel, Beiträge

– see Pagel, Concordanciae

al-Ghazālī, *Tahāfut al-falāsifā*, ed. M. Bouyges, Beirut, 1927

Al-Ghazali's Tahafut al-Falasifah (Incoherence of the Philosophers), transl. S. A. Kamali, Lahore, 1958 (Pakistan Philosophical Congress Publication 3)

H. B. Gottschalk, Aristotelian philosophy in the Roman world from the time of Cicero to the end of the second century AD, in: ANRW II 36,2, Berlin and New York, 1987, pp. 1079–1174

Chr. Habicht, Die Inschriften des Asklepieions, Altertümer von Pergamon VIII 3, Berlin, 1969

R. J. Hankinson, Galen on the foundations of science, in: Galeno: obra, pensamiento e influencia, pp. 15–29

–, Galen's anatomy of the soul, Phronesis 36, 1991, pp. 197–233

–, Galen, On the therapeutic method, books I and II, transl. with an introduction and commentary, Oxford, 1991

G. Harig, Bestimmung der Intensität im medizinischen System Galens. Ein Beitrag zur theoretischen Pharmakologie, Nosologie und Therapie in der Galenischen Medizin, Berlin, 1974 (Schriften zur Geschichte und Kultur der Antike 11)

C. R. S. Harris, The heart and the vascular system in ancient Greek medicine from Alcmaeon to Galen, Oxford, 1973

Th. Heath, Aristarchus of Samos. The ancient Copernicus. A history of Greek astronomy to Aristarchus together with Aristarchus's treatise of the sizes and distances of the sun and moon. A new Greek text with translation and notes, Oxford, 1913 (repr. Bristol, 1993)

G. Helmreich, Galeni περὶ τῶν ἑαυτῷ δοκούντων fragmenta inedita, Philologus 52, 1894, pp. 431–434

Hierokles, Ethische Elementarlehre (Papyrus 9780), nebst den bei Stobäus erhaltenen ethischen Exzerpten aus Hierokles, ed. H. v. Arnim, Berlin, 1906 (Berliner Klassiker Texte IV)

Œuvres complètes d'Hippocrate, ed. and transl. E. Littré, 10 vols., Paris, 1839–1861 (= L.)

Hippocratis Opera quae feruntur omnia, ed. H. Kühlewein, 2 vols., Leipzig, 1894/1902 (= Kw.)

Hippocratis De natura hominis, ed., transl., and comm. J. Jouanna, CMG I 1,3, Berlin, 1975

Hippokrates, Über Entstehung und Aufbau des menschlichen Körpers (Περὶ σαρκῶν), ed., transl., and comm. K. Deichgräber, Leipzig and Berlin, 1935

B. Holmberg, A treatise on the unity and trinity of God by Israel of Kashkar (d. 872), Lund, 1989 (Lund Studies in African and Asian Religions 3)

Ḥunain ibn Isḥāq, Über die syrischen und arabischen Galen-Übersetzungen, ed. and transl. G. Bergsträßer, Leipzig, 1925 (Abh. f. d. Kunde d. Morgenlandes 17,2)

Ioannis Philoponi In Aristotelis De anima libros commentaria, ed. M. Hayduck, CAG XV, Berlin, 1897

Ioannes Philoponus, De aeternitate mundi contra Proclum, ed. H. Rabe, Leipzig, 1899

K. Kalbfleisch, Die neuplatonische, fälschlich dem Galen zugeschriebene Schrift Πρὸς Γαῦρον περὶ τοῦ πῶς ἐμψυχοῦται τὰ ἔμβρυα, aus der Pariser Handschrift zum ersten Male herausgegeben, aus d. Anhang z. d. Abh. d. Königl. Preuß. Akademie d. Wiss., Berlin, 1895

–, Zu Galenos, Philologus 55, 1896, pp. 689–694

–, Parthenios bei Galen, Hermes 77, 1942, pp. 376–379

G. S. Kirk, J. E. Raven, M. Schofield, The Presocratic philosophers, 2nd ed., Cambridge, 1983

P. Kraus, Jābir ibn Ḥayyān. Contribution à l'histoire des idées scientifiques dans l'Islam, vol. II, Cairo, 1942
– see (Galen) *Kitāb al-aḫlāq*
P. Kraus and R. Walzer see Galeni Compendium Timaei Platonis
F. Kudlien, Galen's religious belief, in: Galen: problems and prospects. A collection of papers submitted at the 1979 Cambridge conference, ed. V. Nutton, London, 1981, pp. 117–130
R. Lane Fox, Pagans and Christians, Harmondsworth, 1986
C. J. Larrain see Galens Kommentar
Le opere psicologiche di Galeno. Atti del terzo colloquio galenico internazionale, Pavia, 10 – 12 settembre 1986, ed. P. Manuli and M. Vegetti, Naples, 1988 (Elenchos 13)
G. E. R. Lloyd, Scholarship, authority and argument in Galen's Quod animi mores, in: Le opere psicologiche, pp. 11–42
–, Methods and problems in Greek science, Cambridge et al., 1991
–, Galen on Hellenistics and Hippocrateans: contemporary battles and past authorities, in: Lloyd, Methods and problems, pp. 398–416, and in: Galen und das hellenistische Erbe, pp. 125–143
A. A. Long and D. N. Sedley, The Hellenistic philosophers, vol. 1: Translations of the principal sources with philosophical commentary; vol. 2: Greek and Latin texts with notes and bibliography, Cambridge et al., 1987
LSJ = H. G. Liddell, R. Scott, H. S. Jones, A Greek-English Lexicon, 9th ed., Oxford, 1940
A. Manfron, La biblioteca di un medico del Quattrocento. I codici di Giovanni di Marco da Rimini nella Biblioteca Malatestiana, Cesena, 1998
J. Mansfeld, Doxography and dialectic. The *Sitz im Leben* of the 'Placita', in: ANRW II 36,4, Berlin and New York, 1990, pp. 3056–3229
–, Prolegomena. Questions to be settled before the study of an author, or a text, Leiden, 1994
N. Marinone, Galeno, La dieta dimagrante. Edizione critica del testo e della versione latina, traduzione e commento, Turin et al., 1973 (Historica – Politica – Philosophica. Il pensiero antico – Studi e testi 5)
A. Martini and D. Bassi, Catalogus codicum graecorum Bibliothecae Ambrosianae, Milan, 1906, vol. II
J. N. Mattock, A translation of the Arabic epitome of Galen's book Περὶ ἠθῶν, in: Islamic philosophy and the Classical tradition. Essays presented by his friends and pupils to Richard Walzer on his 70. birthday, ed. S. M. Stern, A. Hourani, V. Brown, Oxford, 1972 (Oriental Studies 5), pp. 235–260
Michaelis Ephesii In Parva naturalia commentaria, ed. P. Wendland, CAG XXII 1, Berlin, 1903
P. Moraux, Der Aristotelismus bei den Griechen von Andronikos bis Alexander von Aphrodisias, 2 vols., Berlin and New York, 1973/1984 (Peripatoi. Philologisch-historische Studien zum Aristotelismus 5; 6)
–, Unbekannte Galen-Scholien, Zeitschrift für Papyrologie und Epigraphik 27, 1977, pp. 1–63
Nemesii Emeseni De natura hominis, ed. M. Morani, Leipzig, 1987
D. Nickel, Untersuchungen zur Embryologie Galens, Berlin, 1989 (Schriften zur Geschichte und Kultur der Antike 27)
V. Nutton, Galen's philosophical testament: 'On my own opinions', in: Aristoteles – Werk und Wirkung, pp. 27–51
–, John Caius and the manuscripts of Galen, Cambridge, 1987 (Proceedings of the Cambridge Philological Society, Supplementary vol. 13)
–, From Democedes to Harvey: studies in the history of medicine, London, 1988
– see Galeni De praecognitione
J. Pagel, Die Concordanciae des Johannes de Sancto Amando, Berlin, 1894
–, Neue literarische Beiträge zur mittelalterlichen Medizin, Berlin, 1896

Pappi Alexandrini Collectionis quae supersunt, ed. F. Hultsch, 3 vols., Berlin, 1876–1878
Flavii Philostrati Opera, ed. C. L. Kayser, 2 vols., Leipzig, 1870/1871
J. Pigeaud, La psychopathologie de Galien, in: Le opere psicologiche, pp. 153–184
M. Plezia see Aristotelis . . . De pomo
Posidonius, I. The fragments, ed. L. Edelstein and I. G. Kidd, Cambridge, 1972 (Cambridge Classical Texts and Commentaries 13)
Procli Diadochi In Platonis Timaeum commentaria, ed. E. Diehl, 3 vols., Leipzig, 1903–1906
al-Rāzī, *Kitāb al-shukūk 'alā Jālinūs*, ed. M. Mohaghegh, Teheran, 1993
RE = Paulys Real-Encyclopädie der classischen Altertumswissenschaft, ed. G. Wissowa, W. Kroll, K. Mittelhaus, K. Ziegler, H. Gärtner, Stuttgart / Munich, 1893–1980
L. Robert, Opera minora selecta. Epigraphie et antiquités grecques, vol. V, Amsterdam, 1989
J. Röhr, Der okkulte Kraftbegriff im Altertum, Leipzig, 1923 (Philologus Suppl. 17,1)
F. Rosenthal, An ancient commentary on the Hippocratic oath, Bulletin of the History of Medicine 30, 1956, pp. 52–87
Œuvres de Rufus d'Ephèse, ed. and transl. Ch. Daremberg and E. Ruelle, Paris, 1879
H. O. Schröder see Galeni In Platonis Timaeum comm.
R. E. Siegel, Galen's system of physiology and medicine. An analysis of his doctrines and observations on bloodflow, respiration, humors and internal diseases, Basle and New York, 1968
as-Sijistānī see Dunlop
M. Simon, Sieben Bücher Anatomie des Galen, ed., transl., and comm., 2 vols., Leipzig, 1906
Simplicii In Aristotelis Physicorum libros quattuor posteriores commentaria, ed. H. Diels, CAG X, Berlin, 1895
P. N. Singer, Aspects of Galen's Platonism, in: Galeno: obra, pensamiento e influencia, pp. 41–55
M. F. Smith see Diogenis Oenoandensis Fragmenta
W. D. Smith, The Hippocratic tradition, Ithaca and London, 1979
R. Sorabji, Time, creation and the continuum, theories in antiquity and the early middle ages, London, 1983
Sorani Gynaeciorum libri IV, ed. J. Ilberg, in: CMG IV, Leipzig and Berlin, 1927
H. v. Staden, Herophilus. The art of medicine in early Alexandria, edition, translation and essays, Cambridge et al., 1989
Ioannis Stobaei Anthologium, ed. C. Wachsmuth and O. Hense, 5 vols., Berlin, 1884–1912
Stoicorum Veterum Fragmenta, ed. H. v. Arnim, 4 vols., Leipzig, 1903–1924
Storia e ecdotica dei testi medici greci. Atti del II Convegno Internazionale Parigi 24 – 26 maggio 1994, ed. A. Garzya, Naples, 1996
G. Strohmaier, Hellenistische Wissenschaft im neugefundenen Galenkommentar zur hippokratischen Schrift „Über die Umwelt", in: Galen und das hellenistische Erbe, pp. 157–164 (repr. in: Strohmaier, Von Demokrit bis Dante, pp. 99–106)
–, Von Demokrit bis Dante. Die Bewahrung antiken Erbes in der arabischen Kultur, Hildesheim, Zurich, New York, 1996 (Olms Studien 43)
A. Stückelberger, Vestigia Democritea. Die Rezeption der Lehre von den Atomen in der antiken Naturwissenschaft und Medizin, Basle, 1984 (Schweizerische Beiträge zur Altertumswissenschaft 17)
SVF = Stoicorum Veterum Fragmenta
O. Temkin, Galenism. Rise and decline of a medical philosophy, Ithaca and London, 1973
Theophrastus of Eresus. Sources for his life, writings, thought and influence, ed. and transl. W. W. Fortenbaugh, P. M. Huby, R. W. Sharples and D. Gutas, 2 vols., Leiden, New York, Köln, 1992 (Philosophia antiqua 54,1. 2)
H. Usener, Epicurea, Leipzig, 1887 (repr. Stuttgart, 1966)

J. T. Vallance, The lost theory of Asclepiades of Bithynia, Oxford, 1990

G. Vlastos, Plato's universe, Seattle, 1975

R. Walzer, Galens Schrift „Über die Siebenmonatskinder", Rivista degli Studi Orientali 15, 1935, pp. 323–357

–, New light on Galen's moral philosophy (from a recently discovered source), Classical Quarterly 43, 1949, pp. 82–96 (repr. in: R. Walzer, Greek into Arabic. Essays on Islamic philosophy, Oxford, 1962 [Oriental Studies 1], pp. 142–163)

A. Wasserstein see Galen's commentary on the Hippocratic treatise

N. G. Wilson, Aspects of the transmission of Galen, in: Le strade del testo, ed. G. Cavallo, Bari, 1987

M. Zonta, Un interprete ebreo della filosofia di Galeno. Gli scritti filosofici di Galeno nell'opera di Shem Tob ibn Falaquera, Turin, 1995 (Eurasiatica 39)

INTRODUCTION

A. The sources for the text

Galen's treatise On my own opinions is unusual in its complex textual history. It is preserved almost entire in a mediaeval Latin translation made from an Arabic translation, and it is this Latin version that, until the last part of the final chapter, serves as the main text on which this edition is based. No manuscript of the Arabic survives, although there are several quotations in Arabic authors, none securely verbatim, but chapter 2 and part of chapter 3 are cited accurately in Hebrew by a Jewish philosopher depending on the Arabic. Of Galen's original Greek there remain only a few extracts, of varying length, until the last three chapters, which are preserved in a continuous text. The last two chapters circulated under the title On the substance of the natural faculties, and it was from this quasi-independent Greek tract that a second Latin translation was made by Niccolò da Reggio in the first half of the fourteenth century. No single branch of the transmission contains the whole of this treatise, but together they permit the recovery of all of Galen's last work.

I. The Greek manuscripts

The Greek manuscripts can be divided into three groups: a series of extracts; quotations in scholia; and manuscripts presenting a continuous text. The extracts are contained in two manuscripts, Parisinus gr. 2332 and Vindobonensis med. gr. 15, and were the first fragments in Greek to be edited and published as coming from On my own opinions.[1]

a) Parisinus gr. 2332

P Paris, Bibliothèque Nationale, fonds grec 2332 (= P) is a badly written paper manuscript of the fifteenth century, 171 mm. by 112 mm. in size, with 24 lines to the page.[2] It has 416 leaves, together with a doublet at fol. 9 and two blank preliminary pages. Many of the leaves have been damaged at the top and bottom and in the outer margin and have been repaired by pasting paper over the damaged area, with the subsequent loss of the opening lines of

1 Helmreich, Galeni fragmenta, pp. 431–434, with corrections by Kalbfleisch, Zu Galenos, pp. 689–694.

2 H. Omont, Inventaire sommaire des manuscrits grecs de la Bibliothèque Nationale, vol. II, Paris, 1888, p. 242.

each page, in some cases of the last lines, and of three or four letters in the left margin. On fols. 199^{v}–201^{v}, it contains the following passages: pp. 64,17 Ἐδείχθη – 66,18 χυμῶν; p. 68,4 τὴν – 7 ἀρίστην; pp. 70,14 περὶ – 72,2 ψυχροτέρου; p. 72,7 Πρῶτον – 27 ἐργάζεται; pp. 74,5 Νομίζεται – 76,17 αἴσθησιν; pp. 84,12 Ἐδείχθη – 90,11 γράμματι; pp. 90,23 νέος – 92,10 ἐμφυομένης; pp. 92,22 οὐ – 94,17 νομίζουσιν.

The same hand corrects some of P's minor errors: p. 86,2 ἁπλῶς ex ἁπλῶν; p. 88,21 ἑκάστω ex ἑκάστου; p. 90,10 τῶ e τὸ. Once the correction mars an otherwise correct text: p. 86,27 ἑαυτῶ ex ἑαυτὸ.

A second corrector (= P^{2}) can also be glimpsed: p. 86,13 ἰδιότητι P: ποσότητι P^{2}. P^{2}

Iota subscript is omitted throughout.

b) Vindobonensis med. gr. 15

An identical selection of extracts is contained in a second Ms., Vienna, Österreichische Nationalbibliothek, med. gr. 15 (= W), on fols. 138^{r}–139^{r}.[1] A paper Ms. of 257 leaves, 280 mm. by 210/20 mm., with 31 lines to the page, it was written in the first half of the sixteenth century and may have been among the 240 Mss. that Busbecq had copied at Constantinople for the Imperial Library in Vienna. It has many peculiar errors: W

1. Omissions: p. 70,18 τῶν om. W; p. 88,24 ἐπί – 26 ἀνθρώπων om. W; p. 92,5 κατὰ om. W

2. Wrong endings: p. 70,15 φαντασία] φαντασίας W; p. 72,18 αὐτό] αὐτοί W; p. 92,5 τὴν] τῇ W

3. Mistranscriptions: p. 72,17 γε] τε W; p. 72,26 οὐκ] οὖν W; p. 86,10 ὠφελούντων] ἐφελούντων W

4. Wrong addition: p. 76,1 post ὀδύνην add. ἐν ἐμοι W

5. Iotacism: p. 94,12 ἔνιοι] ἔνιι W

There are corrections by the first hand: p. 84,19 ἕτερον – 23 δηλητήρια bis scr. et alterum del. W, and by a second, later, hand (= W^{2}): p. 76,3 ναρκώδους e σαρκώδους corr. W, in σαρκ- supra lin. mut. W^{2}. W^{2}

Iota subscript is omitted throughout, and smooth breathings frequently replace rough, e.g. p. 90,25 ἀπάντων; p. 90,27 ἡλικίαν.

The extracts in P and W were made in the correct order of reading, and would appear to preserve the original wording without abridgement.[2]

c) Parisinus suppl. gr. 634

In 1900 G. Helmreich published two small fragments of this treatise he had discovered in a Paris Ms., Bibliothèque Nationale, suppl. grec 634 (= Q), a Ms. of the late twelfth century, which had been brought to Paris by Mynoides Q

[1] H. Hunger, Katalog der griechischen Handschriften der Österreichischen Nationalbibliothek, vol. II, Vienna, 1969, pp. 55–59.

[2] See Nutton, in: CMG V 8,1, p. 15.

Mynas.[1] Its 438 leaves, 290 mm. by 210 mm. in size, have between 30 and 42 lines to the page. Among its collection of scholia to Galen may be found two extracts from On my own opinions. On fol. 23^{v}, the scholiast quotes p. 98,11 ὅτι – 26 χυμούς in commenting on De elem. ex Hipp. sent. 11,2: CMG V 1,2, p. 140,20; and, a few pages later, on fol. 26^{v}, commenting on De temp. III 3: p. 98,19sq. Helmr. = I 666,6–8 K., he adduces pp. 84,19 ἕτερον – 86,9 χρώμεθα.

d) Neapolitanus III.D.15 (229)

An identical group of scholia is contained in another manuscript, Naples,
N Biblioteca Nazionale, III.D.15 (229) (= N), from the late fourteenth century, which has the same fragments on fols. 179^{v} and 182^{v}.[2]

e) Yalensis 234

A second group of scholia contributes only allusions to the text. Yale
Y University, Beinecke Library, 234 (= Y), was written in the thirteenth century. The last section of this composite Ms., fols. 177^{r}–198^{v}, contains scholia to Galen which refer (schol. I A 536 Moraux: ἐν τῷ περὶ ἑαυτῷ δοκούντων) in merely the vaguest of terms to Galen's opinion on the chronological order in which the three main bodily organs are formed, cf. pp. 90,22–94,16.[3]

f) Parisinus gr. 2147

The same group of scholia is contained in a Paris Ms., Bibliothèque Na-
Z tionale, fonds grec 2147 (= Z), fols. 39^{v}–64^{v}, a paper Ms. of the first half of the sixteenth century.[4]

1 G. Helmreich, Zu Galen Περὶ τῶν ἑαυτῷ δοκούντων, Philologus 59, 1900, pp. 316–317; the relevant sections were also reprinted in his Handschriftliche Studien zu Galen, Programm des k. humanistischen Gymnasiums in Ansbach 1909/10, pp. 19; 27. Helmreich dated this manuscript to the late fourteenth century, but Wilson, p. 56, provides evidence for a much earlier date.

2 This group of scholia was brought to light by Moraux, Unbekannte Galen-Scholien, p. 5.

3 B. Shailor, Catalogue of medieval and renaissance manuscripts in the Beinecke Rare Book and Manuscript Library, Yale University, vol. I, Binghampton, 1984, pp. 338–341, who dates it to the early fourteenth century. The earlier dating is offered by Wilson, p. 57. Previous owners include Luigi Celotti, Sir Thomas Phillipps (as Phillipps, no. 890), and Laurence Witten. The scholia were published by Moraux, Unbekannte Galen-Scholien, pp. 9–57. The relevant lines, schol. I A 534–536 Moraux, say: Hippocrates completely omitted to speak about god and providence and about the first part to be formed, as Galen says in On my own opinions. But nowhere in the surviving sections does Galen mention Hippocrates' failure to talk about any of these themes, and he himself says nothing specific about providence. Either the scholiast is totally wrong, or one should delete the comma after μορίου and take the following clause to mean that the scholiast is contrasting Hippocrates' silence with Galen's willingness in On my own opinions to talk about these topics. Even so, unless the clause applies only to the first and last themes mentioned (which is possible), the scholiast has made a mistake.

4 Moraux, Unbekannte Galen-Scholien, p. 3. Since Moraux shows convincingly that Z is a direct copy of Y, and since these scholia contain no direct quotation from On my own opinions, I have not attempted a collation of the relevant passage.

g) Ambrosianus gr. 659

Neither the extracts nor the scholia present a coherent Greek text, which exists only for the last three chapters.

Chapter 13 is found in a single manuscript, Milan, Biblioteca Ambrosiana, cod. graec. 659 (formerly Q 3 Sup.) (= A). This paper manuscript of 272 A
leaves, which measure 210 mm. by 139 mm. in size, was written about 1400.[1] In 1466 it was bought in Thrace by Demetrios Angelos, a student of John Argyropoulos at Constantinople about 1448, and later doctor to the Kral hospital there.[2] It was in Italy in the sixteenth century, when it was used by the Aldine editors and seen by J. J. Scaliger c. 1565 on his Italian journey. In 1611 it was sold at Pisa.[3] The text of On my own opinions is contained on fols. 185^{r}–187^{r}. The action of water has caused many letters at the top of the inner margin on fol. 185^{rv} to become indistinct, and they were subsequently transcribed by a later hand (= A^2), perhaps to be identified with Demetrios, who compiled the A^2
indexes on fol. 2^{v} and 128^{v}. The same scribe added the title Γαληνοῦ περὶ τῶν ἑαυτῷ δοκούντων at fol. 185^{r}. Of greater interest is the insertion, probably by the first hand, at fol. 185^{v} of a heading Γαληνοῦ περὶ τῆς οὐσίας τῶν φυσικῶν δυνάμεων to mark the beginning of the next section. In the two indexes the same heading reappears, as if that section was known as an independent text. There are also a few corrections by the original scribe, none of them significant. There are several scribal errors:

1. Omissions: p. 110,15 καὶ om. A; p. 110,19 ἃ ποιεῖ om. A; p. 118,9 τε — μετεμψυχώσεως om. A
2. Wrong word order: p. 112,14 ἡμῶν αὐτὴν] αὔτην ἡμῶν A; p. 112,18 αὐτῆς ἰδίαν] ἰδίαν αὐτῆς A
3. Wrong ending: p. 108,27 ἀπορῶ] ἀπορῶν A
4. Iotacism: p. 104,26 λέγῃ] λέγει A

1 Martini and Bassi, pp. 738–740; S. Ebbesen, Commentators and commentaries on Aristotle's Sophistici Elenchi, vol. II, Greek texts, Leiden, 1981, p. IX. Notes on this manuscript by Ch. Daremberg are in Paris, Académie Nationale de Médecine, Ms. 480.25, pp. 30–31.

2 For the subscription, see Martini and Bassi, p. 740; H. Diels, Die handschriftliche Überlieferung des Galenschen Commentars zum Prorrheticum des Hippokrates, Abh. d. Königl. Preuß. Akademie d. Wiss., phil.-hist. Kl. 1912, I, Berlin, 1912, p. 31; in: CMG V 9,2, p. X. For Demetrios and his teacher, see Oxford, Bodleian Library, Cod. Barocci 87 (of 1445–1450), with D. J. Geanakoplos, Constantinople and the West, Madison, 1989, pp. 95–99; Demetrios also owned Parisinus gr. 2154, and, in 1442, Ochrid, Ms. 24, see U. Birchler-Argyros, Die Quellen zum Kral-Spital in Konstantinopel, Gesnerus 45, 1988, pp. 425–428. This note corrects and amplifies what I said in: CMG V 8,1, p. 16.

3 See Nutton, in: CMG V 8,1, pp. 40–41; 46. Scaliger consulted a Galenic manuscript "ex s(ancto) Antonio" (see CMG V 8,1, p. 16), probably the Grimani Library at S. Antonio di Castello in Venice, but no entry corresponding to A appears in the surviving library catalogue and the library was not opened until 1525, too late for any of its manuscripts to be used in the Aldine edition, cf. Nutton, John Caius, pp. 52; 67. At the same sale in Pisa, Gratia Maria Gratia bought a Greek medical manuscript formerly belonging to Hieronymus Mercurialis, Ambrosianus L 30 Sup., but there is no proof that A had a similar provenance.

5. Wrong word division: p. 108,2 ἀλλ' ἄχρι] ἀλλὰ χρὴ A
Iota subscript is omitted throughout.

h) Laurentianus gr. 74,5

Three other Greek manuscripts present a continuous text from p. 110,4 until the end. Of these by far the oldest, as well as the most puzzling, is Flor-
L ence, Biblioteca Medicea-Laurenziana, Plut. 74,5 (= L), a product of the scriptorium of Ioannikios in the second half of the twelfth century. It is written on Spanish paper, 290 mm. by 192 mm. in size, perhaps in S. Italy.[1] The sections from On my own opinions are contained on fols. 91^r–92^r, under the title Γαληνοῦ περὶ τῆς οὐσίας τῶν φυσικῶν δυνάμεων. There are the following errors:

1. Repetition: p. 120,24 τὸ δὲ γνωρίζειν bis scr. L
2. Wrong ending: p. 110,20 ἑκάστου] ἑκάστων L
3. Iotacism: p. 124,9 ἐστερῆσθαι] ἐστερεῖσθαι L

Iota subscript is omitted throughout. Occasionally, simple errors of L are corrected by the same scribe.

i) Marcianus gr. 281

The most elegantly written Ms. of this treatise is Venice, Biblioteca Mar-
M ciana, gr. 281 (= M), which formed part of a set of eight volumes copied for Cardinal Bessarion between 1468 and 1472.[2] Under the title Γαληνοῦ περὶ οὐσίας τῶν φυσικῶν δυνάμεων the last chapters of On my own opinions are contained on fols. 75^v–76^v. Its peculiar errors include:

1. Wrong endings: p. 110,24 ἐφεκτικὴν] ἐφεκτικὸν M; p. 116,15 ἀναγκαῖον] ἀναγκαῖα M; p. 122,15 ἀκουστῶν] ἀκουστικῆς M

1 For the importance of this manuscript see Nutton, in: CMG V 8,1, p. 17, and the following studies by N. G. Wilson, A mysterious Byzantine scriptorium: Ioannikios and his colleagues, Scrittura e Civiltà 7, 1983, pp. 161–176; New light on Burgundio of Pisa, Studi Italiani di Filologia Classica, ser. 3,3, 1986, pp. 113–118; Aspects, p. 53; Ioannikios and Burgundio: a survey of the problem, in: Scritture, libri e testi nelle aree provinciali di Bisanzio, Atti del seminario di Erice, 18–25 settembre, ed. G. Cavallo, G. de Gregorio, M. Maniaci, Spoleto, 1991, pp. 447–455. For the paper, see P. Canart, S. di Zio, L. Polistena, D. Scialanga, Une enquête sur le papier de type 'Arabe occidental' ou 'Espagnol, non filigrane', in: Ancient and medieval book materials and techniques, ed. M. Maniaci, P. F. Munafò, vol. I, Rome, 1993 (Studi e Testi 357), pp. 319–324; 334. In his most recent papers, Wilson rules out his earlier suggestion that L was written in Palermo or S. Italy, and wishes to locate its production in Constantinople, perhaps as early as 1150. But J. Irigoin, La tradition de l'Ars medica de Galien dans l'Italie méridionale, Bollettino della Badia Greca di Grottaferrata, n.s. 45, 1991, pp. 85–91, argues strongly for an origin in S. Italy.

2 See Nutton, in: CMG V 8,1, p. 18, with a bibliography of earlier descriptions; E. Mioni, Codices Graeci manuscripti bibliothecae Divi Marci Venetiarum, vol. I, Rome, 1972, pp. 404–405, makes it clear that the omission of Bessarion's name was an oversight on his part, and hence that it was in his possession before 1572. E. Mioni and M. Formentin, I codici greci di medicina nelle tre Venezie, Padua, 1968, pp. 13; 50, assign it to the scribe Giovanni Rhosos, but N. Wilson, personal communication, prefers George Alexandrou. For further details of readers of M, see also Nutton, John Caius, pp. 40–41.

2. Misreading of an exemplar: p. 112,10 ἃ] καὶ M
Iota subscript is always omitted.

j) Parisinus suppl. gr. 35

The same section of text under the same title, Γαληνοῦ περὶ οὐσίας τῶν φυσικῶν δυνάμεων, is also contained in Paris, Bibliothèque Nationale, suppl. grec 35 (= R), on fols. 129^{r}–130^{v}. This paper Ms. of the late fifteenth or early **R** sixteenth century consists of 245 leaves plus two preliminary leaves, 290 mm. by 200 mm., with between 29 and 31 lines to the page.[1] It has many peculiar errors:

1. Omission: p. 124,21 οὐδὲ om. R
2. Wrong endings: p. 110,5 ἐπίστανται] ἐπίσταντες R; p. 112,9 συνθέσεως] συνθέτου R; p. 114,19 βούλομαι] βούλεται R
3. Iotacism: p. 118,10 ἐπιτήδειόν] ἐπιτήδιον R
4. Misreadings of an exemplar: p. 122,13 φυτικῆς] φυσιγῆς R; p. 122,16 ἁπτῶν] ἁπλῶν R; p. 124,11 ἀρκοῦμαι] ἀναγκάσαι R

Iota subscript is usually omitted.

k) Codex Adelphi

Traces of a further Greek manuscript, the Codex Adelphi (= Ad.), can **Ad.** be discerned among the notes of two English medical men with a passion for Galen, John Caius (1510–1573) and Theodore Goulston (1572–1632). Caius, who travelled widely in Italy in the 1540s, inscribed many conjectures and manuscript variants into the margin of his copy of the 1538 Basle edition of Galen, now at Eton College, Berkshire, England, classmark Fc 2 6–8. Among them were many readings taken from a Codex Adelphi or τοῦ ἀδελφοῦ. The readings ascribed to this codex by Caius, and later by Goulston, relate to sixteen tracts, Exhortation to medicine; On the best method of teaching; The best doctor is also a philosopher; On sects; On the best sect; On the constitution of the art of medicine; On temperaments I, II; On the natural faculties; On the formation of the foetus; On the seed; On the opinions of Hippocrates and Plato; On affected parts; On the diagnosis of the passions; On prognosis; On the use of parts and On my own opinions (as On the substance of the natural faculties). This is a remarkable list, in both length and contents, for several of these texts survive in only a handful of Mss. (and the Exhortation to medicine in none), and the whole, if included within one pair of covers, would constitute the largest single medical Ms. known. It is thus tempting to regard the Codex Adelphi not as a manuscript, but as a printed edition (presumably an Aldine or a Basle edition), into which an owner, "Adelphus", had copied marginal notes and emendations. But the generally high quality of the readings ascribed by Caius to this codex is very different from that of the usual aleatory productions of humanist physicians, for they often correspond to correct readings found in Mss. elsewhere or to the (lost) Greek text that lay behind some of the mediaeval translations by Niccolò da Reggio. Hence

[1] H. Omont, Inventaire sommaire des manuscrits du Supplément grec, Paris, 1883, p. 6.

the reports of Caius and Goulston would appear to refer, directly or indirectly, at least to some readings in a manuscript or manuscripts.[1]

John Caius copied only one variant from the Codex Adelphi into the margin of his Basle Galen: p. 124,1 τῆς τρεφομένης, which confirmed one of his own conjectures ("ita enim cast. in adelphi"). Much greater use was made of the Codex by Theodore Goulston, who took notes on it (and also on Caius' Galen) probably around the turn of the century. Since Goulston never travelled abroad, his collations indicate that the Codex was then in England.[2] Some readings were published after Goulston's death by his friend Thomas Gataker in 1640 in the appendix to Goulston's edition and Latin version of On the substance of the natural faculties. Two readings were there specifically ascribed to cod. Adelphi: p. 120,20 πρὶν γνωρίσαι (shared also with A); and at p. 124, 20 ἔτι the wrong ἔστι. The title περὶ τῶν ἑαυτῷ δοκούντων and the chapter heading περὶ φυσικῶν δυνάμεων οὐσίας (sic), were loosely ascribed to "Antiq. Codd." or 'antiquus cod.'; and two readings were given without indication of their source: pp. 110,18 θέμενοι, and 112,6 ἑκάστης. Since for this Galenic fragment, Goulston records only two Mss., the Codex Adelphi and the Codex Londinensis (which is his description of Caius' Galen), and since these readings were not given by Caius, they too must have come from the missing Codex, unless Goulston or his editor had made a mistake, which is not unlikely.[3]

Goulston, however, had taken down more than this, for the marginalia in his copy of the Basle edition, now in the Marsh Library, Dublin, classmark P.3.2.18, reveal other readings:

p. 104,27 διαφωνίας Bas.: διαφωνίαν Goulst.$^{Bas.}$
p. 108,11 ἐρῆταί Bas.: ἐρεῖται Goulst.$^{Bas.}$
p. 114,15 post ὡς add. ἔοικεν Goulst.$^{Bas.}$
p. 122,3 post Πλάτωνος add. et del. ὡς Goulst.$^{Bas.}$

Since some of these marginalia can be parallelled in A or are wrong, it seems more likely that they represent Goulston's collations rather than independent conjectures. Of the fate of this Codex after Goulston's inspection, nothing is known, but if it was an annotated edition of Galen, its continued

1 See, for a full discussion of the Codex Adelphi, Nutton, John Caius, pp. 60–64; 85–86; and The Galenic codices of Theodore Goulston, Revue d'Histoire des Textes 22, 1992, pp. 260–268, correcting the speculations of D. Béguin, L'édition Goulston et les prétendus manuscrits perdus de Galien, Revue d'Histoire des Textes 19, 1989, pp. 341–349. In my article I raise the possibility of identifying the mysterious Adelphus with John Freare or Friar (c. 1499–1563), a doctor and friend of Caius, rather than with my earlier suggestion (see Nutton, John Caius, pp. 63–64), Johannes Adelphus (fl. 1500–1523), an Erasmian physician of Straßburg.

2 It had probably been there since the 1550s, for the hand in which Caius commented on it is more spidery (and, I judge, later) than that in which he made his Italian collations.

3 If Goulston's plural "Antiq. Codd." in connection with the title Περὶ τῶν ἑαυτῷ δοκούντων, which does not appear in any printed book, is to be taken strictly, he may well also have reported the reading of a manuscript identical with, or similar to, A, where the title is added in the upper margin in a later hand, probably that of Demetrios Angelos (see above, p. 17).

existence today, unnoticed and unread within a private library, is far from impossible.

II. The relationship between the Greek manuscripts

The small amount of text available renders dubious any attempt to draw up a stemma of manuscript relationships. The few lines offered by Q and N hardly add anything to the close relationship noted already by Moraux. However, Wilson's radical redating of Q would suggest that N is a copy of Q rather than its twin, and, in the apparatus criticus, since the two share identical readings throughout, I cite only the evidence of Q.[1]

The relationship between the extracts in P and W is likewise close. They share many common errors, e. g.: p. 84,13 τῆς om. PW; p. 86,2 ἁπλῶς] ἁπλῶν PW; p. 94,1 ἤπερ] εἴπερ PW; p. 94,14 τινὲς] τὸν ἐς PW; to which W adds errors of its own, e. g.: p. 72,18 ἐκ om. W; p. 76,1 post ὀδύνην add. ἐν ἐμοι W; p. 88,24 ἐπί – 26 ἀνθρώπων om. W. This suggests that W was copied from P or, less likely, from P's exemplar, and hence can be disregarded in the apparatus criticus.[2] Where the damage to P has been significant, W has been used as source for the text.

The three Mss. L M R form a family distinct from A. Not only do they omit the first chapter of A, but they also share many wrong readings: p. 114,9 εἰδείην – 11 αὐτῆς om. L M R; p. 114,26 τε – 27 ἠθικὴν om. L M R; p. 116,11 μόρια om. L M R. Since neither M nor R has a good reading that is not found in L, and since each has its own selection of wrong readings, one may conclude that both M and R were copied directly from L, although whether this was in Italy or elsewhere remains open to question.[3] I have thus excluded readings of M and R from the apparatus criticus.

Finally, the relationship between A and Ad. is not without interest. The two contain the same chapters, and appear to have had several readings in common. Indeed, if Ad. represents, in part, Ms. collations transcribed into a printed edition of the complete works of Galen, the possibility cannot be entirely ruled out that "Adelphus" was actually copying A. But against this can be ranged strong arguments. Several of the texts included in the Codex Adelphi are absent from A, and, vice versa, many of the works contained in A do not seem to have any readings preserved in Ad. Although one could imagine a variety of reasons why Ad. should not have copied down everything he saw in A, for example, a lack of time or of interest in particular topics, the ab-

1 M. G. Moore, Galen, Introduction to the bones: a critical edition with translation and indices, Diss. University of Michigan, 1969, pp. XIX–XX, also concludes that N is a copy of Q.

2 Cf. also Nutton, in: CMG V 8,1, p. 20, for support for this conclusion from the evidence in On prognosis, and H. Schöne, Markellinos' Pulslehre. Ein griechisches Anekdoton, in: Festschrift zur 49. Versammlung deutscher Philologen und Schulmänner, Basle, 1907, pp. 448–471, esp. p. 451.

3 For the possible dependence of M on L, see Nutton, in: CMG V 8,1, p. 229, the note to p. 140,5–8, modifying the conclusion of ibid., pp. 21–22; for the relationship between R and L, see ibid., p. 22.

sence of anything resembling a close fit between A and Ad. is disconcerting, to say the least. Besides, there is a further pointer away from the notion that A was the source of Ad. The last portion of On prognosis was already lost in A when the index was made by A^2, i.e. by about 1460, but there are many good readings from it attributed by Caius in his Eton notes to Ad.

If a direct dependence of A is excluded, there remain two possible conclusions to be drawn from these readings. The first is that Ad. represents, at least in part, a manuscript of the A family which was still accessible to "Adelphus" (and, although much less likely, perhaps even to Caius and Goulston) in the sixteenth century. The second is that some of the good readings in Ad. are the result of sound conjecture, while others are retroversions into Greek from the Latin of Niccolò. That such a procedure could have been followed in the sixteenth century can be demonstrated from the practice of the editors of the 1538 Basle edition of Galen. But, on the whole, the quality of these hypothetical retroversions is very high, and, given the generally poor quality of sixteenth-century editorial conjectures, one might prefer to place one's faith in the existence of a manuscript that is now lost than in the ability of an unknown "Adelphus". Only the rediscovery of the Codex itself will finally resolve this problem, for the solution may well differ from tract to tract.

Whether the outcome of conjecture, manuscript copying, or both, Ad. did not offer a complete text of On my own opinions. But it at least preserved the correct title of the work, and, like A, it contained the subheading at p. 110,4. The existence of this subtitle within the manuscript tradition (whether inserted deliberately or accidentally, see below, p. 203, the note to p. 110,4–21) would have provided an incentive for a later scribe or scribes to consider the last section as an independent work on its own and hence to copy only the final chapters of the treatise in Greek.[1]

III. The Arabo-Latin translation

Each of the two Latin versions of On my own opinions represents a different stage in the process of the transmission of the Corpus Galenicum to the Latin West. Of the two, the earlier version, taken from the Arabic, is by far the most significant, since it includes the bulk of the treatise and lacks only the last part of the final chapter. In its place is found a section from the pseudo-Aristotelian De pomo, which, since it appears in all the Mss., will have been included in their joint source.[2] Although this section may have been deliberately inserted as a solution to some of the doubts and difficulties expressed in the earlier chapters, the fact that its opening is badly mutilated (as is its ending) suggests that a longer passage from De pomo originally followed a complete text of De sententiis, which subsequently suffered the loss of a leaf

1 The author of the index on fols. 2^v and 128^r in A (see above, p. 17) apparently considered the two parts independent, for both titles are given.

2 The credit for the identification of the ending with De pomo, pp. 58,4–59,2 Plezia, is owed to Einarson, pp. 258–259.

or, if all of De pomo was included, possibly more. Five manuscripts of the Arabo-Latin version survive today, and there are traces of a sixth manuscript once in the possession of the Paris Faculty of Medicine.

a) Parisinus lat. 6865

The oldest manuscript of the Arabo-Latin translation is Paris, Bibliothèque Nationale, fonds latin 6865 (= B)[1], a parchment Ms. of 211 leaves, 385 **B** mm. by 302 mm. in size, written in two columns, each 77 mm. wide. The margin is decorated with coloured filigree work; the initial letters of each tract are multi-coloured; the chapter openings are painted in blue and red, the chapter headings in red; internal divisions within paragraphs and, occasionally, within sentences are made in blue or red. De sententiis, to which a later scribe, B^3, has added the subtitle "ut de fide G(alieni)"[2], occupies fols. 172^r–175^v. There are many marginal drawings, ornaments, and annotations by the original scribe, a scholar using an Italian hand (= B^2), and a third scholar us- **B^2** ing a French hand (= B^3). A later hand (= B^4) adds chapter numbers in the **B^3 B^4** margin, dividing the tract into eight chapters in a manner different from that in Dresdensis Db 92 and Parisinus Academicus 51, and also attempts to bring the conclusion into line with the wording of his text of De pomo. It was written in S. Italy, perhaps at the Angevin court of Naples, between 1345 (the date of the translation of De disnia included in it) and 1353, when a note on fol. 215^v indicates that it was at the Papal court of Avignon.[3] Three hundred years later, it was in the possession of Jacobus Mentelius, a nobleman, physician, and bibliophile of Chateau-Thierry, from whom it may have passed directly into the library of Colbert, and thence into the Royal Library. Orthographically, it is the best of the surviving manuscripts, although it is far from being universally accurate.

b) Malatestianus S.V 4

Cesena, Biblioteca Malatestiana, S.V 4 (= C), is a parchment codex of the **C** late fourteenth century, measuring 417 mm. by 266 mm., in two columns with 56 lines to the page. It has 264 leaves, with an additional blank leaf at the beginning and end, and contains De sententiis on fols. 148^r–150^v. The script is small and crabbed, and hard to decipher because of its many abbreviations and compendia. Corrections and marginalia from at least three hands can be distinguished; the original scribe, and two later owners, Nicolaus de Leonardis (= C^2), and Giovanni Marco da Rimini (= C^3).[4] **C^2 C^3**

1 For the following description see Nutton, in: CMG V 8,1, pp. 26–27.

2 The source is likely to have been the entry in Walter Burley's De vita et moribus philosophorum, see below, p. 41.

3 d'Alverny, p. 363, suggests it was written in S. France, but accepts that it has strong Italian links.

4 To the information given by Nutton, in: CMG V 8,1, pp. 28–29, add Marinone, pp. 14–20, with a photograph of the Ms. at p. 128; Frioli, pp. 117–125; Manfron, pp. 215–219; and T. Pesenti, Professori e promotori di medicina nello studio di Padova dal 1405 al 1509, Padua, 1984, pp. 125–127, for Nicolaus.

c) Dresdensis Db 92

Although much of the beautiful Ms., Dresden, Sächsische Landesbiblio-
D thek, Db 92 (= D), is damaged beyond recall, the pages containing De sententiis, fols. 12^v–16^r, can be read almost entirely, albeit with difficulty. Written on parchment, 455 mm. by 343 mm., in two columns, each 110 mm. wide, it dates from the second half of the fifteenth century, and was illustrated with miniatures painted by a master of the Burgundian school.[1] There are several glosses, either in a smaller hand by the original scribe or by a later annotator
D^2 (= D^2).[2]

De sententiis is divided, as in B, into fifteen chapters, each with its own heading in red, and the whole is preceded by a table of chapter headings, as follows:

Libri Galieni de sententiis sunt quindecim capitula
Capitulum primum. de comparatione actoris huius libri ad bethenem uersificatorem.
Capitulum II. de hiis que sentit actor circa mundi durationem et ambitum eius et creatorem omnium.
Capitulum III. de hiis que sentit circa animam et uirtutes eius.
Capitulum IIII. de hiis que sentit actor circa corpora inferiora et calorem eorum et genera febrium.
Capitulum V. de complexionibus corporum, temporum et etatum et de comparatione earum adinuicem.
Capitulum VI. de primo membro sensibili et uirtute eius et modo sui influxus et cui magis influit uel neruo uel carni.
Capitulum VII. de habitudine anime ad corpus et de natura corporis et spiritus.
Capitulum VIII. de moribus quorundam circa iudicia et de triplici principio in nobis secundum tres motus.
Capitulum IX. de modis qui de modis quibus alteratur corpus et de medicinis proportionaliter illis modis alterantibus corpus; et de diuisione operationum naturalium secundum hos modos.
Capitulum X. de utilitate epatis et uirtute eius et de comparatione dispositionis sue uirtutis ad dispositionem uirtutum cerebri et cordis et de errore male intelligentium corpus nostrum regi a tribus principiis.
Capitulum XI. de uirtute formatiua embrionis et plantarum et de ordine formationis membrorum et quid format membra.
Capitulum XII. de humoribus et habitudine medicinarum laxatiuarum ad eos.
Capitulum XIII. quod cor est fons caloris animalium; et de comparatione dicti

1 A reproduction of the initial miniature of De sententiis, alas not in colour, is given by E. C. van Leersum and W. Martin, Miniaturen der lateinischen Galenos-Handschrift der Kgl. Öffentl. Bibliothek in Dresden Db 92–93 in phototypischer Reproduktion, Leiden, 1910, p. XIX, no. 4. It shows Galen debating with the poet Parthenius, a misunderstanding of Galen's introduction.

2 See Nutton, in: CMG V 8,1, pp. 27–28; K. Assmann, Sächsische Landesbibliothek Dresden, 1556–1956, Leipzig, 1956, pp. 30–34; 144; 191; and V. Nutton, Galeno salvato dalle acque, Kos 1, 1984, pp. 33–49.

caloris ad calorem naturalem inuentum in plantis et nobis. et de diuersitate platonis super animam, scilicet quibus communicatur corporibus, et de differentia inter animalia et plantas.

Capitulum XIIII. de substantia uirtutum et de opinionibus circa substantiam anime.

Capitulum XV. de hiis quorum habetur certa noticia in medicina et de hiis quorum non. et de quibus non est cura.

d) Parisinus Academicus 51

Like D, Paris, Académie Nationale de Médecine 51 (= E), forms part of a large collection of Latin versions of Galen. It is a paper manuscript, 260 mm. by 205 mm. in size, written in a single column, with 31 lines to the page. De sententiis is contained on fols. 211^{v}–222^{v}, and is preceded by a list of chapters on fol. 211^{rv}.[1] The initial letters of sentences and the chapter headings are in red, and there are several corrections and marginalia, either in the hand of the first scribe or in that of a later glossator (= E^2). It was written in the second half of the fifteenth century in Northern France or Flanders, where E^2 glossed at fol. 219^{r} the (to him unintelligible) word "ysore" as ".i. busbo", the Middle Dutch word for "box tree" or the caper tree (capparis spinosa).[2] **E** **E^2**

e) Biturigensis 299 (247)

Bourges, Bibliothèque de la Ville 299 (247) (= O) is a parchment Ms. of 180 leaves. Written in the late fourteenth century, it is 410 mm. by 270 mm. in size, and contains De sententiis on fols. 140^{v}–144^{v}.[3] There are no chapter numberings or chapter headings. In addition to corrections by the original scribe, there are two brief marginal comments at pp. 64,21 and 78,8 by a later hand (= O^2). **O** **O^2**

f) The lost Paris manuscript

Already in 1395 the Paris Faculty of Medicine owned a "volumen magnum" of Galen (= F), which was handed down from one Dean of the Faculty to another. According to a detailed list of 1470, it contained 22 works of Galen, including, in Wickersheimer's transcription[4], a "liber qui dicitur medicus **F**

[1] The wording of the list is the same as in D, except that, in the heading for chapter 3, E^2 adds the word "actor" above "sentit".

[2] For this Ms. see Nutton, in: CMG V 8,1, pp. 30–31; V. Nutton, A forgotten manuscript of Galenus Latinus, in: Studia Codicologica, Berlin, 1977 (Texte u. Untersuchungen 124), pp. 332–340; and d'Alverny, p. 364, who notes that the paper comes from Champagne or N. E. France, and suggests that it may have been written in the last quarter of the century.

[3] H. Omont, Catalogue général des manuscrits des bibliothèques publiques de France, Départements, vol. IV, Paris, 1886, p. 72.

[4] See E. Wickersheimer, Commentaires de la Faculté de Médecine de l'Université de Paris, 1395–1516, Paris, 1915, p. 2 (1395) and p. 252 (1470). The volume was also mentioned in 1415 (p. 87), 1440 (p. 168) and 1455 (p. 203).

introductivus de sententiis medicorum et credulitate seu fide Galieni"[1]. However, the editor or the scribe erred here in conflating a version of the pseudo-Galenic Introductio sive medicus with De sententiis, and thereby obscured the significance of the latter work and of its subtitles. All knowledge of this volume then disappears for three centuries, a period during which the Faculty library saw much disruption and many losses. In 1745, a note on the Library described it as "très incomplet: trois cahiers en mauvais ordre", and consisting only of On crises and On critical days, the first two tracts in the volume. Between then and Franklin's study of the library in 1864, even these remnants were lost.[2]

But all trace of this Ms. and of its readings has not disappeared entirely, for it (or, much less likely, a direct copy) was cited by Pierre Gas (Petrus de Sancto Floro), who took his M.B. at Paris in 1342 and who in 1349 became a Regent Master of the Medical Faculty.[3] His major work was an expansion of the Concordanciae of Jean de St. Amand, which was finished by 1363, when the captious Guy de Chauliac described it as "non est diu". To Jean's Medical Dictionary, Gas added many new citations from Galen, taken in particular from the new translations by Niccolò da Reggio and including some from De disnia, finished only in 1345.[4] Eight of his entries contain material from a work which is variously entitled in Pagel's transcription: de sententiis medicorum; de credulitate Galieni; de medicorum sectis; de sententia medicorum sive credulitate Galeni; de credulitate Galeni vel de sectis; de sectis; and de credulitate Galeni.[5] There can be little doubt that these variants correspond to the title as given in F, which alone has the addition "de credulitate". A further proof of the identity of Gas's source, if one were needed, comes from the fact that five of the quotations attributed to this text are taken from the Introductio, which preceded De sententiis in the Faculty Ms. and whose title was somehow shared with it.[6] Only three of the entries are, in fact, taken from De sententiis, but they are sufficient to show that F is very likely to have contained the whole of the present text as it has come down to us. Gas quotes it

1 It would be tempting to claim that this manuscript was the source of the entry De fide sua in Walter Burley's De vita et moribus philosophorum, see below, p. 41, but this is far from certain.

2 For the later history of the manuscript, see A. Franklin, Recherches sur la bibliothèque de la Faculté de Médecine de Paris, Paris, 1864, p. 64, and, for the library's losses, A. Boinet, Catalogue général des manuscrits des bibliothèques publiques de France: Paris, tome I, Paris, 1909, pp. 216; 218.

3 Biographical details in E. Wickersheimer, Dictionnaire biographique des médecins de France au Moyen Age, Paris, 1936, pp. 634–635. See also D. Jacquart, Les Concordances de Pierre de St. Flour et l'enseignement de la médecine à Paris dans la seconde moitié du XIVe siècle, in: The vocabulary of teaching and research between Middle Ages and Renaissance, ed. O. Weijers, Turnhout, 1995, pp. 172–183.

4 The text was somewhat confusingly edited by J. Pagel, initially as a series of glosses to Jean, see Pagel, Concordanciae, pp. XXIV–LIII; and Beiträge, pp. 1–120.

5 Respectively, Pagel, Concordanciae, p. XLII (twice); Beiträge, pp. 26; 49; 67 (twice); 119.

6 Respectively, Pagel, Concordanciae, p. XLII = cap. 10: XIV 704,7–9 K.; Beiträge, p. 49 = cap. 13: XIV 729,9 K.; p. 67 = cap. 1: XIV 674,3–675,5 K.; p. 67 = cap. 5: XIV 685,3 K.; and p. 119 = cap. 1: XIV 676,8–10 K.

three times. To explain "cor", he cites chapter 11,2: pp. 90,22–92,3, a passage also preserved in the Greek extracts; and he makes up the initial entry on "complexio" out of three sections of chapter 5,1. 2. 3: pp. 66,26–68,2. 4–7. 16–17. The most striking of the three quotations relates to "Deus", for here Gas copies part of the (spurious) final chapter, pp. 122,11–124,9, but refers his readers, not to the "Eight Books" of Aristotle, but to the first eight books of the Megategni, The Method of healing.[1] Even allowing for authorial adjustments to give a continuous text, there is no doubt that, in part at least, Gas's quotations preserve some trace of F.[2]

IV. The relationship between the Latin manuscripts

Although there are links between B and F, not least in the addition of a subtitle, it is unlikely that either was copied from the other. The range of texts in the two Mss. differs, and, although both were written at almost the same time, a descent from a common parent (= δ) is perhaps more probable δ
than any direct dependence.[3]

The same conclusion applies also to the relationship between D and E: they share the same chapter headings and many wrong readings: p. 54,12 et – expositionis *om.* DE; p. 54,17 in – secundum *om.* DE; p. 56,15 dicam quod *om.* DE; p. 72,7 nos *om.* DE; p. 90,19 illud – 20 sit *om.* DE.

There are also separative errors that would seem to indicate that neither was copied directly from the other: p. 66,9–10 magis minus] maior est et minor E; p. 82,17 addiscere] addicere E; p. 66,23 sed – 24 humidi^{II} *om.* D; p. 80,4 uoluit *om.* D; p. 92,20 ueraciter – 22 non *om.* D; p. 96,3 quam – libro^{II} *om.* D; p. 102,8 antequam – 9 fuerunt *om.* D.

This suggests that both D and E were copied from the same exemplar (=
ε), which circulated in N. France or Belgium in the middle of the 15th centu- ε
ry.[4]

It is indeed tempting to associate all the French Mss., B(F)ODE (= β), to- β
gether against the Italian C, for the latter presents many good readings that are not found elsewhere, as well as many wrong readings: p. 54,5 Ait Galienus] inquid Galienus noster C; p. 56,14 uel – extra^{II} C: *om.* β; p. 56,17 habeam scientiam C: debeam scire β; p. 58,7 et – operationibus *om.* C; p. 66,21 nouem *om.* C; p. 116,9 quatuor – 10 commixtio C: *om.* β. Such a conclusion agrees

1 Respectively, Pagel, Concordanciae, p. XLII; Beiträge, p. 26 (where, line 9, the words "et subdit infra" are commentary by Gas, not part of the Galenic quotation); and Concordanciae, p. XLII.

2 Given that it included several translations by Niccolò, e.g. De typo and De subtiliante dieta, F can be assumed to have been written between 1309 and 1360, and even before 1340 if Burley saw it, see below, p. 41.

3 It should perhaps not be forgotten that Pierre Gas came from a town not too remote from Avignon, where B was for a time.

4 See M. R. McVaugh, Armengaud Blaise as a translator of Galen, in: Texts and contexts in ancient and medieval science. Studies on the occasion of John E. Murdoch's seventieth birthday, ed. O. Sylla and M. R. McVaugh, Leiden et al., 1997, pp. 114–133, esp. pp. 116–117.

with what has been found for On prognosis and for On the slimming diet, but it says little about the internal relationships within the French group.[1]

O is often very close to B: p. 54,11 dicendo] dicentem BO; p. 68,9 nam *om.* BO; p. 70,20 dicitur] dicet BO; p. 102,19 Plato *om.* BO, but, at the same time, O does not always follow B in its errors: p. 62,4 in quibus] et B; p. 62,5 qua^{I} – uirtus^{II} *om.* B; p. 76,12 accidit *om.* B; p. 84,9 qualitatum^{I} – duarum *om.* B, which excludes the descent of O from B. Any descent of B from O is ruled out by palaeographical dating, the different selection of tracts, and wrong readings in O, e.g. p. 60,5 non *om.* O; p. 94,11 quidam dicunt] dicunt quidam O; p. 96,2 huius] hius B: minus O. But B and O undoubtedly descend from the
γ same manuscript (= γ). Many of their differences are only trivial or orthographic: e.g. p. 56,8 et *om.* O; p. 68,21 hyemem] yemem O; p. 108,4 quod^{II} *om.* O. In general, O shares more good readings with C DE than does B, and may have been a more faithful copy than B of the exemplar of the French group.

Similarly the omissions in B already noted at pp. 76,12 and 84,9, would seem to exclude a dependence of the ancestor of DE on B, and those at pp. 60,5 and 108,4, a similar dependence on O.

A stemma of the manuscripts may thus be drawn up as follows:

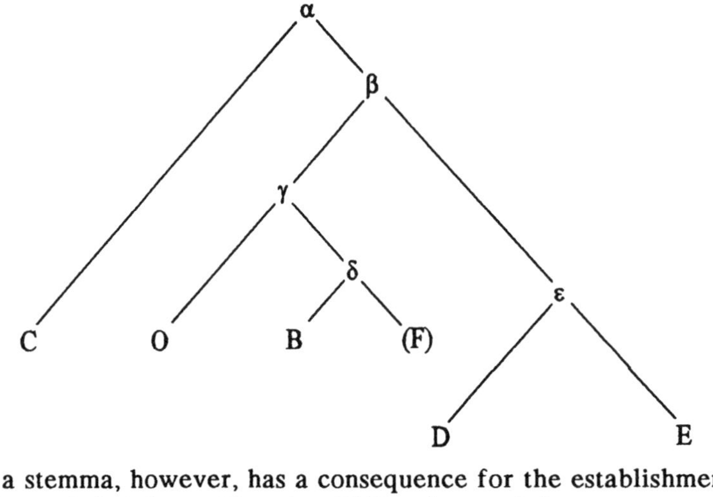

Such a stemma, however, has a consequence for the establishment of the text that demands brief consideration. If C and one of the groups γ or ε agree in a reading, then that reading is likely to have stood in the copy from which
α the surviving manuscripts derive (= α). But often ε presents a reading that is apparently superior to that of all other manuscripts. Sometimes this superiority may well be illusory, the product of scribal emendation to give a smoother text. But sometimes, as at p. 88,4 ἕκαστον] unumquodque ε: *om.* C γ; p. 92,8 ἐπὶ τὴν καρδίαν] ad cor (line 11) ε: *om.* C γ; p. 98,24–25 et quod omnium aliorum humorum ε: scilicet omnes alii (-os C) tres humores C γ, ε agrees with the Greek text in a way that is unlikely to be the result of emendation or chance.

One possible explanation for the presence of good readings only within

[1] See Nutton, in: CMG V 8,1, p. 32; Marinone, p. 17.

the two late manuscripts DE is that the stemma codicum is tripartite; in other words, that C, the direct common ancestor of BO(F), and the lost source of DE each had independent access to the same original. But B(F)ODE agree so often in error against C that such an explanation is unlikely, especially as it also runs counter to what has been suggested for other treatises of Galen. A better explanation for the agreement of C in error with γ or with ε is to suppose that the source of B(F)ODE retained many of the abbreviations of the common source of all the surviving manuscripts. If the argument, above, pp. 22–23, is correct that the mutilation of the ending of this treatise and of the opening of De pomo is the result of the loss of a leaf or leaves, this lost source cannot have been copied before the 1260s (cf. below).[1] To judge from the frequent errors within the manuscript tradition, it was badly written and heavily abbreviated, and bore occasionally alternative versions (cf. p. 62,14; p. 88,24; p. 96,16 plus magis; p. 98,24–25). A copy was made from it, itself poorly written, heavily abbreviated and containing doublets and interlinear alternatives, and was taken to France, where it became the ancestor of all the French Mss. The source manuscript remained in Italy, where it was seen and copied by the scribe of C. Any errors shared by C with any of the other Mss. would thus derive from misreadings of similar, although not identical, manuscripts, both with substantial abbreviations, and both liable to be misunderstood and miscopied in the same way.

V. Date and authorship of the Arabo-Latin translation

The proof of an Arabic origin for De sententiis is simple – the presence of many words transliterated from the Arabic and of constructions that correspond to the Arabic, but in the absence of any Arabic manuscript, it is impossible to say which of the versions and recensions the translator used.[2] Nor is it clear when and where he was active. At first sight a comparison with the specimens of mediaeval Latin translations of Aristotle from the Arabic suggests links with Gerard of Cremona and the early members of the "School of Toledo" in the late 12th century, and such forms as p. 84,5 reubach = *riwāq* (cf. also p. 62,14) and p. 70,5 Elguefete = *al-wāfida* hint at a Spanish origin.[3] But the earliest manuscripts come from Italy, and the presence of the mutilated ending from De pomo, translated from the Hebrew for (or by) an Italian ruler, the emperor Manfred (regn. 1258–1266), in all the manuscripts, might argue for an origin in S. Italy around the middle or end of the thirteenth century.[4] Linguistically, too, the words "briga" (p. 58,8) and "branca" (p. 88,14)

[1] Unless, of course, De pomo was added to an already existing manuscript. The ending of this section from De pomo is also badly corrupt.

[2] For the Arabic versions and the possibility that a Hebrew version intervened between the Arabic and the Latin, see below, pp. 39; 31–33.

[3] I base this tentative judgment on G. Lacombe, Aristoteles Latinus, Codices, vol. I, Rome, 1939, pp. 113–223.

[4] The ungrammatical beginning of De pomo and the general agreement of the manuscripts of De sententiis with the readings in Plezia's edition militate against the possibility that

are found relatively frequently in Italian authors, according to the compilers of the Mittellateinisches Wörterbuch, and the latter especially is found in Salernitan medical texts.[1] But this is hardly strong evidence, and the movement of translators from Spain to Sicily and S. Italy, and vice versa, makes any decision on date and origin extremely hazardous.

VI. The Arabo-Latin translation and the Greek original

In part the difficulty of assigning a date and place to the translation is the result of the generally poor performance of the translator. His version at times is imprecise; he uses terms that have a specific meaning within medicine in a somewhat confusing way; e.g. pp. 58,5; 90,13. 14. 16 regimen (= διοίκησις); pp. 70,19; 80,3. 5 membra radicalia (= στερεὰ σώματα). Both philosophical and medical terms are left in transcription: e.g. p. 84,5 reubach (= *riwāq*) for the Stoics (cf. also p. 62,14); p. 70,5 Elguefete (= *al-wāfida*) for the Epidemics; p. 98,2 listilia (= *al-istisqā'*) for dropsy, with consequent confusion in the manuscript tradition. The result is that at times it is very hard to penetrate behind the Latin version to the original Greek, and some Greek words, particularly proper names, are almost unrecognisable (e.g. p. 80,4 Elumerephilis; p. 86,1 guibentirie = δηλητήρια).[2] The order and structure of Galen's Greek, changed once to suit the demands of an Arabic grammar and syntax, is further altered by the intervention of the Latin translator to produce something at times almost unintelligible.

But many difficulties of comprehension are removed by an acquaintance with the standard procedures of the mediaeval Latin translators from the Arabic. The following are among the most obvious features:

1. Since both Syriac and Arabic lack adverbs *sensu stricto,* Greek adverbs have to be translated in a variety of ways. Most common is the *figura etymologica,* the repetition in a different grammatical form of some portion of the verb: p. 58,14 significat significatione manifesta; p. 96,19 demonstratum est demonstratione manifesta.

Occasionally, the phrase itself can be recast: p. 110,9–10 αἰσθανομένων τε πολυειδῶς] in sensu nostro diuersarum rerum (sentientibus multiformiter Nic.).

2. Both Arabic and Latin translators frequently use hendiadys, duplication and parallelism, of both words and phrases, to convey the force of the

the translator was working from a text containing both On my own opinions and De pomo in an already mutilated form.

1 See Mittellateinisches Wörterbuch bis zum ausgehenden 13. Jahrhundert, ed. Bayer. Akademie d. Wiss. and Deutsche Akademie d. Wiss. zu Berlin, vol. I, Munich, 1967, col. 1562 s. v. branca; col. 1582 s. v. briga; cf. p. 110,21 in zarolis, and below, p. 206, the note to p. 110,21–24.

2 J. Ruska, Turba philosophorum. Ein Beitrag zur Geschichte der Alchemie, Quellen und Studien zur Geschichte der Naturwissenschaften und der Medizin 1, Berlin, 1931, pp. 18–30, offers a valuable guide to the vagaries of the transcription of Greek proper names via Arabic into mediaeval Latin. J. D. Latham, Arabic into Medieval Latin, Journal of Semitic Studies 17, 1972, pp. 30–67, esp. pp. 31–38, is also useful.

original: p. 54,16 infecta siue destructa; p. 56,3 declarati uel manifestati; p. 70,2–3 conuersionem hore unius horarum anni; p. 70,6 in hac dispositione dispositionum aeris; p. 104,14 ἀρκεῖται] sufficiet ... et hoc sufficit ei; p. 112,17–18 εἶναί τινα ὕπαρξιν αὐτῆς ἰδίαν] sit ens existens per se et diuisum ab alio.

At times this duplication may be regarded as an intrusive gloss, whether in the Arabic or in the Latin alone: p. 56,20 deitas, id est uirtus deitatis.

3. "qui est" is frequently used to indicate a relationship expressed in other ways in the Greek: p. 60,2–3 occasionem que est motus uoluntarii (= genitive); p. 60,17 perceptio que est omnium sensibilium (= genitive).

4. "hoc est quod" corresponds to γάρ or γοῦν: pp. 72,7; 86,8–9. 22; 104,15.

5. "esse" + present participle corresponds to a Greek present: p. 78,9 non est existens; p. 116,5 sum sciens.

6. Comparatives are usually expressed with "magis"; superlatives either in the same way or with the addition of "omnibus".

7. The use of a personal pronoun before the verb is more likely to derive from an Arabic idiom than from Galen's own usage: p. 72,8 ἐδείξαμεν] nos manifestauimus C γ: manifestauimus ε; p. 84,12 ἐδείχθη] et ego demonstraui.

When these changes are taken into consideration, much of the Latin becomes more intelligible, and Galen's thought, if not his Greek, can be reconstructed. But we are still far from the pedantic accuracy of Niccolò, or the stylish genius of Ḥunayn, and in many places the Latin is only a crude approximation of the original Greek. How crude can best be seen from a comparison of the Latin with the surviving Greek fragments or with the original Greek texts to which Galen is alluding. Although, in general, the translator succeeds in retaining the sense of the original Greek, it would be very hard to reconstruct its wording. Unhappily often, he has obscured Galen's meaning or misunderstood either Galen or his Arabic exemplar, and confusion may well have been increased by copyists who misread or miscopied his abbreviations, e.g. at p. 122,4 γένος] genus *scripsi*: igitur α. Without the very many parallel passages in other Galenic texts much of De sententiis would remain incomprehensible or delusory. Unlike Niccolò's versions, whose Greek original can often be reconstructed precisely, the Arabo-Latin translation brings almost nothing of value to the constitution of the Greek text, where that exists, and in turn it often requires the help of the Greek for its understanding and elucidation.

VII. The excerpt in Hebrew translation

The second chapter and the beginning of the third, pp. 56,12–60,7, are also preserved in the first part of the Sefer ha-Mebaqqesh (The book of the seeker) written in 1263 by the Spanish Jew Shem Tob ben Yosef Ibn Falaquera (ca. 1225 – after 1290). Ibn Falaquera was acquainted with many of the philosophical and ethical texts of Galen, as well as with a whole range of writers on ethics in Arabic as well as in Hebrew. Although this popular encyclopaedia was first printed in Hebrew as long ago as 1778 and an English

Fal.

version of the first part appeared in 1976, its significance was not revealed to students of Galen until 1995, when M. Zonta published his important study of Galenic philosophy in mediaeval Hebrew.[1] As well as drawing attention to new fragments from the Protrepticus and De indolentia, Zonta provides, pp. 103–106, an edition of the Hebrew passage based on a collation of the 1778 DH editio princeps (= DH), pp. 35,16–36,1, with two manuscripts, New York, Jew- NY ish Theological Seminary, microfilm 2306 (= NY), fols. 23^{v}–24^{r}; and London, L British Library, or. 1484 (= L), fols. 22^{v}–23^{r}. The Hebrew text is not only given an Italian translation, but compared with a facing text of De sententiis based partly on my earlier collations and partly on Zonta's own readings of B and C.[2] The importance of this evidence for the text of De sententiis is further discussed by Zonta on pp. 107–108. Although my conclusions differ somewhat from his, his pioneering work forms the basis for this section. The Hebrew text, as edited by Zonta, has been integrated into the present edition.[3]

While Ibn Falaquera clearly derives his dating for this tract from a secondary source, perhaps Rhazes, see below, p. 37, he expressly claims to be quoting Galen's own words, a claim easily born out by a comparison with the text of De sententiis. As Zonta amply demonstrates, Ibn Falaquera thus offers a way back to the (lost) Arabic that is independent of the Latin tradition. His text preserves traces of Arabic idiom, and confirms at times variants in the Latin that might otherwise be doubted, e.g. at pp. 56,16 (manifestum est ε); 56, 23 (ipse). In particular, he proves that the difficulty in the Latin at p. 58,8–9 goes in part back at least to the Arabic, but has been made worse by further confusion within the Latin tradition.

Zonta, pp. 107–108, also raises the intriguing possibility that De sententiis was a translation made from a Hebrew intermediary, and that Ibn Falaquera was not himself translating from the Arabic, although he knew it fluently, but was copying from an already existing Hebrew translation. Two arguments are advanced to support this hypothesis; the presence in the Latin tradition of part of De pomo, which had been translated into Hebrew by Abraham ibn Chasdai of Barcelona around 1200 before its translation into Latin in S. Italy around 1260.[4] And, secondly, that the possible translation error "apparuerunt", p. 58,9, is slightly better explained as a corruption of the Hebrew than of the Arabic.[5] But against this, Zonta himself admits that there is otherwise no trace whatsoever of this Hebrew version, and that the transla-

1 See Zonta, pp. 25–26; 152. I am grateful to him for sending me a copy of his book.

2 Not all of Zonta's collations are correct, especially as he is unfamiliar with the difficult abbreviations in C.

3 The variant readings carefully recorded by Zonta do not alter significantly the sense of the passage, with the exception of the name Protagoras NY: Pythagoras L DH (Pictagoras, p. 58,1). The English translation is based on those kindly prepared for me by G. Bos, N. Serikoff, and G. Strohmaier.

4 See M. Steinschneider, Die hebräischen Übersetzungen des Mittelalters und die Juden als Dolmetscher, Berlin, 1893, pp. 267–270; F. E. Peters, Aristoteles Arabus, Leiden, 1968, p. 65. For the date and origin of the Latin version, see Plezia, pp. 20–24.

5 One might consider also the possibility that the mutilation at the end of the book and the beginning of De pomo occurred within the process of transmission in Hebrew.

tion "apparuerunt" could be derived from the Arabic through a corrupt exemplar. Furthermore, if Ibn Falaquera was simply copying out mechanically an existing Hebrew version, one would have to conclude that it was a text that had reached him with some differences from that which formed the basis of De sententiis; e.g. the omission of "et hoc expertus sum egoipse", p. 58,15–16; and the longer "et accipere – uideo quod est", p. 58,19–22; and the addition of "and are attributed to Him", p. 58,1, "blessed be He", p. 58,9, and, for "predicare", p. 58,18, the doublet "exalt and praise". None of the transcriptions found elsewhere in the Latin suggests a Hebrew intermediary, and the mutilated section from De pomo corresponds sufficiently closely to the Latin of Plezia's edition to exclude the possibility that the translator was working from a Hebrew text that already included that ending.

On balance, therefore, it is easier to assume that Ibn Falaquera was making his own version from an Arabic text as he went along than that he was copying an existing Hebrew translation whose text differed in part from that used by the translator of De sententiis. It cannot, of course, be excluded that Ibn Falaquera himself was responsible for these divergencies, perhaps working from memory or deliberately rewriting as he went along, but, until a Hebrew manuscript of On my own opinions comes to light, the existence of a lost Hebrew intermediary is very far from being proved.

VIII. The Graeco-Latin translation of chapters 14—15 (= De substantia)

In the first half of the fourteenth century, a second version was produced by the S. Italian physician and translator, Niccolò da Deoprepio da Reggio (fl. 1308–1345).[1] Entitled De substantia virtutum naturalium, it covered only the last two chapters of On my own opinions, which, as we have already seen, were given a separate sub-heading in some Greek Mss. and also circulated independently before the end of the twelfth century. De substantia (= Nic.) is **Nic.**
found in seven Mss., two of which have already been described.

a) Parisinus lat. 6865

Paris, Bibliothèque Nationale, fonds latin 6865[2] (= Nic.^{b}), contains De **Nic.^{b}**
substantia on fols. 117^{v}–118^{r}.

b) Malatestianus S.V 4

Cesena, Biblioteca Malatestiana, S.V 4[3] (= Nic.^{c}), includes De substantia **Nic.^{c}**
on fols. 26^{v}–27^{r}.

1 To the bibliography on Niccolò given by Nutton, in: CMG V 8,1, p. 23, add G. Pezzi, La vita e l'opera di maestro Nicolao da Reggio, Atti della IX Biennale della Marca e dello studio Firmano per la storia dell'arte medica, Fermo, 1971, pp. 229–233. To his list of non-medical translations by Niccolò, add Sextus Empiricus, Venice, Marcianus lat. 3460.

2 See above, p. 23.

3 See above, p. 23.

c) Malatestianus S.XXVI 4

Nic.^{g} Cesena, Biblioteca Malatestiana, S.XXVI 4 (= Nic.^{g}), a parchment codex of 242 leaves, 312 mm. by 227 mm. in size, was written c. 1465 by a scribe at the Malatesta court, and, like Nic.^{c}, once formed part of the library of Giovanni Marco da Rimini. De substantia is to be found on fol. 14^{rv}.[1]

d) Matritensis lat. 1978

Nic.^{h} Madrid, Biblioteca Nacional, codex lat. 1978 (= Nic.^{h}), a parchment manuscript of 136 leaves, 385 mm. by 265 mm., written in Spain about 1375, has two columns to the page, and contains De substantia on fols. 101^{v}–102^{r}.[2]

e) Monacensis lat. 490

The only dated Ms. of De substantia is Munich, Bayerische Staatsbiblio-
Nic.^{i} thek 490 (= Nic.^{i}), a paper Ms., which was copied by Hartmann Schedel at Rentzenhoff in autumn 1488, "dum aucupio operam dedi". De substantia is found on fols. 17^{r}–19^{v}.[3]

f) Neapolitanus VIII D 38

In 1981, R. J. Durling drew attention to two further manuscripts that had escaped the notice of earlier cataloguers and compilers.[4] Naples, Biblioteca
Nic.^{j} Nazionale VIII D 38 (= Nic.^{j}), is a manuscript of the fourteenth century, 230 mm. by 320 mm., written in S. Italy in two columns of 45 lines to the page. It was formerly in the Franciscan convent of S. Bernardino at L'Aquila in Central Italy. De substantia occupies a single leaf, fol. 51$^{ra\text{-}va}$, badly worn on the back.[5] The numerous comments on the argument and on the meaning of particular words, written in a contemporary or slightly later hand, show that at least one reader thought the text of some interest.

g) Wellcomensis 286

The final Ms. of De substantia is itself incomplete. London, Wellcome

1 See Nutton, in: CMG V 8,1, p. 29; Marinone, pp. 16–17; Manfron, pp. 238–240. On Giovanni Marco, see G. Baader, Die Bibliothek des Giovanni Marco da Rimini, in: Studia Codicologica, Berlin, 1977 (Texte u. Untersuchungen 124), pp. 43–97; Frioli, pp. 171–179.

2 See J. L. de Toro, Inventario general de manoscritos de la Biblioteca Nacional, vol. V, Madrid, 1959, pp. 394–397.

3 See C. Halm, G. Meyer, S. Riezler, Catalogus codicum manu scriptorum bibliothecae regiae Monacensis, 2nd ed., vol. III 1, Munich, 1892, p. 138. For the subscription, see R. Stauber, Die Schedelsche Bibliothek, Freiburg i. Br., 1908, p. 72.

4 See R. J. Durling, Corrigenda and addenda to Diels' Galenica, Traditio 37, 1981, p. 378. I am grateful to Dr. Rita Masullo for providing me with photographs of this manuscript.

5 The section is not identified in the detailed description of the manuscript given by C. Cenci, Manoscritti francescani della Biblioteca Nazionale di Napoli, vol. II, Grottaferrata, 1971, p. 833, no. 468. The verso of the leaf, beginning at p. 122,13 οὐ μετεχούσης (non participante), is badly worn and stained, and hence difficult to read. For a similar error about the content of the text by a modern cataloguer, see below, p. 35 n. 1.

Institute Library codex 286 (= Nic.^{k}), is a parchment manuscript of 178 folios, 390 mm. by 260 mm. in size, written in Italy c. 1348. Of its Latin versions of Galen four, On crises, On critical days, On the small ball, and On affected places, are ascribed either to Niccolò or to a "nova translatio". On the natural faculties, book III, breaks off at the bottom of fol. 173^{r}, and is then followed by two blank pages. The text begins again at the top of the first column on fol. 174^{v} with:]icut animam habemus (p. 110,4–5), the opening of De substantia, and continues to the end of the column, where it breaks off at: corpus subsepturum animam. alterato vero ... (p. 118,11–12).[1] The reason for these gaps is easily explicable. The Ms. was originally intended to be illustrated with historiated miniatures at the beginning of each book, and with rubricated initials at the beginning of individual chapters, but this was never fully carried out. Some illustrations were completed in colour, e.g. fols. 11^{r}, 27^{v}, 84^{r}, 132^{r}, 133^{v}; others were left in outline, e.g. fol. 1^{r}; and here space was left free for the scribe and artist to work in, and, perhaps, also to include missing sections if they could be found. The curious way in which De substantia breaks off suggests that the scribe had a larger text from which to copy, and, for whatever reason, failed to complete his task, leaving sufficient space to come back and finish without interfering with the next tract, which is rubricated but lacks the opening initial. This Ms. is also of considerable interest because of its origin close to the Angevin court, for among the many marginalia are several references to Giovanni da Penna, d. 1348, a physician colleague there of Niccolò, and the text itself exhibits many italianisms.[2] On fol. 64^{r} is a note referring to illnesses and deaths occurring in 1361, which indicates that the Ms. itself was produced almost in the lifetime of Niccolò. Nic.^{k}

IX. The relationship between the Latin manuscripts of De substantia

Not enough material survives to draw up a conclusive stemma codicum, and only a few points can be made here. There is no doubt, as Marinone and I have argued, that Nic.^{g} is a direct copy of Nic.^{c}.[3] The Ms. from which Schedel copied Nic.^{i} must be presumed lost, for the selection of texts in Schedel's volume in no way corresponds to that of any other surviving group.[4] Nor can any

1 See S. A. J. Moorat, Catalogue of western manuscripts on medicine and science in the Wellcome Historical Medical Library, vol. I: Mss. written before 1650, London, 1962, pp. 180–183, wrongly identifying it, p. 183, as an unfinished tract on the soul. This entry silently corrects Moorat's fallible description in several places. De substantia is not the only text in this volume that seems to have been left incomplete by the scribe, e.g. fol. 117^{v}–118^{r} contain the beginning of Galen, On semen; see De Lacy, in: CMG V 3,1, p. 17.

2 See R. J. Durling, Burgundio of Pisa's translation of Galen's Περὶ κράσεων, 'De complexionibus', ed. (Galenus Latinus I), Ars Medica II 6, 1, Berlin – New York, 1976, pp. XVI–XVII. The role of Giovanni da Penna, the recipient of Niccolò's version of On critical days, fol. 68^{r}, is stressed by R. Weiss, Medieval and humanist Greek, Padua, 1977, pp. 134–135.

3 See Nutton, in: CMG V 8,1, pp. 31–32; Marinone, p. 17. Cf. the following coniunctive errors: p. 112,5 ἐνεργεῖν] agere Nic.: *om.* Nic.^{cg}; p. 122,4 αἰσθήσεως] sensus Nic.: *om.* Nic.^{cg}.

4 In view of the history of De sententiis, and its identification in F with [Gal.], Introd. s.

direct link be proved between the other four surviving Mss., despite their early date and a possible Angevin connection, although the presence of such shared readings in Nic.[k] and the badly copied Nic.[j] as p. 110,7 διὰ] per Nic.: propter Nic.[jk]; p. 112,1 ἐκπονήσαντες] laborauerunt Nic.: laborauerit Nic.[jk] might well indicate that both were copied from the same source.

X. Authorship of the Graeco-Latin translation

Although this version is ascribed to Niccolò only in Nic.[i], there can be little doubt that this fragment comes from him or, less likely, his school.[1] Its presence alongside other new translations of his in Nic.[k] only adds weight to what might be gained from a study of the peculiarities of the translation. It was made directly from a Greek original (note such words as p. 110,13 ἀξιώματος] anxiomate; p. 112,1 θεωρίαν] theoria; p. 120,1 εὐκρασίας] eucrasia) by a competent translator who kept close to the details of the original Greek syntax. The Greek is translated "de verbo ad verbum", with only occasional words omitted, paraphrased or transposed, and the choice of particles and other stylistic features correspond closely to those found in De consuetudinibus, De morborum temporibus and De victu attenuante.[2] There is thus no compelling reason to challenge Niccolò's authorship.

XI. The Graeco-Latin translation and the Greek manuscripts

The remarkable ability of the translator to reproduce many of the fine details of his Greek original means that it is relatively easy to determine its worth. The fact that it contained only the last two sections offers an obvious link with L and its derivatives rather than with A.[3] It also shared some interesting and significant errors with them: p. 112,17 μηδὲ om. L Nic.; p. 116,13 οὐσιῶν] οὐσῶν L, existentibus Nic.; p. 116,22 κεραννυμένη] κεραννῦν ψυχῆς L, confunditur, animamque Nic.; p. 120,21 μέν τι] μὲν A: μέντοι L, quidem nimirum Nic. At the same time, it had some good readings not in L: p. 114,9–11

med. and Gal., De sectis ad eos qui introd. (see above, pp. 25–26), it may not be without interest to note that in Nic.[i] De substantia follows immediately on the Liber introductorius vel de sectis. The following bad readings might suggest that Nic.[i] and Nic.[h] were related: p. 118,20 θερμαινομένου] calefacto Nic.: calefactio Nic.[hi]; p. 118,24 δὲ] autem Nic.: *om.* Nic.[hi]; p. 122,17 μόνον] solum Nic.: solorum Nic.[hi], but they are far from conclusive.

1 L. Thorndike, Translations of works of Galen from the Greek by Niccolò da Reggio (c. 1308–1345), Byzantina Metabyzantina 1,1, 1946, p. 230, labels it as dubious, perhaps under the influence of a Renaissance editor who identified it with Gal., De sequela potentiarum anime (= Quod animi mores corp. temp. sequ.), cf. p. 229.

2 Galeni De consuetudinibus, ed. J. M. Schmutte, CMG Suppl. III, Leipzig and Berlin, 1941; I. Wille, Die Schrift Galens Περὶ τῶν ἐν ταῖς νόσοις καιρῶν und ihre Überlieferung, Diss. Kiel, 1960 (typescript); Galeno, La dieta dimagrante, ed. N. Marinone, Turin et al., 1973.

3 Although the fact that the last sections are similarly subtitled in A and were perhaps regarded by A^2 or Demetrios as forming a separate tract means that this is not as cogent as might at first sight appear.

εἰδείην τὴν ἐν αὐτοῖς ἀλήθειαν, τῶν δὲ ἄλλως οὐδὲν αὐτῆς A: sciui eam que in eis ueritatem, horum autem quoniam nichil de ea Nic.: om. L; p. 114,26–27 τε καὶ τὴν ἠθικὴν A Nic. (et secundum moralem): om. L; p. 116,11 μόρια A Nic. (particulas): om. L; p. 122,18 αὐτὴν A Nic. (eam): om. L. On two occasions Nic. would appear to have preserved a good reading otherwise lost in the Greek tradition (unless it derives from the very act of translation): p. 114, 11 ὡς] quoniam Nic.: ἄλλως A: corr. Ald.: deest L; p. 122,10 παραπλήσια] proximas (passiones) Nic.: παραπλησίαν L A Ald.

From this one may conclude that Nic.'s exemplar did not come from the same family as A, and sometimes preserved a better text than L.[1] Its agreement with A may thus help to settle the text in favour of A in three places where A and L differ stylistically: p. 110,7 ante τὰ add. καὶ L: non hab. A Nic.; p. 118,10–11 χρὴ τὸ σῶμα A Nic. (oportet corpus): τὸ σῶμα χρὴ L; p. 120,15–16 ὁπόσαι τέ εἰσι καὶ ὁποῖαι A Nic. (quot sunt et quales): εἰσι post ὁποῖαι trsp. L. But in general Nic. sides with L, and thus contributes relatively little that is significant to the establishment of the Greek.

B. The textual history of De propriis placitis

Having surveyed the manuscript evidence for On my own opinions, we are now able to describe its various vicissitudes, at least in outline. There can be no doubt whatsoever about its authenticity. The very many cross references, the style, and the doctrines it contains, to say nothing of any external evidence, are conclusive. That it is not mentioned in any of Galen's own bibliographies is no problem, for it was among the very latest, if not the last, of his writings. The allusion in chapter 1 to De libris propriis dates the text to the late 190s, at the very earliest, and possibly a decade or more later. This book's avowed purpose, to provide a guide to Galen's own opinions, finds a strong parallel in his attempt in De libris propriis to authenticate his writings by means of a bibliography, and, on those grounds alone, one would be prepared to put it at the end of Galen's life. There is no reason to disagree with Rhazes, who said, "it is well known to all those who have read the works of Galen that he only composed this book ... after exhaustive investigation and confirmation of his opinions, and that it was the last of his books and compositions."[2]

A more precise date may perhaps be furnished by an Arabic quotation from the *Ṣiwān al-ḥikma* ascribed to Abū Sulaymān al-Sijistānī (died c. 985). According to this source, "when, at the end of his life, he [Galen] wrote a book on what he believed as simply opinions, he included these topics [i. e. the eternity of the world, the nature of the soul ...], and he confessed his ig-

1 In this relatively short text the precise relationship with L is hard to determine, but conjunction in error suggests a descent from the same archetype.

2 Al-Rāzī, *Shukūk*: p. 4,2–4 Mohaghegh. I am grateful to L. I. Conrad for translating this passage for me.

norance and his incertainty, and acknowledged his inability in matters that exercised the philosophers. Thereupon Alexander of Aphrodisias remarked that Galen had taken eighty years of his life to come to the conclusion that he did not know, notwithstanding his labours in his own art, an art based upon rational deductions as well as experience, which he had carried out to the benefit of mankind."[1] But is this an authentic contemporary reference to Galen and his book? Or has the author (or compiler) of the Ṣiwān al-ḥikma made up his story out of a genuine allusion to On my own books and the dispute at De praecognitione 5,9–16: CMG V 8,1, p. 96,5–98,11, between Galen and Alexander of Damascus, whom Arabic authors identified with Alexander of Aphrodisias?

Three arguments suggest that we are dealing with genuine material. Firstly, Alexander of Aphrodisias, although conceding that Galen was ἔνδοξος, In Arist. Top. comm.: CAG II 2, p. 549,23–24, vigorously opposed his views on a variety of philosophical themes. Secondly, despite the hyperbolic praise of Galen's medical art, this passage must originally come from a hostile Greek philosophical source, and, in both manner and argument, Alexander is a far better candidate for authorship than Simplicius, Themistius, or Philoponus, let alone any Arabic writer. Thirdly, Galen's refusal to commit himself in this treatise to any answer to many philosophical problems, especially on the nature of the soul, his *Nichtwissen,* could very easily be interpreted by an opponent as a confession of ignorance. 'I do not know enough to make up my mind' can easily be represented in polemic as 'I know nothing at all'. All this suggests that the Arabic author has preserved that great rarity, a genuine contemporary criticism of a work of antiquity.

Whether he is also right to date this treatise to, at the earliest, 209/210 is harder to decide. The traditional date for Galen's death, supplied by the Suda, would have him dying aged 70, i.e. in 199/200. But there are strong grounds for believing that this date rests on a misunderstanding, and that in its original context the seventy years referred only to Galen's activity as writer and doctor. Besides, De theriaca ad Pisonem, which would appear to be a genuine work of Galen, cannot have been written before 204, and probably not before 207 at the earliest.[2] Nonetheless, one cannot exclude the possibility that Alexander was exaggerating for rhetorical effect, and was himself ignorant of Galen's exact age. But even if the question of the date of Galen's death is left open, there can be little doubt that the story of their quarrel was

1 As-Sijistānī, lines 98–101. The reference in al-ʿĀmirī is more fanciful, see A Muslim philosopher on the soul and its fate: Al-ʿĀmirī's Kitāb al-Amad ʿalā l-abad, ed. E. K. Rowson, New Haven, Conn., 1988 (American Oriental Series 70), pp. 74–75, cf. the commentary pp. 214–216.

2 For arguments that De ther. ad Pis. was genuine and composed around 207, see S. Swain, Hellenism and Empire, Oxford, 1996, Appendix D, pp. 430–432; V. Nutton, Galen ad multos annos, Dynamis 15, 1995, pp. 25–39; Galen on theriac: problems of authenticity, in: Galen on pharmacology. Philosophy, history and medicine, Proceedings of the Vth International Galen Colloquium, Lille, 16 – 18 March 1995, ed. A. Debru, Leiden, New York, Köln, 1997 (Studies in Ancient Medicine 16), pp. 133–151.

widely circulated in the Islamic world and that it contained at least a kernel of truth.[1]

Direct knowledge of On my own opinions then ceases for many centuries. The late-antique commentators on Aristotle, Themistius, Philoponus and Simplicius, may have derived their understanding of some of Galen's philosophical beliefs from this tract, but it is perhaps more likely that they took them from other treatises, in particular from the now lost On demonstration.[2] Given the philosophical orientation of On my own opinions, it is hardly surprising that no excerpts from it appear in the Greek medical encyclopaedic tradition from Oribasius onwards, or that it should have attracted no attention from the first wave of oriental translators in the sixth century. Only with the succession of translations produced in the middle years of the ninth century was this silence broken.

Ḥunayn ibn Isḥāq, in his remarkable list of Galenic versions, writes as follows[3]: "His book about his personal beliefs: This treatise consists also[4] of one book. In it he tells what he knows and what he does not know. Ayyūb had translated it into Syriac. I translated it into Syriac for my son Isḥāq. Thābit ibn Qurra translated it into Arabic for Abū Jaʿfar Muḥammad ibn Mūsā.[5] ʿĪsā ibn Yaḥyā translated it into Arabic. Isḥāq collated it with the original and I corrected it for ʿAbdallāh ibn Isḥāq." Since we have only the Latin translation and a handful of Arabic quotations and allusions to go on, it would be foolish to decide whose Arabic version lies behind the Latin translation. The fact that in 987 the bookseller Ibn al-Nadīm, followed later by Ibn al-Qifṭī,[6] named Thābit as the sole translator into Arabic, may indicate no more than that he was drawing on recension B of Ḥunayn's Risāla (cf. n. 5), which omits the reference to ʿĪsā.

Through one or both of these Arabic versions, On my own opinions became accessible to the Arab world. If Holmberg is right in his attribution of a treatise On the unity and trinity of God to Israel of Kashkar, d. 872, Galen's agnostic view of the soul in this treatise was being discussed among Chris-

1 On this see Temkin, pp. 71–94; V. Nutton, Galen in the eyes of his contemporaries, Bulletin of the History of Medicine 58, 1984, pp. 315–324 (repr. in: Nutton, From Democedes to Harvey, no. III); and Galen's philosophical testament, pp. 45–49; R. W. Sharples, Alexander of Aphrodisias, On time, Phronesis 27, 1982, pp. 58–81. The closer the first evidence for the story of the quarrel comes to the era of the translation of the works of Galen and Alexander, the more likely it is that this pretty story had some textual basis.

2 Nemesius of Emesa, who strongly attacked Galen's views on the soul and who was aware both of his agnosticism and his later shift towards an identification with some form of mixture, De nat. hom. 2: pp. 23,24–24,4 Morani, took his information from De demonstratione, not De propriis placitis.

3 Ḥunain, no. 113. Cf. Bergsträßer, no. 152, where Ḥunayn included it among the genuine works of Galen absent from the autobibliographies.

4 Ḥunayn had just described De optimo medico cognoscendo, in one book.

5 Here the text of recension B ceases. The following passage is preserved only in recension A; see Bergsträßer, p. 32, col. 3.

6 Ibn al-Nadīm, *Kitāb al-fihrist*, ed. G. Flügel, vol. I, Leipzig, 1871, p. 291,5 (transl. B. Dodge, vol. II, New York, London, 1970, p. 685); Ibn al-Qifṭī, *Taʾrīkh al-ḥukamāʾ*, ed. J. Lippert, Leipzig, 1903, p. 131,13–14.

tians within Ḥunayn's lifetime.[1] As well as mentioning in passing Galen's declaration of his agnosticism in De placitis Hippocratis et Platonis, Israel claims that Galen was perplexed about the soul, and that, in general, in discussing it he was prepared to follow the guidelines laid down by Plato.[2] Although Israel appears to be quoting the actual words of this treatise directly – "he said in the book entitled The book on his opinions ..." –, he is merely summarising one of its main themes, and combining the reference to Plato and Aristotle (p. 102,18–19) with the wider acceptance of Plato's views in the final chapters. The same procedure is followed by a variety of other doctors and philosophers. Rhazes, Jābir, Averroes, al-Ghazālī, Maimonides, and Ibn Falaquera, all take issue with Galen's refusal to commit himself on the nature of the soul or on the eternity of the world, but only Ibn Falaquera appears to quote Galen directly.[3] The rest offer merely a brief statement of his agnosticism, which they need not have derived from a personal reading of this book. Nonetheless, they were engaging with him as a respectable, if misguided, scholar, whose ideas were not confined to the principles of therapy.[4]

By contrast with this occasional interest, in the world of Byzantium there is little trace of any response whatsoever. The text as a whole was still accessible in Greek in the ninth century, when Ḥunayn and his followers translated it, and possibly even later, if the scholia were compiled then, and if, as seems likely, the ordered selection of extracts is to be placed in the Byzantine intellectual renaissance of the tenth and eleventh centuries. The text may already by this time have been divided into chapters, perhaps with section headings,

1 Holmberg, ch. 53: Arabic, p. 17. Alternative attributions to Yaḥyā ibn ʿAdī or a second Israel of Kashkar, rejected by Holmberg, would place this treatise a century later.

2 Holmberg, ch. 41: Arabic, p. 13. To be added to the references made by Arab authors to De plac. Hipp. et Plat. at CMG V 4,1,2, pp. 42–46; 613–614.

3 Al-Rāzī, *Shukūk*: pp. 3,22–4,7; 6,20–7,1; 7,22; 14,17–18; 15,10–11; 32,10–11 Mohaghegh; Jābir, *Kitāb al-baḥt̲*, quoted in: Kraus, p. 329 n. 7; al-Ghazāli, *Tahāfut al-falāsifā*, pp. 21–22 Bouyges (transl. p. 13 Kamali); Averroes, *Tahāfut al-tahāfut*, transl. S. van den Bergh, London, 1954, vol. I, pp. 74–75; idem in: Aristotelis Opera cum Averrois commentariis, fol. 17^{va}6–16 (cf. Kalbfleisch, Zu Galenos, p. 694, who cites as source R. Chartier, Hippocratis Coi, et Claudii Galeni Pergameni ... Opera, ed., Paris, 1679, vol. II, p. 71); Maimonides, Guide for the perplexed II 15: Le guide des égarés, transl. S. Munk, new ed., Paris, 1963, vol. II, p. 127; Aphorisms, XXV 59: J. Schacht and M. Meyerhof, Maimonides against Galen on philosophy and cosmogony, Majalla kulliyyati l-ādāb bi-l-jāmiʿati l-miṣriyya 5, 1937, p. 66; Ibn Falaquera, see above, pp. 31–33. The whole question is elegantly surveyed by Bürgel, pp. 276–290.

4 Not all the Galenic opinions attacked by these Arabic scholars are to be found in this treatise, e.g. those on motion, time, and place. But to argue from this that the work was never finished is unjustified, for an alternative reading suggests that they regarded these views as additional to what was contained in On my own opinions. The list of references to Arabic and Jewish authors in Zonta, pp. 15–16, does not distinguish between engagement with this text and knowledge that Galen had held these views, which the author may have taken from another treatise. E.g. Kraus, p. 330, and Kraus and Walzer in the introduction to Galen's Compendium Timaei Platonis, London, 1951, p. 11, attribute to On my own opinions a quotation more likely to come from the lost De demonstratione; and Averroes, in: Aristotelis Opera cum Averrois commentariis, fol. 17^{va}6–16, quotes Galen's De demonstratione as well as On my own opinions.

for when L and the exemplar of Niccolò were written, the last section was already circulating as an independent treatise with a different title. Niccolò's translation into Latin made this part accessible to the West, but with little effect. Although several near-contemporary copies survive to show at least a brief flurry of interest in the newly available work, I have found no citations from it in medical authors of the fourteenth and fifteenth centuries.[1]

The picture of reactions to De sententiis is only slightly less dark. We cannot be certain when or where the translation was made from the Arabic, or how the section from De pomo came to circulate with it, and Pierre Gas appears to be alone in quoting from it.[2] It is missing from the lists of Galenic writings made by Vincent of Beauvais in the thirteenth century and by Jacobus Philippus Forestus of Bergamo in the last years of the fifteenth, although the latter does note Niccolò's version, albeit under the slightly altered title of De substantia virtutum.[3] However, both versions are contained in the list of books appended by the Oxford scholar Walter Burley (1275–1345) to his account of Galen in his Liber de vita et moribus philosophorum, although they are missing from some of the manuscripts, translations and printed editions of this popular work.[4] Burley's citation of Niccolò's version as De substantiis virtutum needs no comment, but his reference to a treatise De fide sua is potentially significant in the light of the titles in B and F. While that in B is a later addition, one cannot exclude entirely the possibility that F had been seen by Burley, himself trained at Paris, when he was writing his book towards the

1 Gentile da Foligno, ob. 1348, in his little treatise De divisione librorum Galieni, printed in the Articella, Venice, 1483, fol. 210^{v}, includes De substantia naturalium facultatum among the works that Galen had devoted to the formal cause. Since he refers also to De disnia, it is likely that his list was compiled after 1345 (see above, p. 23), and with knowledge of a manuscript of these works, but there is no evidence that Gentile had read them – indeed, his description suggests that he had not. His apparent reference, ibid., to a Latin version of De plac. Hipp. et Plat. derives from a cross-reference to this tract within a translation of the Ars medica.

2 Gentile, ibid., does not mention De sententiis at all, although he knows of De demonstratione, and, as we have seen, mentions Niccolò's version of De substantia. Neither De substantia nor De sententiis appears in the list of Galenica in Wiesbaden, Ms. 24, of c. 1400, see K. Sudhoff, Eine Liste von Galenschriften aus dem Anfang des 15. Jahrhunderts, Archiv f. Geschichte d. Medizin 17, 1925, p. 140.

3 Vincent of Beauvais, Speculum Historiae, of c. 1254, cited from the Douai edition of 1624, where the list appears on pp. 400–401. I doubt that De sententiis, even with its incorrect ending, can be identified with the otherwise unknown tract on alchemy entitled De ramo pomi congelati, or with De proprietate, which, from its place among the drug books, would appear to be a pharmaceutical work. These curious works, as well as De substantia virtutum, appear in the list given by Jacobus Philippus Forestus, Supplementum chronicarum ad annum 1490, Venice, 1490, fol. 118^{v}, under the year 147 A.D.

4 Gualteri Burlaei liber De vita et moribus philosophorum, ed. H. Knust, Tübingen, 1886, p. 390. Knust cites them only in the apparatus criticus, but, as J. O. Stigall, The manuscript tradition of the De vita et moribus philosophorum of Walter Burley, Medievalia et Humanistica 11, 1957, p. 53, pointed out, the best Mss. consistently follow readings left by Knust in the apparatus. That these (and other) texts were added later in the manuscript tradition is highly unlikely.

end of his life somewhere on the Continent.[1] But the order of titles in F does not correspond to those in Burley, nor is his title exactly the same, and De fide sua appears at the end of his list along with titles of works preserved today only in Arabic, like De examinatione medici and De nominibus medicinalibus, or derived by misunderstanding of passages elsewhere in Galen, as De magnanimitate Antoni(n)i. Rather than Burley obtaining his information from F or a similar but now lost, manuscript, his reference to De fide sua is more likely to have come from his own reading or from his acquaintance in S. France or Spain with scholars who knew of it through Arabic.

One such was Ramón Martí (c. 1230 – c. 1285), head of the Dominican Studium Hebraicum at Barcelona and teacher of Arnald of Villanova, whose reference to De sententiis derives avowedly from Rhazes' *Shukūk*, although Martí's Latin does not correspond exactly either to the text of Rhazes as printed by Mohaghegh or to the wording of 2,1: p. 56,12–13.[2] His title, Quid credidit Galenus et quid sibi opinatus est, is also anomalous.

It is not surprising therefore to find that De sententiis did not survive the transfer from the age of manuscript to the age of print. Niccolò's version, however, appeared in the edition of the Latin Galieni Pergamensis ... Opera published in Venice in 1490 by Philippus Pincius and prepared by the Brescian physician Diomedes Bonardus (= Bon.), vol. I, sig. bb. VI^{v}–VII^{r}. What manuscripts he used for this edition remains a puzzle. Nic.^{j} and Nic.^{k} are unlikely because of their incompleteness, Nic.^{h} because it seems to have been always in Spain, and Nic.^{i} because it remained in Schedel's possession. The presence of a shared wrong reading, as at p. 118,1 τοῖς σώμασι (corporibus Nic.)] corporalibus Nic.^{cg} Bon., would appear to indicate the use of one of the Cesena Mss., which, on other grounds, not least the absence of De sententiis from Nic.^{g}, is likely to have been Nic.^{g}.[3] There are no shared errors of significance between Bon. and Nic.^{b}, but there are a few good readings that might indicate that Bonardus had access to Schedel's source Ms.: p. 110,14 καθ'] secundum Nic.^{hij} Bon.: sed Nic.^{cg}: .s. Nic.^{b}; p. 112,11 ἄναρμα] anarma Nic.^{ci}: anarama Bon.: anarina Nic.^{g}: anarnia Nic.^{j}: enarma Nic.^{h}: *om.* Nic.^{b}; p. 116,20 μὴν] demum Nic.^{i} Bon.: deinde Nic.^{b}: demonstratum Nic.^{h}: *om.* Nic.^{cgjk}. Bonardus' text was reprinted, with a mixture of correction and added error, in the edition of Pavia, J. de Burgofranco, 1515, vol. I, fol. CXLII^{r}, and in the first Juntine edition, Venice, 1528, vol. I., fol. CIII^{rv}. By the latter date, however, a new Greek text was available and possibly even a new Latin translation, by Guinther of Andernach, based on the Greek.[4]

1 For the date and place, see A. Uña Juárez, La filosofia del siglo XIV. Contexto cultural de Walter Burley, El Escorial, 1970, pp. 83–89.

2 C. Burnett, Encounters with Razi the Philosopher: Constantine the African, Petrus Alfonsi and Ramón Martí, in: Homenaje a Horacio Santiago-Otero, ed. J. M. Soto Rábanos, Madrid, 1997 (in press). Martí's text reads: fateor me omnino nescire utrum mundus sit antiquus vel novus.

3 Cf. also Nutton, in: CMG V 8,1, p. 35. It is hard to be sure of such wrong readings as p. 120,21 τὸ] quod Nic.: *om.* Nic.^{bg} Bon.

4 De facultatum naturalium substantia. Quod animi mores corporis temperaturam sequuntur. De propriorum animi cuiusque affectuum agnitione & remedio, Paris, S. de Colines,

The first edition of the complete Galen in Greek had finally appeared, **Ald.** after many years of expectation, at Venice in April, 1525, and contains De substantia in vol. I, fol. 167^{rv}. For the first chapter, the Aldine editors could rely only on A, which they corrected in a few places from their own ingenuity or from the rewritings of A^2 in the margin: p. 108,2 ἀλλ' ἄχρι] ἀλλὰ χρὴ A: corr. Ald.; p. 108,27 ἀπορῶ] ἀπορῶν A: corr. Ald.; p. 104,7 ἀκριβ . . . ις A: ἀκριβέστερόν τις A^2 (in marg.) Ald.; p. 104,13 θε . . . ρὸν A: θερμὸν ἢ ψυχρὸν A^2 (in marg.) Ald. At p. 104,8–9 they appear to have filled in the gap in A with the unsuccessful conjecture τῆς ἐσχάτης ἐπιστήμης, see the commentary, below, pp. 193–194 to p. 104,7–14. For the rest of the text, the omissions in A at, e.g., pp. 112,3; 116,21; 118,3. 9 were supplemented from a manuscript of the L family, either M, despite the difficulties of obtaining access to the Marciana collections, or, as has been recently suggested, R.[1] The later editors of Galen's Opera omnia added little. I have recorded one minor correction from the edition Galeni Pergameni ... Opera omnia ..., ed. J. Camerarius, L. **Bas.** Fuchs and H. Gemusaeus, Basle, 1538, vol. I, pp. 342–343: p. 112,7 γε om. L Ald.: hab. A, add. Bas.; orthographic variants at pp. 114,22 and 120,7, and a shared correction at p. 124,1 from that of R. Chartier, Hippocratis Coi, et **Chart.** Claudii Galeni Pergameni ... Opera, Paris, 1679, vol. V, pp. 3–6; and three emendations, at pp. 104,26; 108,5; and 120,21, from that of C. G. Kühn, Claudii Galeni Opera omnia, Leipzig, 1822, vol. IV, pp. 757–766. Other scholars have made only minor improvements to the text: pp. 110,18; 124,1 Janus Cornarius (in the notes to his Aldine, now at Jena); p. 108,14 Schröder, in: CMG Suppl. I, p. 41; pp. 104,8; 112,22 an anonymous renaissance annotator. Nor can much profit be gained from the sixteenth-century translators, whose Latin versions, however elegant, only reflect the base text of the Aldine edition.[2] Trincavelli commented in the margin at p. 114,11–12 that the Greek text was "valde depravatus", although he still continued to follow the reading of the Aldine and Basle editions. Likewise Rasarius at p. 122,13 printed in his margin an excellent emendation, anima stirpium, a reading also to be found in L (τῆς φυτικῆς), although his translation follows the incorrect vulgate, τῆς φυ-

1528. I have consulted this translation in Galeni Varia opera, Paris, S. de Colines, 1534, pp. 1–3.

[1] For the circumstances of the production of the Aldine edition, see Nutton, John Caius, pp. 38–50. That the editors used some of the Marciana Bessarion manuscripts is certain, and D. Béguin, Sur la méthode de travail suivie dans la préparation de l'édition aldine des Opera omnia de Galien (1525): analyse du De sectis ad introducendos, in: Storia e ecdotica, pp. 31–42, has argued strongly that R was also available to them, having been copied for Aldus around 1500 as part of his original plan to print the Greek works of Galen.

[2] For details of the translations by Guinther, Sylvanius, Trincavelli, and Rasarius, see R. J. Durling, A chronological census of renaissance editions and translations of Galen, Journal of the Warburg and Courtauld Institutes 24, 1961, p. 288. I have consulted the version of Sylvanius in Galeni Opera omnia, vol. I, Basle, 1542, pp. 833–834; that of Trincavelli in Galeni De naturalibus facultatibus, Lyons, G. Rouille, 1550, pp. 170–178 (an edition not noted by Durling); that of J. B. Rasarius, in Galeni Opera omnia, vol. I, Venice, 1562, fols. 47^{v}–48^{r}.

σικῆς.[1] There is, however, one small exception to this lack-lustre list. Theodore Goulston's edition and translation, for all its failings, made a considerable advance on those of his predecessors, not least because of his use of the "codex Adelphi". It was perhaps unfortunate that his work appeared at a time when Galenism was distinctly out of fashion, and when the editing of classical medical texts had long fallen out of favour. As an emender and translator Goulston was at best an honest workman, but, in the context of what other editors have done, that modicum of praise sets him above the rest.[2]

For all the efforts of the sixteenth-century translators, their work passed largely unread. De substantia naturalium facultatum remained a fragment, with neither context nor commentary, and only the most devoted of Galenists cited it in their writings.[3] Interest in On my own opinions began to revive again only at the end of the nineteenth century, when Georg Helmreich and Karl Kalbfleisch published the fragments in P and Q.[4] It was Kalbfleisch who, in 1902, first identified the *membra disiecta* and showed, by using A, that De substantia was indeed part of Galen's lost philosophical autobiography.[5] He had planned to edit the whole text as part of the Berlin Corpus, but he had published a text, with a parallel Greek retroversion, only of the opening story of Parthenius[6] before death took him and before bombs destroyed his home and library at Gießen. Benedict Einarson, the learned editor of Theophrastus, then took up the challenge, and published the conclusion of De sententiis, which he brilliantly identified as coming from De pomo.[7] His plans for a future edition likewise came to naught, but he was gracious enough to supply me with a microfilm of O and to discuss some of the textual problems with me. The first substantial survey of the text and its contents, along with a preliminary edition of chapter 2, had to wait until 1987, when it appeared in a volume of Aristotelian studies dedicated to the memory of Paul Moraux, who had himself brought to light the fragments in Y and V.[8] That survey was

1 At p. 108,18 ὀνομάζω, Sylvanius, Trincavelli, and Rasarius all use a main verb, but their sentence structure does not make it clear whether they had made in passing the simple emendation adopted in the text.

2 For Goulston and his edition, see above, pp. 20–21, and Nutton, John Caius, pp. 61–63; 96–99.

3 L. D. Richardson, The generation of disease, in: The medical renaissance of the sixteenth century, ed. A. Wear, R. K. French, I. M. Lonie, Cambridge, 1985, p. 177, is triply wrong in asserting that a commentary on De substantia by J. B. Montanus was published posthumously in 1554. Montanus' Methodus ... de elementis appeared first at Vienna in 1553 (and again, as Periocha methodica, at Venice in 1560 as an appendix to the Isagoge ad medicinam of Johannes Crato von Crafftheim); Montanus' discussion is avowedly a summary of Galen, not a commentary; and, most serious of all, the Galenic text in question is the far more significant De facultatibus naturalibus, not De substantia. The latter was known to Montanus, but neither he nor any other scholar wrote specifically about it.

4 See above, pp. 14–16.

5 See K. Kalbfleisch, Griechische Miscellen, in: Festschrift Theodor Gomperz dargebracht zum siebzigsten Geburtstage, Vienna, 1902, p. 98.

6 See Kalbfleisch, Parthenios, pp. 376–379.

7 See Einarson, pp. 258–259.

8 See Nutton, Galen's philosophical testament, pp. 27–51.

made in ignorance of the evidence of Ibn Falaquera (see above, pp. 31–33) which, although printed as long ago as 1778, was not brought to the attention of historians of medicine until 1995. This present volume, which brings together for the first time all the various texts and traditions, is thus a partial *editio princeps,* whose novelty is only slightly eroded by the undoubted truth that, as might be expected from the title, very few of the ideas and opinions contained herein are not already known from surviving writings of Galen.

C. Editorial principles

Editing a text in mediaeval Latin presents a series of problems unfamiliar to an editor of classical Latin, and almost any decision on orthographical consistency can be challenged. I have chosen to follow the manuscripts in keeping forms in -e instead of regularising them to -ae (e.g. que for quae; anime, not animae), as well as such spellings as gramaticos (p. 54,7); superhabundat (p. 60,19); nichil (p. 110,12) and michi (p. 54,5). However, the manuscripts are often divided over the spelling of such words as sententia (or -cia), enuntio (or -ncio or -mptio), and exercitium (or -cium). Here, although the oldest manuscripts tend to prefer the -ci- form, I have chosen to standardise and to print the forms in -ti- throughout. Orthographical variants of this kind (e.g. oppinor/opinor; philosophia/phylo-; attrahere/atraere; diu/dyu; demonstrare/demostrare) have usually been ignored in the apparatus criticus, but such variants as id/illud are recorded there.

With a text that has gone through so many versions, it is frequently difficult to decide whether errors in the Latin derive from miscopyings within the Latin tradition, from mistakes in translation into Latin, or from corruptions that have occurred earlier in the process of transmission. When I have become convinced that an error derives solely from within the Latin tradition, I have emended the text to what I believe the translator to have written. Elsewhere, I have been more cautious, putting suggestions for possible improvement into the apparatus rather than the text.

In such places, where the Latin translation presents either a transcription of the Arabic or a dubious reading dependent on a misunderstanding of the Arabic intermediary, the English equivalent is given in italics. An English translation of what would have been Galen's original Greek or of the Arabic version if rightly understood is given at the foot of the page.

D. De propriis placitis and Greek autobiography

Galen was never reluctant to reveal details of his own life or his own opinions. It is a rare book indeed that does not contain some reminiscence of a past achievement or some comment on the society in which he found himself. His medical tracts are occasionally structured around a story from his own practice in order to show how advice given in theory can be applied to the real world of medicine.[1] Indeed, one whole treatise, On prognosis, is made up of examples taken from his career in order to show friends, potential patients, fellow physicians, and others more sceptical, that prognosis in the manner prescribed by Hippocrates was both possible and effective. One of his ethical treatises, unfortunately no longer extant, On slander (see Gal., De libris propr. 12 [13]: Scr. min. II 122,2 Müller = XIX 46,5–6 K.), also included many incidents from his own life, perhaps in response to the complaints of his enemies that he details elsewhere.[2] In On my own books, he provided a biographical introduction to a bibliographical survey of his own writings in order to offer a means to guarantee the authenticity of his works in circulation.

On my own opinions presents a variant on this approach. Except for the story in the preface, which owes at least as much to literary invention as to an actual event, Galen refers to no incident in his own life, offers no comment on contemporary life and society, and with the single exception of a reference to his change of heart in chapter 11,2, gives no indication of the chronology of any of his writings and ideas. This treatise presents a picture of almost total consistency: it reports scarcely any change in Galen's main ideas throughout his life, from his student days until old age.[3] That is why he can use the criteria of his doctrines, just as in On my own books he had listed his writings, in order to establish the authenticity of works circulating under his name. We need not doubt that such supposititious works existed, see below, p. 127, the commentary on p. 54,5–18, for the chaotic nature of ancient 'publishing' lent itself to such confusion, to say nothing of the ease with which in ancient and mediaeval manuscripts works by different authors could become almost inextricably jumbled together.[4]

But while still accepting Galen's own explanation for why he wrote this treatise, one may note that no other ancient author was so obviously concerned to ensure his own survival in the manner he would have wished. Not only did he list his writings for posterity, but in On the order of my own books he carefully explained to his readers just how those writings should be studied and in what order. In the opening chapter of Anatomical procedures, I 1: pp.

1 See V. Nutton, Galen and medical autobiography, Proceedings of the Cambridge Philological Society 198, 1972, pp. 50–62 (repr. in: Nutton, From Democedes to Harvey, no. I); Style and context in the Method of healing, in: Galen's Method of healing, pp. 1–25.

2 For complaints about his wealth, see Meth. med. VIII 3: X 561,1–5 K.; for assistance to others, see the fragment from On how to profit from one's enemies, in M. Meyerhof, Autobiographische Bruchstücke Galens aus arabischen Quellen, Archiv f. Geschichte d. Medizin 22, 1929, p. 84.

3 It is perhaps worth noting that the one great change in Galen's life, his move to medicine, was the result of a vision sent by Asclepius to his father, not to Galen himself, and he views his whole life story as a natural progression under the god's guidance. The 'conversion-experience' was Nicon's, not his.

4 For a brief survey of ancient book-production and distribution, see P. E. Easterling and B. M. W. Knox, The Cambridge history of classical literature, I. Greek literature, Cambridge, 1985, pp. 1–41. W. Speyer, Die literarische Fälschung im heidnischen und christlichen Altertum. Ein Versuch ihrer Deutung, Munich, 1971 (Handb. d. Altertumswiss. I 2), is a masterly account of the opportunities for deliberate or accidental forgery in Antiquity, and of the ways used to secure authentication.

1,1–5,10 Garofalo = II 215,5–218,15 K., he set out his debts to other anatomists in order to emphasise his own position within the Alexandrian tradition of anatomical dissection. On examinations by which the best physicians are recognized (CMG Suppl. Or. IV), a tract ostensibly to help the patient find a good doctor, becomes a celebration of what Galen believes to be essential for medical practice and of his own superiority. On my own opinions thus is not unique in offering the reader a view of Galen as Galen wanted to be seen by posterity – as a consistent thinker, even in his agnosticism, and even when, as with his ruminations on the soul (see below, pp. 140–141, the commentary on pp. 58,22–60,6), his uncertainties and hesitations are far more insistent than he perhaps would have wanted to acknowledge. What psychological reasons lay behind this desire for consistency, certainty, and authenticity one cannot say. But, equally, one cannot fail to come away with the impression of a man whose outward rigidity of doctrine was a defence against all difficulties and dangers, personal and social as well as professional.

In its avowed aim as a guide to authenticity, On my own opinions is unusual as a presentation of personal beliefs. The closest ancient parallel is perhaps provided by Epicurus, whose Κύριαι δόξαι (pp. 120–137 Arrighetti), Basic doctrines, offered a summary of his ethical thought for the benefit of future generations, although at what stage of his life this book was written is hard to determine, and it in no way covered the whole of his philosophy.[1] But, leaving aside the stylistic contrast between the maxims of the philosopher and the more extended account of the physician, Galen's exposition differs significantly from that of Epicurus in two ways. First, it is far from systematic in its choice of topics or in the way in which they are developed; some are covered in a chapter or more, others in a few lines, others not at all. Its emphasis is on theory, with no reference to practical treatment. Galen mentions the ideas that underlie his dietetics and pharmacology, but not those that might have guided his surgical practice, and he considers the changes brought about by bodily processes only in the most general of terms. Within the treatise, the argument in general simply leads directly on from one topic to the next (for an exception, see below, pp. 182–183, the note to p. 94,18–21) without a strong controlling structure. Indeed, the final sections end in what is at best a clarification of a problem in Plato's Timaeus. As a guide to what Galen believed, this treatise is far from perfect, showing, as it does, a weakening of its author's powers of organisation in his old age.

Secondly, Galen's presentation is, for him, unusually tolerant, at least at the level of epistemology, for it refers from time to time to views which he had himself elsewhere rejected. In On my own opinions Galen operates on a triple schema of knowledge: things that he knows to be certain, things that he regards as plausible but as yet unproven, and things on which he can not yet make up his mind, even to the extent of assenting to any proposition, e.g. the

1 Ancient claims that this was the 'crowning achievement' of Epicurus might indicate that it was composed late in life, but this is far from assured. For a characterisation, emphasising its fragmentary nature, both physical and doctrinal, see C. Bailey, in: Epicurus, The extant remains, ed., Oxford, 1926 (repr. Hildesheim and New York, 1970), pp. 344–346.

nature of the soul or the ultimate constituents of matter. This last group he dismisses as irrelevant and inessential both to medical practice and to ethics, but merely to mention such topics entails the inclusion as possibilities of ideas that Galen rejects elsewhere in his medicine, e.g. the atomism of Democritus and Asclepiades. For the sake of a wider argument about the different types of knowledge Galen is prepared to countenance, albeit within a restricted context, ideas that he mentions elsewhere only to condemn. His sketch of the second, 'more plausible' group is not entirely free from this difficulty, and involves a further problem as well. In terms of a proper epistemology, Galen emphasises the importance of sound, sure, and certain knowledge, derived empirically and logically by means of scientific apodeictic. Only knowledge obtained in this way qualifies for certainty. But, in practical terms, there is often no difference between this knowledge and what Galen regards as merely plausible, and in many of his writings Galen takes as a starting point doctrines that he here ascribes only to this second category. Nor is it entirely clear just how this category at times differs from the first or the third, except at an abstract level of epistemology, and one may justifiably wonder at an author who so frequently confesses his agnosticism and yet equally frequently accepts in practice a standard school answer to the very same problem (see below, p. 132, the note to p. 56,12–20).

Although, as has been suggested, there are no convincingly close ancient parallels to what Galen is here attempting, one further consideration is not inappropriate. Almost a century ago, Georg Misch, in his History of autobiography, endeavoured to set the bio-bibliographical tracts of Galen within the wider story of autobiography as the discovery of self, a process that culminated in late Antiquity with the Confessions of St. Augustine.[1] Far more than Galen's bio-bibliographies, On my own opinions fits neatly into this picture of a growing self-awareness, of an individual trying to define his own place within the universe, and, as his frequent return to the question of the soul shows, wrestling with his uncertainties even as he attempts to define the certainties of his own beliefs.

In his desire to make public his own opinions, and to reveal to future generations his guiding principles Galen was not alone. As studies of the cultural, religious, and social history of the second century have amply demonstrated, his age was an age of creeds and credos, publicly asserted and preserved both in manuscript and on inscriptions. We need not believe that Galen must have been influenced by public pronouncements of Jews or, still more, Christians eager to proclaim their individual message – although he was well acquainted with both communities in Rome, see e.g. De puls. diff. II 4: VIII 579,16 K. His fellow-pagans were not averse to making their own philosophical views known to their fellow-citizens in a dogmatic form. At some point in the second century A.D., Diogenes of Oenoanda had his Epicurean beliefs inscribed on the wall of a stoa in his home town for all to read and

1 G. Misch, History of autobiography, 3rd ed., London, 1950, pp. 328–332. The collection of essays, Jewish and Christian self-definition, ed. B. F. Meyer and E. P. Sanders, London, 1982, offers further food for thought on this topic.

"for the salvation of men, now and in the future".[1] On the town wall of the same town at the same period another inscription displayed lines from an oracle that expounded the wisdom of God to those who "questioned about his nature", lines familiar from a more literary collection, the so-called Theosophia Tubingensis.[2] On the nature of the gods, and on many of the themes that his contemporaries and fellow inhabitants of Asia Minor treated so confidently, Galen takes up a more sceptical position than they. They declared their unshakeable faith, Galen only his agnosticism. But Galen's ardent wish to ensure that the world knew what he himself truly believed cannot entirely be dissociated from theirs, even if, ultimately, an explanation is to be found in coincidence rather than in any spirit of the age. All had a message, all were convinced that they had a key that would resolve the problems of others, and all were concerned that what they had to say should be transmitted to and for posterity.

The preparation of the *editio princeps* of On my own opinions has occupied Galenic scholars for over a century, and this editor intermittently for almost thirty years. If any excuse is needed for this tardiness, one can point to the complicated nature of the transmission of the text and, above all, to Galen's own range and prolixity. One can at times only marvel at the many-sidedness and the ingenuity of the doctor from Pergamum. In the commentary I have endeavoured not only to explain and justify the readings adopted in the text, but also to relate what Galen says to the debates and culture of his own day. Those who preceded me in struggling with this text, Georg Helmreich, Karl Kalbfleisch, and Benedict Einarson, laboured manfully, and only a fellow editor can appreciate what they managed to achieve. Without their work, this edition would have been even longer in the making.

It is a pleasure also to acknowledge the help I have received over the years from fellow Galenists. Much information on the manuscripts and editions was given me by Daniel Béguin, Richard Durling, Benedict Einarson, Stefania Fortuna, and Nigel Wilson, and Rita Masullo helped me obtain a photograph of the Naples copy of Niccolò's translation. Any understanding I have of Galen's philosophical theories has been gained from conversations and correspondence with Matthias Baltes, Jonathan Barnes, Myles Burnyeat, Phillip De Lacy, Silvia Fazzo, Jim Hankinson, Geoffrey Lloyd, Paul Moraux, and Richard Sorabji, and from criticisms of audiences in Cambridge, London, and Berlin. Owsei Temkin and Luis García Ballester were always ready to compare their visions of Galen with mine. Arabist colleagues at the Wellcome Institute over the years, Gerrit Bos, Larry Conrad, A. Z. Iskandar, and Nikolai

1 M. F. Smith, Diogenes of Oinoanda, The Epicurean inscription, Naples, 1993, supersedes all previous editions. Diogenes, like Galen, wrote his 'confession' at the end of his life, to inform others "as if I were actually present". Note also D. Clay, The philosophical inscription of Diogenes of Oenoanda: new discoveries 1969–1983, in: ANRW II 36,4, Berlin and New York, 1990, pp. 2446–2559.

2 On this see L. Robert, Un oracle gravé à Oinoanda, in: Comptes rendus de l'Académie des Inscriptions 1971, pp. 597–619 (repr. in: Robert, Opera minora selecta, pp. 617–639); Lane Fox, pp. 169–171; Athanassiadi, pp. 45–62, esp. pp. 49–55.

Serikoff responded generously to my importunings. Preliminary drafts of the whole edition were read by Elizabeth Craik, James Longrigg, and Bob Sharples, who together eliminated many errors and infelicities, and made valued suggestions. As well as thanking formally the Libraries and Librarians who have allowed me to use their facilities and to work on their manuscripts, I must offer a special word of appreciation to the staff of the Wellcome Institute Library, who have for many years provided me with a splendid range of facilities and who have uncomplainingly struggled with mighty tomes of the renaissance Galen. Their support, and that of the Wellcome Trust, has been invaluable. Two further acknowledgments are in order. I am grateful to the Berlin-Brandenburgische Akademie der Wissenschaften for publishing this volume in the Corpus Medicorum Graecorum. The officers of the CMG in Berlin, Jutta Kollesch, Gotthard Strohmaier, and Diethard Nickel, have become friends as well as colleagues, and their advice and encouragement has been greatly appreciated; only those who have worked with them know how much their editorial labours contribute to the accuracy of their editions. Finally, my wife and family have lived with Galen, and with On my own opinions, for more years than they would care to remember. They are to be thanked for their patience, and for their affectionate interest that has, I trust, prevented this editor and Galenic biographer from developing all the faults of his subject.

The Wellcome Institute for the History of Medicine, London
January 1997

Vivian Nutton

ΓΑΛΗΝΟΥ

ΠΕΡΙ ΤΩΝ ΕΑΥΤΩΙ ΔΟΚΟΥΝΤΩΝ

GALEN

ON MY OWN OPINIONS

LIBER GALIENI

DE SENTENTIIS

GALEN

ON OPINIONS

CONSPECTVS SIGLORVM ET COMPENDIORVM

Codices textus Graeci

A = Ambrosianus gr. 659; s. XIV/XV
A^2 = eiusdem codicis corrector
L = Laurentianus gr. 74,5; s. XII
P = Parisinus gr. 2332; s. XV
Q = Parisinus suppl. gr. 634; s. XII
Ad. = codex Adelphi, nunc perditus

Codices versionum Latinarum

C = Malatestianus S. V 4; s. XIV
B = Parisinus lat. 6865; s. XIV
B^2, B^3, B^4 = eiusdem codicis correctores
O = Biturigensis 299; s. XIV
O^2 = eiusdem codicis corrector
D = Dresdensis Db 92; s. XV
D^2 = eiusdem codicis corrector
E = Parisinus Academicus 51; s. XV
E^2 = eiusdem codicis corrector

α = consensus codicum CBODE
β = consensus codicum BODE
γ = consensus codicum BO
ε = consensus codicum DE

Nic. = Nicolai versio Latina; s. XIV
$Nic.^b$ = Nicolai versio codice Parisino lat. 6865 s. XIV tradita
$Nic.^c$ = Nicolai versio codice Malatestiano S. V 4 s. XIV tradita
$Nic.^h$ = Nicolai versio codice Matritensi lat. 1978 s. XIV tradita
$Nic.^i$ = Nicolai versio codice Monacensi lat. 490 a. 1488 tradita
$Nic.^j$ = Nicolai versio codice Neapolitano VIII D 38 s. XIV tradita
$Nic.^k$ = Nicolai versio codice Wellcomensi 286 s. XIV tradita

Fontes excerpti Hebraei

Fal. = excerptum Hebraeum, quod Ibn Falaquera e Galeni libro sumpsit
L = Londiniensis Or. 1484

NY = New York, Jewish Theological Seminary, microfilm 2306
DH = editio Den Haag, a. 1778

Editiones

Ald.	= editio Aldina, Venetiis, a. 1525
Goulst.	= editio Goulstonii, Londinii, a. 1640
Chart.	= editio Charterii, Lutetiae Parisiorum, a. 1679
Kühn	= editio Kühnii, Lipsiae, a. 1822
Helmreich	= Helmreich, Galeni fragmenta
Zonta	= editio excerpti Hebraei, quam Zonta, p. 103–105, curavit
Arist.	= [Aristotelis] liber De pomo, ed. Plezia, p. 58sq.

Caius	= I. Caius in editionis Basileensis exemplari suo nunc bibliothecae collegii Etonensis proprio
Corn.	= I. Cornarius in editionis Aldinae exemplari suo nunc bibliothecae universitatis Ienensis proprio
Gas	= Petri de Sancto Floro (P. Gas) excerpta (v. supra, p. 26sq.)
Goulst.$^{Bas.}$	= Th. Goulston in editionis Basileensis exemplari suo (v. supra, p. 20)

ΓΑΛΗΝΟΥ

ΠΕΡΙ ΤΩΝ ΕΑΥΤΩΙ ΔΟΚΟΥΝΤΩΝ

LIBER GALIENI

DE SENTENTIIS

1. Ait Galienus, quia michi accidit prout dicitur quod accidit Bertheni uersificatori, quod dicitur quod uersus sui peruenerunt in uita sua ad aliquos. et cum transiret per terram illorum inuenit duos gramaticos in loco scolarum altercantes de sententia suorum uersuum, unus quorum exponebat uersus secundum quod Berthenis uersificator intellexit cum eos composuit,
2 alter uero exponebat contrario modo. Berthenis autem incepit reprobare expositionem illius qui exponebat non secundum quod ipse uoluit, dicendo ipsum errare et sententiam illorum uersuum contrariam sententie sue expositionis. qui cum noluisset recipere dictum eius, respondit eidem: „Ego audiui Berthenem uersificatorem exponere ipsos uersus secundum sententiam quam modo narro.“ et cum ille noluisset recipere uerba sua secundum quod ipse dixit, ait: „Timeo quod ymaginatio mea sit infecta siue destructa, cum indigeam inducere istos familiares meos in testimonium secundum quod sim Berthenis.“

3 Et uidetur quod accidit michi simile huius propter defectum studentium in arte medicine et philosophie, quia nos uidemus multos non esse exercitatos

19–56,5] *cf.* Gal. Adv. eos qui de typis scrips. 3: VII 486,16–18 K. De alim. fac. I 1,3: CMG V 4,2, p. 202,17–20 Meth. med. I 1: X 2,7–10; 5,3–6; 8,9 K. De fac. nat. III 10: Scr. min. III 230,23–231,6 Helmr. = II 179,4–11 K. De animi cuiusl. pecc. dign. et cur. 2,8: CMG V 4,1,1, p. 44,21–28

1sq. Γαληνοῦ – δοκούντων *add. in marg. sup.* A² 2 *ante* Περὶ *add.* ἐν τῷ P 3 *ante* Liber *add.* Incipit γ 3sq. Liber – sententiis *om.* C: Libri Galieni de sententiis sunt quindecim capitula ε 4 *post* sententiis *add.* medicorum B, ut de fide G(alieni) B³ *(v. supra, p. 23; 25sq.; 41sq.)* 5 *ante* Ait *add.* Capitulum primum de comparatione actoris huius libri ad bethenem uersificatorem ε Ait] inquid C *post* Galienus *add.* noster C quia *om.* D: *in textu om., in marg. add.* E: quod C *post* quod *iter. et del.* dicitur quod B betheni β: *corr. Kalbfleisch, Parthenios, p. 377*: e/bertenis C 6 quod[I] *om.* ε: quia C 7 gramantes B: gramantes uel guarrulentes O: garrulantes ε B² *in marg.* 8 alterantes *in* -cantes *corr.* O suorum] illorum β 9 bethenis O ε: thebenis B uersifficatorum C 10 bethenis β probare B 11 dicens ε: dicentem γ 12 et – expositionis *om.* ε sententiam] sententia O contrariam] erat contraria O: est contraria C sue] qua C B 13 *ante* qui *add.* tunc O cum *e* cumque *corr.* B: cumque O *post* cum *add.* ille C uoluit O 14 bethenem ε: *corr. Kalbfleisch, Parthenios, p. 377*: berthem C: beth` γ uersus *om.* C 15 cum] tunc O noluit β 16 ait *om.* B, *in marg. add.* B² Timeo *om.* C 17 famulares C in – secundum *om.* ε secundum *om.* C O bethenis ε: *corr. Kalbfleisch, Parthenios, p. 377*: beth` γ: bertheni C 19 *post* uidetur *add.* mihi O simile *om.* C hius B: hoc C: *om.* D defectuum γ

GALEN
ON MY OWN OPINIONS

GALEN
ON OPINIONS

1. Galen says: There happened (once) to me an incident similar to one that allegedly befell *Berthenis* the poet; as the story goes, his poems were widely read during his lifetime. And once, as he was on a journey overland, he found two schoolmasters arguing in school about the meaning of his poems; one of them was interpreting the poems in the way *Berthenis* the poet had intended when he composed them, the other in the opposite manner.
Berthenis began to criticise the exposition of the master who was not in- 2
terpreting them in the way he had intended, saying that he was wrong and that the meaning of this poem was contrary to the meaning of his exposition. When he found him unwilling to accept this advice, he went on: "I have heard *Berthenis* the poet expounding these lines in the way I have just explained." When the man still refused to accept this interpretation as he had given it, he said, "I am afraid that my intellectual powers are failing or gone, since I must call in friends of mine to prove that I am *Berthenis*."

I seem to have found myself in a similar situation to his through the fail- 3
ings of those who study the art of medicine and philosophy, for we see many

6. 9. 11. 15. 18 Orig.: Παρϑένιος (Parthenius)

in arte gramatice. et non sunt sic exercitati quod uenirent ad complementum, sed ipsi potuerunt addiscere artem cum difficultate propter defectum intellectus in libris quos composuimus, quamuis sint in ultimo declarati uel manifestati illis qui sunt exercitati in primo exercitio super libros quos composuerunt
4 antiqui. et differentia inter sermonem meum et sermonem Berthenis, quia Berthenis indiguit conuocare in testimonium familiares suos, sed ego conuoco in testimonium illud quod composui de meis libris et probaui quod sciui de scientia uirtuosa et [de] hoc quod probaui quod sciui secundum uiam sufficientie et illud quod est †in ipso† non habeo notitiam cum dixerim quod non sum firmus scientie sue. et ego uideo quod ego debeam ante exponere narrationem istarum rerum quas narrauimus in fine.

2. אמר אין לי ידיעה אם העולם מהווה אם לא ואם יש אחריו דבר מחוץ או אם אין דבר אחריו ומאחר שאני אומר שאין לי ידיעה באלו הדברים מהמבואר כמו כן שאין לי ידיעה ביוצר כל מה שיש בזה העולם אם הוא גוף או זולתי גוף ואי זה מהמקומות מקומו ואמנם האלהים והכחות האלהיים והם הכחות אשר פעליהם נמצאים בעולם אי אפשר שיהיו אלא מצד הבורא ועל כן הם מורים עליו

2. Igitur dico quod non habeo scientiam utrum mundus sit generatus et utrum aliquid sit extra uel non aliquid sit extra. et cum dicam quod non habeam scientiam istarum rerum, igitur manifestum est quod non habeam scientiam de creatore omnium istarum rerum que sunt in mundo, utrum sit corporeum aut incorporeum et in quo loco sit locatum scilicet deitas, id est uirtus deitatis. et illa est uirtutes quarum operationes repeRiuntur in hoc mundo operationibus que non possunt esse nisi a creatore: ergo ipse deum

7 quod^{I} – libris] *v.* Gal. De libris propr.: Scr. min. II 91–124 Müller = XIX 8–48 K. De ord. libror. suor.: Scr. min. II 80–90 Müller = XIX 49–61 K. quod^{II} – 10] *cf. infra,* p. 108,25–110,1; 114,8–11 De plac. Hipp. et Plat. IX 9,3: CMG V 4,1,2, p. 598,7–9 12 Igitur – 20] *cf.* Gal. De animi cuiusl. pecc. dign. et cur. 3,4; 7,5–11: CMG V 4,1,1, p. 46,23–25; 66,15–68,4 De plac. Hipp. et Plat. IX 6,21; 7,9: CMG V 4,1,2, p. 576,29–578,1; 588, 7–15 De locis affectis III 5: VIII 159,2–7 K. De exper. med. 19,3: p. 122sq. Walzer al-Rāzī, Shukūk: p. 3,22–4,7; 6,20–7,1; 15,10 Mohaghegh

12 אמר אין] ואין L 13 יש *om.* L 14 *post* דבר^{I} *add.* אחר L NY אם *om.* NY 14sq. אחריו דבר L 18 שיש] שהוא NY 23 מורים] מודים NY

1 in *om.* C 2 poterunt β discere C: addicere O: *om.* B artem *om.* ε intellectum γ 3 siue manifesti ε 4 in *om.* C 5 *post* differentia *add.* est O ε bethenis ε: *corr. Kalbfleisch, Parthenios, p. 377*: beth` γ: uersuum C 6 bethenis ε: beth` O: b` B inuocare ε testiōīum O 7 illud] id β posui C libris meis ε, *fort. recte* *post* probaui *add.* et O ε quod^{II} – 8 probaui *om.* C quod^{II} *supra lin. add.* O 8 et *om.* O de^{II} *secl. Kollesch et Nickel* *ante* sciui *add.* et ε 9 illud] id B: illius ε in ipso] *cruces posui; fort.* in obscuro <de quo> *scribendum est* dixi ε 10 firmus *ex* infirmus *corr.* B sue *om.* C deberem β ponere C 11 fiñ C 12 *ante* Igitur *add.* Capitulum secundum de hiis que sentit actor circa mundi durationem et ambitum eius et creatorem omnium. ε 13 *post* generatus *sec. Fal.* (אם לא) *fort.* uel non generatus *addendum est* 14 uel – extra^{II} *om.* β 15 dicam quod *om.* ε habebam B 16 manifestum est] manifestius C γ 17 habeam scientiam] debeam scire β 18 mundo] medio O ε 19 aut] uel C quo loco *e* loco quo *corr.* E 21 uirtus D 22 operibus B 23 ergo] igitur ε ipsum β

who lack any training in the art of grammar. They are not so well trained as to acquire a full understanding but they have been able to pick up the art (of medicine only) with difficulty as a result of their lack of understanding of the books I have written, although they are extremely clear or obvious to those who have first been trained in the writings of the ancients. The difference 4
between my story and that of *Berthenis* is that *Berthenis* had to call on his friends to vouch for him, whereas I bring as my witnesses what I have written about my own books and proved that I have known for certain and that which I have proved that I have known to the extent of sufficiency, and that which is ... I have no knowledge, when I say that I have no secure knowledge about it. But I see that I must first explain what I have said last.

2. He said: I have no knowlege if the world is generated or not, and if there is something after it outside, or if there is nothing after it. And since I say that I do not have knowledge about these things, it is also clear that I do not have knowledge about the creator of everything that is in this world, whether he is a body or incorporeal, and which of the places is his place, namely God and the divine powers. These are the powers whose activities are found in the world which can only be from the side of the Creator, therefore they

2. Thus I say that I do not know whether the universe is created and whether there is anything outside (the universe) or not. And since I say that I have no knowledge of these things, then it is obvious that I have no knowledge about the creator of everything in the universe, whether it is corporeal or incorporeal and where it is located, namely the deity, or rather the power of the deity. This (power) is identical with those powers whose workings are revealed in this world by acts that can only come from a creator: thus they themselves indi-

6 Orig.: Παρθένιος (Parthenius)

2 ומיוחסים אליו ואין אני אומר בהם כמו שאמר פרטאגורס אני איני יודע מענינם כל עיקר אלא אני אומר שאין לי ידיעה בעצמם אבל שהם נמצאים אני יודע זה מפועליהם ומאלו הפעלים הרכבת בעלי חיים ומה שיראה בניחוש ובעוננות ובראיית החלומות וממעשי השם ית׳ וית׳ אשר יורו על כחו והשגחתו ביצורים שרפא אותי ממחלה היתה בי ומה שיראה בים מהצלת היורדים בו באניות אחר שחשבו להשבר ולשקוע בים באות אשר יראו אותו ויבטחו ויושעו יורה ראיה ברורה על כח
3 נפלא ואין אני רואה שיזיק לבני אדם שלא ידעו מה הוא עצם הכחות האלהיים ועל כן ראיתי לגדלם ולהללם כפי מה שיחייב הדת

3. ואני יודע שיש לנו נפש כמו שיודעים כל בני אדם וזה כי

2 significant. et non dicam sicut dixit Pictagoras recusando se de ipsis scire; sed ego dico quod nulla scientia est in me de substantia earum; sed quod ipse sunt, scio per operationes earum quoniam ab ipsis est regimen animalium et inueniuntur in diuinationibus et in sompniis. sed de operationibus dei in nobis in contraria briga †misi magis quam† apparuerunt per uirtutem suam, quod curauerit me semel de una infirmitate quam habui et quod uidetur in mari ⟨in⟩ liberatione illorum qui sunt propinqui pati naufragium per signa que uident et firmiter credunt liberari. et significat significatione manifesta uirtutem mirabilem et hoc expertus sum
3 egoipse. et non uideo quod noceat hominibus si nesciant substantiam deitatis, et uideo quod debeam predicare et sequi in hoc legem et accipere illud quod precepit Socrates qui de hoc precepit firmius. et istud est quod habeo de deitate.

3. Sed de anima uideo quod est. de ipsa scio quod habemus animam secundum quod

1 Pictagoras] Protagoras, B 4: II, p. 265,7–9 D.-K. (*cf.* A 2,2; 3; 12: p. 255,23sq.; 256, 2sq.; 257,38–258,1 D.-K.) 3sq. de substantia earum] *cf.* Gal. De plac. Hipp. et Plat. IX 7,13; 9,3: CMG V 4,1,2, p. 588,22–25; 598,7sq. 6sq. in diuinationibus et in sompniis] *cf.* *e.g.* Gal. In Hipp. Epid. VI comm. VIII: CMG V 10,2,2, p. 485,30–486,12 De ord. libror. suor. 4: Scr. min. II 88,15–17 Müller = XIX 59,9–11 K. 10sq. curauerit – habui] *cf.* Gal. De cur. rat. per venae sect. 23: XI 314,18–315,7 K. De libris propr. 2: Scr. min. II 99,9–11 Müller = XIX 18,18–19,3 K. 19 quod precepit Socrates] *v.* Xenoph. Memor. I 1,11–16 *cf.* Gal. De plac. Hipp. et Plat. IX 7,3sq.: CMG V 4,1,2, p. 588,25–29

2 פרוטאגורט NY: *corr. Zonta*: פיטאגארש L DH 8 והעוננות L NY והמלחמות L DH 9 ומעשי L יורו] יורה L NY DH: *corr. Zonta* 10 ביצורים] ביכורים L 14 אותו *om.* NY 15sq. כחו הנפלא DH 17 שהוא NY 19 שיתחייב L NY 23 *post* שיודעים *add.* זה L NY

4 eorum C: rerum O sed – 5 earum *in textu om.*, *in marg. add.* E sint γ scio *om.* γ 5 quoniam *om.* B, *in marg. add.* B[2] 6 diuinationibus] dei actionibus B 7 et – operationibus *om.* C sompnis B 8 in^{II} *om.* C misi – 9 quam] *cruces posui*: mihi magis palam *coni. Mazzini per litt.*: missis quanto magis *coni. Kollesch et Nickel* misim γ: misissem ε 9 quam] que O E quod] quam O 10 curauit C O una] mea ε 11 uidetur *sec. Fal.* (שיראה) *scripsi*: uir C γ: uirum ε in liberatione *sec. Fal.* (מהצלת) *scripsi*: liberaueris C: liberauerit B ε: liberauit O 12 illorum] eorum ε 13 per] uel ε: que O firmiter *ex* infirmiter *corr.* B 14 significant C 16 hominibus *om.* C 17 si nesciant] siue sciant O non sciant ε substanticiam B: sciam (= scientiam) O 18 legem in hoc ε 20 qui *om.* C γ precipit O E firmius] minus ε 22 *ante* Sed *add.* Capitulum III. de hiis que sentit (actor *supra lin. add.* E[2]) circa animam et uirtutes eius. ε: ca^{m} 2^{m} *in marg. add.* B[4] set B uideo *post* est *trsp.* C quid α: *correxi* 23 habens C

refer to Him and are attributed to Him. I do not say of them as Pro- 2 tagoras said: "I do not know about them anything at all" but I say that I have no knowledge of their substance, but that they exist I know from their activities, and to their activities belongs the composition of animals, and what becomes visible through divination, augury, and in visions in dreams. And of the actions of God, blessed and praised be He, which indicate his power and his providence for the creatures are that He healed me from a disease that was in me and what can be seen at sea from the rescue of those who put out to sea in ships; after having expected to break up and to sink in the sea (they were rescued) by the sign which they see whereupon they trusted and were saved. It gives a clear indication of wonderful power, and I do not see that it is harm- 3 ful to people that they do not know what is the substance of the divine powers. Therefore I thought that I should exalt and praise them as ordained by religion.

3. And I know that we have a soul as all mankind knows, and this because I see that everyone calls

cate God. I shall not speak as *Py-* 2 *thagoras* did in denying that he has any knowledge of them; but I say that I have no knowledge of their substance; but that they exist, I know from their acts since the organisation of (all) living beings comes from them and they are revealed in divination and dreams. Concerning the workings of God in us +having come+ into deep trouble, +how much clearer+[1] have they appeared in their power! Inasmuch as he cured me once of an illness I had, and inasmuch as it can be seen at sea in the salvation of those who are about to suffer shipwreck, (when they are saved) by the signs that they see and thereupon firmly believe that they will be saved. Clearly this signifies some wondrous power, and indeed I have experienced it myself. But I do not 3 see that men are harmed if they do not know the substance of the deity, and I see that I should declare and follow the law in this and accept the teaching of Socrates on this – for his view was quite definite. That is what I have to say about the deity.

3. But as far as the soul is concerned, I see that it exists. I know about it that we have a soul,

1 *Pythagoras*] orig.: Πρωταγόρας (Protagoras)

1 +having come+ ... +how much clearer+: see the app. crit.

אני רואה כי כל בני אדם קוראים לסבה אשר בה תהיה התנועה הבחירית וההרגש במה שישיגו בעלי חיים נפש אבל עצם הנפש אני מודה שאין לי ידיעה בו וכל שכן שלא אדע אם היא מתה או זולתי מקבלת המות

scit uniuersaliter populus. nam uideo quod omnes homines denominant occasionem que est motus uoluntarii et sensus animam. substantiam autem anime renuncio scire, et quanto magis ego non debeo scire utrum sit mortalis.

2 Et ego composui in Sententiis Y p o c r a t i s et P l a t o n i s librum uolens
quod esset michi defensio et memoria in senectute, que est domina obliuionis,
sicut ait P l a t o. et non iudicaui in aliquo ipsorum de anima utrum sit morta-
3 lis aut immortalis et utrum sit corporea aut incorporea. principium autem tri-
um motuum, unum a cerebro, secundum a corde, tertium ab epate, et demon-
straui in hac re demonstrationibus meis in libro Y p o c r a t i s et P l a t o n i s.
et demonstraui in isto eodem libro quod debeam proponere demonstrationes
manerierum rationis et memorie quibus percipiuntur ea que sunt in scientia
loyce. et motus uoluntarius uadit unicuique membrorum istorum ab hoc mem-
bro, et ita perceptio que est omnium sensibilium procedit quod hec percipian-
4 tur sensibilia extra posita. probaui etiam quod cor sit principium motus opera-
tionis pulsus, quod est in ipso et in arteriis et quod superhabundat a calore na-

2sq. occasionem – animam] *cf.* Gal. De fac. nat. I 1: Scr. min. III 101,1–5 Helmr. = II 1,3–6 K. De plac. Hipp. et Plat. II 3,4: CMG V 4,1,2, p. 110,1sq. Adv. Iul. 5,4: CMG V 10,3, p. 48,20–22 3sq. substantiam – scire] *cf. e. g.* Gal. Quod animi mores corp. temp. sequ. 3: Scr. min. II 38,20–23 Müller = IV 776,1–4 K. In Hipp. Epid. VI comm. V 5: CMG V 10,2,2, p. 271,19–272,25 De foet. form. 6: IV 701,14–702,4 K. De plac. Hipp. et Plat. VII 3,19–22; 7,25; IX 9,1–7. 8: CMG V 4,1,2, p. 442,37–444,11; 474,22–27; 598,1–28; 600, 4–8 al-Rāzī, Shukūk: p. 14,17sq.; 15,10sq.; 32,10sq. Mohaghegh 8 Sententiis – Platonis] Gal. De plac. Hipp. et Plat.: CMG V 4,1,2 10 Plato] *cf.* Plat. Phaedr. 276 d Gal. De puls. diff. III 3: VIII 657,10sq. K. Meth. med. VII 1: X 456,10sq. K. 11–13] *v.* Gal. De plac. Hipp. et Plat. VI–VII: CMG V 4,1,2, p. 360–478 *cf.* Gal. In Plat. Tim. comm. III 2: CMG Suppl. I, p. 11,21–12,21 Meth. med. VII 13: X 527,4–7 K. 14 demonstraui – libro] *cf.* Gal. De plac. Hipp. et Plat. IX 1,6–13; 6: CMG V 4,1,2, p. 540,20–542,20; 572, 16–586,6 16–18] *cf.* Gal. De plac. Hipp. et Plat. II 7,1–21: CMG V 4,1,2, p. 152,9–156, 19 In Hipp. Epid. VI comm. V 5: CMG V 10,2,2, p. 271,7–9 18–62,1] *cf.* Gal. De plac. Hipp. et Plat. II 4,49; 6,9sq.; 8,24; VI 8,74sq.: CMG V 4,1,2, p. 128,2–4; 150,3–9; 160,37–162,2; 422,28–424,4 In Hipp. Epid. VI comm. III 18; IV 25; V 5: CMG V 10,2,2, p. 152, 24sq.; 237,2sq.; 274,4sq.

2 תהיה] חטה L 3 שישיגוהו L

1 uniuersalis *Zonta* nam] etiam B: sed C 2 qui γ 3 uoluntarius C γ anima C O substantia O 5 non *om.* O *post* debeo *add.* aliud γ, illud ε sciens O: sciens sciens B *post* scire *add.* scilicet ε 6 *post* mortalis *sec. Fal.* (או זולתי מקבלת המות) *fort.* aut immortalis *addendum est* 9 senetute C 10 et *om.* C indicaui O *post* aliquo *add.* loco C ipsorum] de ipso O B, *in* ipsorum *corr.* B^2: de ipiso C 11 aut immortalis *om.* ε aut^{II}] an C E principium] p^m C 12 et *om.* ε 13 *post* meis *add.* m^i C 14 isto et O: ipso C: uno et B delibeam prius ponere C 16 membrorum] membro B ε 18 exposita β, extra posita *supra lin.* E^2 motus *om.* C 19 *ante* pulsus *add.* et B $quod^I$ *om.* B et^{II} *om.* C superabundant *in* -dat *supra lin. corr.* E

the cause by which exists voluntary movement and the sense with which animals perceive "soul". But the substance of the soul, I admit that I have no knowledge about it; and all the more so do I not know if the soul is mortal or immortal.

inasmuch as everyone everywhere acknowledges it. For I see that all men call the cause of voluntary motion and sensation "the soul". Yet I make no claim to know the substance of the soul, and hence how much more difficult it is for me to know whether it is mortal.

I (once) wrote a treatise (called) On the opinions of Hippocrates and 2
Plato, intending it to be a safeguard and a memorial for me in old age, the
mistress of forgetfulness as Plato says. And I did not decide in any of these
(books) whether the soul was mortal or immortal, corporeal or incorporeal.
That it was the source of three movements, one coming from the brain, one 3
from the heart and one from the liver, I proved also in this matter by my
proofs in my book (On the opinions) of Hippocrates and Plato. And I
showed in that same book that I had to put forward proofs of the type of reason and memory by which is perceived whatever is included in the science of
logic. Now from this part (of the body) voluntary motion goes to every other
part, and our perception of all sensible things proceeds in this way that these
external sense objects are perceived. I also proved that the heart is the source 4
of the movement of pulsation because (this movement) is in it and in the ar-

turali. et in omnibus tamen ⟨de⟩ hoc est parua quantitas et aliquo indiget iuuamine caloris delati a corde, quod accenditur in hora ire.

5 Et ego dico quod in plantis est principium motus et uirtutis regitiue in ipsis regentis eas. et narraui hoc in tribus dictionibus in quibus probaui quod inuenitur in plantis uirtus qua attrahit ei conuenientia et uirtus qua expellit sibi contraria et uirtus digestiua qua digerit illud quod attrahit de nutrimento et uirtus retentiua qua retinet sibi similia. operatio autem uirtutis digestiue facit augmentum in puero postquam ortus est. sed uirtutem que format embrionem in matrice non determinaui in aliquo loco utrum substantia sua sit substantia istarum quatuor uirtutum, id est uirtutis appetitiue, uirtutis retentiue, uirtutis digestiue et uirtutis expulsiue, uel substantia alia magis subtilis. et narraui hoc
6 in dictione quam scripsi de formatione embrionis. sed de substantia regente plantas dico quod cum sumitur secundum socios Platonis philosophi, nomino eam animam prout nominauit eam Plato, et cum sumitur secundum reuac nomino eam naturam. ego nominaui etiam uirtutes que sunt in hac anima naturam in libro De uirtutibus naturalibus, quia in hoc libro communicaui cum medicis popularibus.

4. Corpora uero que sunt super terram, quia de corporibus celestibus recuso me habere scientiam, demonstraui quod Ypocras fuit primus qui iudicauit quod hec sint creata ex temperamento ignis terre aque et aeris. et ipse ueraciter iudicauit de hoc quod iudicauit de hiis rebus et reprobauit similiter illos qui dicebant quod elementa corporum non recipiebant alterationem in

3sq.] *cf. infra*, p. 108,4–8 Gal. Adv. Iul. 5,4: CMG V 10,3, p. 48,18–21 In Hipp. Epid. VI comm. V 5: CMG V 10,2,2, p. 272,27–273,1 4–7] *v.* Gal. De fac. nat.: Scr. min. III 101–257 Helmr. = II 1–214 K. 7sq.] *cf.* Gal. De fac. nat. I 7: Scr. min. III 112, 11–13 Helmr. = II 16,6–8 K. 10sq. istarum – expulsiue] *cf.* Gal. In Hipp. Epid. III comm. I 17: CMG V 10,2,1, p. 46,12–15 11sq.] *cf. infra*, p. 90,18–20 Gal. De foet. form. 6: IV 700,5–702,4 K. 12–14 Plato] *cf. infra*, p. 102,17–19 Gal. In Hipp. Epid. VI comm. V 5: CMG V 10,2,2, p. 272,25–273,4 De foet. form. 3. 6: IV 665,3–17; 700,6–10 K. De plac. Hipp. et Plat. VI 3,7: CMG V 4,1,2, p. 374,13–19 15–17] *v.* Gal. De fac. nat. I 1: Scr. min. III 101,1–15 Helmr. = II 1,3–2,5 K. 18sq. de – scientiam] *cf.* Gal. De plac. Hipp. et Plat. IX 6,21sq.; 7,9–12: CMG V 4,1,2, p. 576,27–578,2; 588,7–22 Adv. Iul. 5,3. 5: CMG V 10,3, p. 48,13sq.; 49,1–5 19sq. demonstraui – aeris] *v.* Gal. In Hipp. De nat. hom. comm. I 13: CMG V 9,1, p. 27,22sq. De elem. ex Hipp. sent. 5,32; 9,25: CMG V 1,2, p. 100,19–24; 134,13–15 21 reprobauit] *cf.* Gal. De fac. nat. I 2: Scr. min. III 103, 25–104,11 Helmr. = II 5,1–11 K.

1 *post* omnibus *add.* plantis C tamen] cum B ε de *add. Kollesch et Nickel* parue quantitatis C *ante* aliquo *add.* in O indigent adiuuamine C 3 Et *om.* β ergo γ uirtutes C 4 regentia C γ eas *om.* γ: ipsas C in quibus] et B 5 qua[I] – uirtus[II] *om.* B qua[I]] que C O ε: *correxi* eis C uirtus[II]] uirtas O qua[II]] que C ε 6 qua] quam B: que O illud] id C B E: et D 7 qua] que β facit *om.* C 8 est] natus C 9 sua *in textu om., in marg. add.* B 10 id est] et B 10sq. digestiue ... retentiue ε 11 ex/expulsiue C 12 digõe C descripsi β 13 quod *om.* C O B, *supra lin. add.* B^2 14 animam *om.* ε nominat C reuac *scripsi (cf. infra, p. 84,5)*: rem ueram C: rationem β 16 hoc libro] s. presenti *in marg. ut interpretamentum* B^2 18 *ante* Corpora *add.* Capitulum quartum de hiis que sentit actor circa corpora inferiora et calorem eorum et genera febrium. ε corporea B supracelestibus γ E: superioribus D 19 me] modo ε fuerit E D, *ut vid.* 20 creata *bis scr.* B: creatio O *ante* aque *add.* et C 21 de[I] – iudicauit[II] *om.* O ε *ante* iudicauit[II] *add.* ueraciter B 21sq. illos similiter C

teries and because it enjoys an excess of natural heat. And yet in all (other parts) there exists a small quantity of this (heat), and it needs some additional heat transferred from the heart because (heat) is fired (in the heart) with anger.

I also say that in plants there is a source of movement and of a govern- 5
ing faculty governing them within them. I described this in three books in which I proved that there is found in plants a faculty by which it attracts what is suitable for itself, and another by which it removes what is unsuitable for itself, a digestive faculty by which it digests what it attracts from the food, and a retentive faculty by which it retains whatever is like itself. The working of the digestive faculty is responsible for growth in a child after birth. But as for the faculty which forms the embryo within the womb, I have nowhere decided whether its substance is identical with that of these four faculties, i.e. appetitive, retentive, digestive and expulsive, or if it is another more subtle substance. I explained this in a tract which I wrote on the formation of the foetus. But as for the substance which governs plants, I say that 6
when the matter is understood in the manner of the followers of Plato, the philosopher, I call it "soul", just as Plato (himself) called it, but when it is understood in the manner of *reuac*, I call it "nature". I have also called the faculties within this soul "nature" in my book On the natural faculties, because in this tract I was dealing with ordinary doctors.

4. As for bodies in this world, since I refuse all claim to knowledge of celestial bodies, I showed that Hippocrates was the first to declare that they were created from a mixture of fire, earth, water and air. In his judgment that he passed on these matters, he came to the right decision, and he similarly (rightly) criticised those who claimed that the elements of these

19 *reuac*] orig.: οἱ Στωϊκοί or οἱ ἀπὸ τῆς Στοᾶς (the Stoics)

qualitatibus eorum. ego uero posui probationem de hiis rebus in meo libro De elementis secundum sententiam Ypocratis et in commento libri sui De humana natura in tribus dictionibus, et demonstraui in ipso quod in omnibus libris sit eadem sententia.

2 Et demonstraui quod nomen caliditatis significat rem simplicem, non commixtam sui contrarii de qualitatibus, secundum quod est unum elementorum, et significat illud quod superhabundat secundum istud elementum. et significat similiter aliud diuersum ab hiis duabus rebus, et est illud quod de consuetudine est nominare calorem naturalem, et temperantia sua in omni genere
3 animalium est prima temperantia. et demonstraui in uno librorum et in dictione in qua reprobaui Boelium de hoc quod fuit contrarius Ypocrati in libro Amphorismorum dicenti: „Que crescunt plurimum habent innatum calorem et cetera“, cum oppinatus est quod diceret „plurimum calorem innatum habent“ quod calor sit magis fortis quam possit esse, non superhabundans in propria substantia caloris naturalis, que est sperma et sanguis, quia generatio nostra non est nisi ab hiis duobus et ab hiis etiam procedit.

4 Ἐδείχθη δὲ καί, ὅπως λέγεται τὸ «πλεῖστον» ⟨...⟩ οὐ γὰρ κατὰ τὴν τῆς ποιότητος ἐπίτασιν, ἀλλὰ τῷ μέτρῳ πλέον ἀκούειν χρή. ἐδείχθη ⟨...⟩ τῷ μὲν ἐμφύτῳ θερμῷ θερμοτέρους εἶναι τοὺς παῖδας τῶν ἀκμαζόντων,

4 Et demonstraui etiam quot modis aliquid dicitur esse „plurimum“ quoniam erratur in significatione istius. quia non debemus intelligere in dictis suis „plurimum“ hoc est fortis in qualitate sua sed quod sit superhabundans in substantia. et

1 in – 3 dictionibus] Gal. De elem. ex Hipp. sent.: CMG V 1,2 In Hipp. De nat. hom. comm.: CMG V 9,1, p. 3–113 *cf.* Gal. De san. tuenda I 2,3: CMG V 4,2, p. 4,8–12 De diff. febr. I 3: VII 281,7–9 K. 5–7] *v.* Gal. De elem. ex Hipp. sent. 6,23; 8,1: CMG V 1,2, p. 108,11–13; 122,4–9 De temp. I 1: p. 1,11–19 Helmr. = I 510,2–11 K. In Hipp. De nat. hom. comm. I 14: CMG V 9,1, p. 28,20–23; 29,9–16 nomen caliditatis] *cf.* Gal. In Hipp. Aphor. comm. I 14: XVII B 404,13–407,12 K. 7–10] *cf.* Gal. De trem., palp., convuls. et rig. 6: VII 616,4–617,2 K. De marcore 3: VII 675,13–16 K. 10 demonstraui – librorum] *v.* Gal. In Hipp. Aphor. comm. I 14: XVII B 404,8–415,6 K. 10sq. in^{II} – Boelium] *v.* Gal. Adv. Lycum: CMG V 10,3, p. 3–29 *cf.* Gal. In Hipp. Aphor. comm. I 14: XVII B 414,14–415,6 K. 12sq.] Hipp. Aphor. I 14: IV 466,8 L. 13 cum – 15 naturalis] *cf.* Gal. Adv. Lycum 6,13–15. 17–19: CMG V 10,3, p. 22,1–16; 23,5–22 15 que – 16] *cf.* Gal. Adv. Lycum 2,3; 7,2. 4: CMG V 10,3, p. 5,11–13; 24,15–20; 25,1 19 κατὰ – ἐπίτασιν] *cf.* Gal. Adv. Lycum 6,1. 11: CMG V 10,3, p. 18,20sq.; 21,12–21 23 et – 66,7] *v.* Gal. De temp. II 2: p. 47,3–56,9 Helmr. = I 582,18–598,5 K. *de calore innato puerorum nihil in libro* Gal. De elem. ex Hipp. sent. *inveni; sed cf.* Gal. In Hipp. Epid. VI comm. I 5; III 15: CMG V 10,2,2, p. 20,9–13; 146,11–17 In Hipp. De nat. hom. comm. II 13; III 7: CMG V 9,1, p. 79,16–28; 95,8–13

3 in^{III} *om.* β 7 illud] id B ε secundum *om.* C γ significat^{II}] significant O 8 similiter] super illud ε aliud] aliquid B illud] id B ε 10 uno librorum] primo <commento> libr<i amphorism>orum *coni. Kollesch* uno] un^{i}o O: libro in unum *in* unum *mut.* B: n$\overset{2}{u}$o (= neruo?) C dictione] demostratione C 11 boelius C: *correxi*: bethenem ε: beth´ γ 12 amfforismorum C dicens C γ qui γ habent calorem innatum C: calorem innatum habent B, *fort. recte*: innatum calorem habent O 13 est *supra lin. inser.* B 14 habent *om.* ε *post* non *add.* est C 15 natuturalis E que *om.* C quia] quod E 18 dicitur aliquod ε: debet aliquid γ 20 illius ε debetur C 21 „plurimum“] hic exponit G(alienus) istam dictionem plurimum quomodo intelliguatur *in marg.* O^{2}

bodies never suffered any change in their qualities. I provided the proof of this in my book On the elements according to Hippocrates and in my three volume commentary on his work On the nature of man, where I showed that the same opinion is found in all his writings.

I also demonstrated that the word "heat" means something simple, not a 2
mixture of opposing qualities, inasmuch as it is one of the elements and means where there is a superabundance according to that element. But there is also another meaning which differs from these two, namely what we usually call natural heat, whose mixture in every kind of animal is its prime mixture. I 3
showed this in one of my books as well as in the treatise in which I criticised *Boelius* for opposing the view of Hippocrates in his Aphorisms that "Growing beings have most innate heat and so on", since he thought that "have most innate heat" meant that the heat was stronger than ever possible, not that there was a predominance of natural heat in its own substance, which is seed and blood, for our birth comes only from these and proceeds from them.

It was also shown what is 4
meant by "most" ... one should understand it not as an increase in quality but as one in measure. It was shown ... that children are warmer than adults in their

I also demonstrated in how many 4
ways something is said to be "most" since there are mistakes in its meaning. For we should not understand "most" in his writings as strong in its quality but that it is superabundant in

11 *Boelius*] orig.: Λύκος (Lycus)

τῷ δ' ἐπικτήτῳ τοὺς ἀκμάζοντας τῶν παίδων, ὥσπερ γε καὶ τοὺς ὑγιαίνοντας τῶν πυρεσσόντων πλέον ἔχειν τὸ ἔμφυτον ϑερμὸν καὶ τοσούτῳ χείρονα τὸν πυρετὸν ὑπάρχειν, ὅσῳπερ ἂν ἔλαττον ᾖ κατὰ τὸ τοῦ ζῴου σῶμα τὸ ἔμφυτον ϑερμόν. εἶναι γὰρ τὸ μὲν ἐπίκτητον ἀηδές τε καὶ δακνῶδες, ἄδηκτον δὲ καὶ ἄλυπον τὸ ἔμφυτον ϑερμόν. καὶ [κατά γε τὸ] κατὰ τὴν τροπὴν [τε] τῆς ἐμφύτου ϑερμασίας γεννᾶσϑαι τοὺς πυρετούς, ὧν ἔδειξα τρία γένη εἶναι τὰ πρῶτα, ὀνόματα δ' αὐτῶν ἓν μὲν τῶν ἐφημέρων, ἕτερον δὲ τῶν ἑκτικῶν καὶ τρίτον τῶν ἐπὶ σήψει χυμῶν.

demonstraui in libro meo De generibus complexionum et De elementis secundum sententiam Ypocratis quod calor innatus est plus in pueris quam in consistentibus, licet calor acquisitus sit in consistentibus plus quam in pueris; secundum quod in sanis est calor naturalis plus quam in febricitantibus; et febris, quanto magis minus est calor naturalis in corpore, tanto deterior, quia calor acquisitus est nocitiuus et mordicatiuus ⟨...,⟩ quia generatio febrium est de alteratione caloris naturalis. et demonstraui quod genera prima febrium sunt tria. et nominaui primum effimeram, secundum ethicam, tertium quod accidit ex putredine humorum et locutus sum in meo libro Febrium de generibus febrium.

5. Et demonstraui in meo libro Complexionum quod modi complexionum sunt nouem, quatuor simplices et quatuor composite et una equalis. et ipsa est dignior, quia modi simplicium complexionum accidunt ex dominio unius elementi, aut calidi aut frigidi aut sicci aut humidi. sed compositi accidunt ex dominio aut frigidi et humidi simul aut calidi et sicci uel calidi et humidi uel ex dominio frigiditatis cum siccitate. uerumptamen omnes isti modi complexionum sunt illaudabiles; sed dignior modus complexionum omnibus hiis est in

2 ὥσπερ – 11] *cf.* Gal. In Hipp. Aphor. comm. I 14: XVII B 407,10–410,17 K. 19 in – Febrium] Gal. De diff. febr.: VII 273–405 K.; *v. imprimis* I 7–9: 296,16–313,10 K. *cf.* Gal. In Hipp. Epid. III comm. I 6: CMG V 10,2,1, p. 29,17–21 20sq.] *v.* Gal. De temp., *imprimis* I 2sq.; II 1: p. 2,4–8,27; 40,3–10 Helmr. = I 510,16–522,1; 572,5–573,1 K. *cf.* Gal. In Hipp. Aphor. comm. III 2: XVII B 565,10–566,2 K. De constit. artis med. 9,2: CMG V 1,3, p. 82,13–19 26 sed – 68,2 alterum] *haec verba citat* Gas: Pagel, Beiträge, p. 26 *cf.* Gal. De temp. I 8: p. 29,4–32,4 Helmr. = I 554,13–559,9 K.

3 πυρεττόντων *Helmreich* 5 τοσούτω *e* τοσοῦτο *corr.* P 11 κατά γε τὸ *seclusi*: κατά<δηλον> τὸ *Helmreich* 12 τε *seclusi* 13 γενᾶσϑαι P

1 meo libro ε 3 *ante* sententiam *add. et del.* sbam B 4 quia B in *om.* C 5 licet – 8 naturalis *om.* B, *in marg. add.* B^{2} licet] sed C 6 adquisitus O: aquisitus C est C O 8 erit *in marg.* B^{2} 9 febricitatitibus B 9sq. magis mius C: maior est et minor E 11 quia *supra lin. inser.* B: quod O 12 mordicatiuus et nocitiuus ε et] nec C mordiuatiuus B 13 *lac. indicavi* 14 *ante* et *in marg. add.* ca^{m} 3^{m} B^{4} 15 quod] quia β generatio B, *corr.* B^{2} 17 secundam E 18 humorum *om.* β 19 Febrium *om.* ε genere ε 20 *ante* Et *add.* Capitulum quintum de complexionibus corporum, temporum et etatum et de comparatione earum adinuicem. ε libro meo B ε, *fort. recte* 21 nouem *om.* C compositi C B D, *ut vid.* 23sq. sed – $humidi^{II}$ *om.* D 24 aut^{I} *om.* γ E simul *om.* C aut^{II}] uel C uel^{I}] aut E 26 hiis *om.* E *Gas*

innate heat, adults more so than children in their acquired heat; similarly, those who are well have greater innate heat than fever-sufferers, and fever is more dangerous, the less innate heat there is in the body of the individual. For acquired (heat) is unpleasant and biting, innate heat does not bite and is trouble-free. Fevers are caused by a change in the innate heat and I showed there are three main types of them, and their names are ephemeral, hectic and those that are caused by corruption of the humours.

its substance. And I demonstrated in my books On types of temperaments and On the elements according to Hippocrates that there is more innate heat in children than in adults, although there is more acquired heat in adults than in children; as there is more natural heat in the healthy than in fever-sufferers; and fever is the more dangerous, the lesser the natural heat in the body, for acquired heat is harmful and biting . . . ; for the generation of fevers comes from an alteration of the natural heat. And I showed that the main types of fever are three. And I called the first ephemeral, the second hectic, the third that which comes from the putrefaction of humours, and in my book of Fevers I spoke about the types of fevers.

5. I also showed in my work On temperaments that there are nine types of temperament, four simple temperaments, four mixed, and one balanced. And this one is best because the types of simple temperaments derive from the dominance of one element, the hot, the cold, the dry or the wet. But the mixed (types) derive from the dominance of the cold and the wet together, or of the warm and the dry, or of the warm and the wet, or of the dominance of coldness and dryness. All these types of temperaments deserve scant praise; but far better than all these is that type of temperament in which none of the

quo non est dominium alicuius quatuor elementorum, uerumptamen omnia sunt mixta cum temperamento et nullum superat alterum.

2 Et locutus sum multum in eodem libro de complexione calida et humida.

τὴν θερμὴν καὶ ὑγρὰν κρᾶσιν ἀρίστην ἀπεφήναντο πολλοὶ τῶν ἰατρῶν τε καὶ φιλοσόφων, οὐκ οὖσαν ἀρίστην.

et illa est complexio de qua iudicauerunt multi philosophorum et medicorum quod sit dignior omnibus aliis modis complexionum. uerumptamen non est dignior modis complexionum, cum intellexerimus quid significant calidum et humidum cum superant. nam secundum quod uolunt quod intelligatur ab eis cum dico complexio calida, complexio frigida, complexio sicca, complexio humida, hoc est quod uincit unum istorum, eodem modo contingit ut intelligatur ab ipsis cum dicunt complexionem calidam et humidam quia illa est complexio in qua caliditas et hu-
3 miditas excedunt temperamentum. et dixi quod non ob aliud dixerunt medici et philosophi quod complexio calida et humida est dignior modis complexionum nisi quia inuenerunt corpora nostra quando sunt in existentia eorum naturali sunt magis humida et magis calida corporibus mortuorum et plantarum. iudicauerunt ergo de corporibus cum sint in eorum habitudine naturali est calida et humida natura istorum corporum.

4 Eodem modo dixerunt uer inter tempora anni quoniam facta comparatione ad estatem inuenitur humidius ea, facta autem comparatione ad hyemem inuenitur calidius ea. uerumptamen si consideretur complexio ueris in seipsa, inuenietur temperata inter caliditatem et frigiditatem et siccitatem et humidi-
5 tatem. et oportet quod complexio in qua superat caliditas frigiditatem et hu-

3 in eodem libro] *v.* Gal. De temp. I 3: p. 8,3–10,3 Helmr. = I 520,10–523,17 K. 4 et – 7 complexionum] *haec verba citat* Gas: Pagel, Beiträge, p. 26 5sq. πολλοὶ – φιλοσόφων] *v.* Gal. De temp. I 3: p. 8,28–10,3 Helmr. = I 522,1–523,17 K. *cf.* Arist. De generat. anim. II 1: 732 b 31sq. Theophr., fr. 335; 336 Fortenbaugh 14–17] *v.* Gal. De temp. I 3. 5: p. 9,13–20; 18,5–9 Helmr. = I 522,15–523,4; 536,15–537,3 K. 16 nisi – 17 plantarum] *haec verba citat* Gas: Pagel, Beiträge, p. 26 20–24] *cf.* Gal. De temp. I 4: p. 10,7–12,7 Helmr. = I 524,3–527,6 K. 24 oportet – 70,2 Epidimiarum] *haec verba citat* Gas: Pagel, Beiträge, p. 26

7 ἀστίστην P: *corr. Kalbfleisch, Zu Galenos, p. 691*

1 dominium *bis scr. et alterum del.* E elementorum] humorum C uerum ε: sed *Gas* 2 temperato *Gas* suparat D 3 in – libro *om.* ε 3sq. et – illa *om.* O 4 et – 6 quod] multi medicorum et philosophorum judicauerunt quod complexio calida *Gas* 8 complexionum *om.* C 9 intelleximus C qui C: quod O significat β cum superant. nam] nam calidum et humidum cum superant C nam *om.* γ 10 quod[II]] ut γ intelligantur O *post* complexio *add. et del.* complexio sicca E 11 quod] quia C 12 contingit ut] conuenit quod C 13 et[I] *bis scr. et alterum del.* C complexio est β 14 dixi] dixit O: dicit B ob *ex* ab *corr.* E *ante* aliud *add.* hoc O 15 calida et *om.* C γ *ante* modis *add.* aliis O 17 sunt *om. Gas* *ante* calida *add. et del.* mortuorum E 18 ergo] idem γ: enim C sint in eorum] sunt ab eadem C *post* naturali *add. et del.* quod E esse C 19 istarum B 20 in uere C γ anni tempora quod C 21 estatem – ad[II] *om.* C ε estatem *ex* estantem *corr.* O humidius *e* humidus *corr.* B yemem O 23 inuenitur C caliditatem] siccitatem B 24 quod] ut *Gas*

four elements predominates, but where all are in a balanced mixture and none dominates another.

I spoke a great deal in that book about the warm and wet temperament. 2

Many doctors and philosophers have declared that the warm and wet temperament is the best, although it is not so.

That is the temperament about which many philosophers and doctors have declared that it is better than all other types of temperaments. But it is not better than (the other) types of temperaments
if we consider what is meant by a predominance of the hot and the wet. For
just as they want to understand the meaning of my "hot temperament", "cold
temperament", "dry temperament", "wet temperament" as indicating the pre-
dominance of one of these things, so they should understand that their "warm
and wet temperament" refers to a temperament in which warmth and wetness
predominate over an even mixture. I declared that the only reason why doc- 3
tors and philosophers believed a warm and wet temperament to be the best
type of temperament was that they found our bodies in their natural state to
be wetter and warmer than the bodies of the dead and of plants. They there-
fore considered that bodies in their natural condition possess a warm and wet
nature.

Similarly they favoured the spring among the seasons of the year be- 4
cause it is found to be wetter by comparison with summer and warmer by
comparison with winter. But if the temperament of spring were to be consid-
ered by itself, it will be found to be balanced between warmth and coldness
and dryness and wetness. Indeed, a temperament in which warmth predomi- 5

miditas siccitatem sit complexio pessima secundum quod dicit Y p o c r a s in secunda dictione libri sui Epidimiarum quod cum narrauit conuersionem hore unius horarum anni que est estas in caliditate et humiditate, sed in tertia dictione eiusdem libri quod cum narrauit conuersionem totius anni in caliditatem et humiditatem, dicens in principio secunde dictionis eiusdem libri sui Elguefete in hac dispositione dispositionum aeris hoc dictum: „fuerunt multe pluuie cum forti caliditate in tota estate“. et dixit in secunda dictione hoc dictum: „Et fuit constitutio anni australis et pluuiosa sine uentis“. post hoc narrauit quod acciderunt in hiis duabus dispositionibus dispositionum anni egritudines mortales.

6 Secundum autem quod oppinatur per equiuocationem nostram quod inter ipsum sum et illos qui uolunt quod sit dignior modus modis complexionum in corporibus animalium calidum et humidum et in temporibus anni complexio ueris, eodem modo potest percipi diuersitas in temporibus [anni] senectutis, cum aliquis dicet quod hec complexio etatis est humida, et alius quod sit complexio sicca, quod non est ita, quoniam cum dicitur quod complexio membrorum radicalium senum sit complexio sicca uerum dicitur; sed ratione complexionis humorum in corporibus eorum membra eorum sunt humida, quoniam fleuma in ipsis superhabundat multum et est humor frigidus 7 et humidus. eodem modo cum dicimus

περὶ ⟨τῆς⟩ τῶν γερόντων ἡλικίας ἔσται τις φαντασία διαφωνίας, ἐὰν ὁ μέν τις αὐτὴν ὑγράν, ὁ δὲ ξηρὰν εἶναι λέγῃ· κατὰ μὲν γὰρ τὴν αὐτῶν τῶν στερεῶν σωμάτων κρᾶσιν ὀρθῶς ἂν λέγοιτο ξηρά, κατὰ δὲ τὴν τῶν ὑγρῶν περιττω-
7 μάτων ὑγρά ⟨...⟩ οὕτω κἀν τῷ φάσκειν ἡμᾶς τὰ μὲν νεῦρα τῆς ψυχροτέρας εἶναι κράσεως, εὐαισθητότερον δὲ

1sq. Ypocras – Epidimiarum] Hipp. Epid. II 1,1: V 72,3–7 L. *cf.* Gal. In Hipp. Epid. II comm. I: CMG V 10,1, p. 156,2–157,7 3sq. in^{II} – libri] *cf.* Hipp. Epid. III 2: I 224,7 Kw. = III 66,14 L. *cf.* Gal. In Hipp. Epid. III comm. III 1: CMG V 10,2,1, p. 110,14–112,10 6sq.] Hipp. Epid. II 1,1: V 72,3sq. L. 8] Hipp. Epid. III 2: I 224,7 Kw. = III 66,14 L. 14 eodem – 25] *cf.* Gal. De temp. II 2: p. 45,9–46,14 Helmr. = I 580,5–582,3 K. De san. tuenda V 3,2; 9,19: CMG V 4,2, p. 141,6sq.; 154,19–21 De simpl. med. temp. et fac. I 8: XI 395,16–396,3 K. In Hipp. Aphor. comm. III 31: XVII B 650,10–15 K. [Gal.] Def. med. 104; 107: XIX 374,6–9; 375,1–4 K. 22 οὕτω – 25 κράσεως] *cf.* Gal. De temp. I 9: p. 37,18sq. Helmr. = I 568,8sq. K.

14 τῆς *add. Kalbfleisch, Zu Galenos, p. 691* 17 λέγει P: *corr. Helmreich*

1 secundum – Ypocras] sed C secundum – dicit] sicut narrauit *Gas* 2 diuisione *Gas* quod] et B: *om.* ε narrauerit γ 3 *fort.* caliditatem ... humiditatem *scribendum est; cf. lin. 4sq.* et humiditate *in textu om., in marg. add.* B 4 quod *om.* ε caliditate B 5 principio] prima O D E, *supra lin. add.* parte E^2: prim᾽ B dictionis secunde β elgufeit O ε: elgufert B: i. epidimiarum *ut interpretamentum supra lin.* E^2 8 Et] etiam ε constitutus D E, *corr.* E^2 9 accidit C γ 11 oppinatum est C per] propter B nostram] nequa C 12 sunt et illos C: et illos sunt β: *corr. Kollesch et Nickel* modis *om.* E 13 *ante* animalium *add.* cum C, est γ ani C complexio – 15 anni *om.* C B, *in marg. add.* B^2 complexio] constructio B^2 E *(deest* D*)* 14 eo E 15 anni *seclusi*: etatis B^2 ε 16 hec complexio] complexio huius C humida est O 17 aliud O *post* alius *add.* dicet O ε 18 ita *supra lin. inser.* B 19 *post* complexio *add.* sicca B 20 sicca] humida C γ uero ε dicet γ 23 ipsis] eis O 24 humorum O

nates over cold and wetness over dryness should be a very bad one according to the opinion of Hippocrates in the second book of his Epidemics when he described the change of one of the seasons of the year, the summer, into warmth and wetness, and in the third book of the same treatise when he described the change of a whole year towards warmth and wetness: in the beginning of the second book of his *Elguefete* he said about this state among the states of the atmosphere, “there occurred much rain and strong heat throughout summer”. In the second passage he said, “The climate of the year was southerly and rainy and windless.” He then described how at these two particular times of the year there occurred deadly illnesses.

Just as it can be deduced from my hesitation that I take a position between him and those who believe that the best temperament in animal bodies is the warm and wet and among the seasons of the year the temperament of spring, 6

there will be an apparent difference of opinion about old age, one saying that it is wet, another that it is dry. For according to the temperament of solid bodies in the elderly, it could rightly be termed dry; according to that of their moist residues, it could be termed wet ... Similarly, 7
when we say that nerves are of a colder temperament, and, on the other hand, that a hot

so it is possible to observe a difference of opinion about old age, one saying this complexion of the age is wet, another that it is a dry temperament, which is not so, since when it is said that the complexion of the fundamental parts of the old is a dry complexion, it is truthfully said; but from a consideration of the complexion of the humours in their bodies, their members are wet, because there is a great superabundance of phlegm in them and it is a cold and wet humour. In the same way, when we say 7

6 *Elguefete*] orig.: Ἐπιδημίαι (Epidemics)

τὸ θερμὸν σῶμα τοῦ ψυχροτέρου.

quod complexio membri sit complexio frigida et quod magis sit sensus in corporibus calidis quam in corporibus frigidis, oportet quod tu intelligas in hoc postquam bene intellexeris et fueris bene perscrutatus quod demonstraui in hiis duabus complexionibus sunt ea dicta que dixi.

6. Πρῶτον μὲν γὰρ αἰσθητικὸν ἐδείξαμεν εἶναι τὸ μόριον, ὡς καὶ τοῖς παλαιοῖς ἔδοξεν εἶναι, ⟨ἐν⟩ ᾧ τὸ τῆς ψυχῆς ἡγεμονικόν ἐστιν· ἐπιρρεῖν γοῦν ἀπ' ἐκείνου διὰ τῶν νεύρων ἐπὶ πάντα τοῦ σώματος τὰ μόρια δύναμιν αἰσθήσεώς τε καὶ τῆς καθ' ὁρμὴν κινήσεως – ἐρρέθη δέ, ὅτι καθ' ὁρμὴν ἢ προαίρεσιν λέγειν οὐ διοίσει –. ταύτην δὲ τὴν δύναμιν εἴς γε ἕκαστον μόριον ἀφικνουμένην αἰσθητικὸν ἀποτελεῖν αὐτό. τὴν δὲ ἐκ τῆς δυνάμεως ἀλλοίωσιν ἑτοιμότερον δέχεσθαι τὰ θερμότερα μόρια καὶ διὰ τοῦτο αἰσθητικώτερα γίνε-
2 σθαι τῶν φύσει ψυχροτέρων. ἡ δὲ διὰ τῶν νεύρων ἰοῦσα δύναμις οἱονεὶ δι' ὀχετῶν αἰσθανόμενα μὲν ποιεῖ καὶ τὰ νεῦρα, μᾶλλον δ' αἰσθανόμενα τῆς σαρκώδους οὐσίας οὐκ ἐργάζεται.

6. Et hoc est quod nos manifestauimus quod primum membrum sensibilium secundum sententiam antiquorum sit membrum in quo est pars regitiua partium anime et quia fluit ab isto membro per neruos ad remota membra corporis uirtus sensitiua et uirtus motiua uoluntaria. et cum hec uirtus expergitur ad unumquodque membrum, efficitur sensibile. et receptio que est particularis corporis est calidior propter alterationem istius uirtutis. et ideo sunt iste partes magis sensibiles partibus que habent complexionem na-
2 turaliter frigidam. et uirtus influens in membris est sicut aqua que currit in cursu et ministrat neruis sensum. uerumptamen non ministrat magis neruis quam carni.

7 Πρῶτον – 18] *cf.* Gal. De plac. Hipp. et Plat. VII 5,13–15; 6,12; 8,2–12; VIII 1,3–5: CMG V 4,1,2, p. 456,5–17; 464,24sq.; 476,1–37; 480,16–26 De usu part. III 11: I 178,3–11 Helmr. = III 242,14–243,4 K. De locis affectis V 1: VIII 299,16–300,5 K. 9 τοῖς παλαιοῖς] *cf.* Gal. De plac. Hipp. et Plat. VII 6,12: CMG V 4,1,2, p. 464,24–26 *(de Platone)*; 3,6–12: p. 440,20–442,11 *(de Erasistrato)*; VIII 1,6: p. 480,24–30 *(de Hippocrate, Erasistrato, Eudemo, Herophilo et Marino)* 14 ἐρρέθη – 16] *cf.* Gal. In Hipp. Progn. comm. II 6: CMG V 9,2, p. 266,22–24 In Hipp. Epid. III comm. I 4: CMG V 10,2,1, p. 18,21sq. 22–24 ὀχετῶν] *cf.* Gal. De sympt. causis I 8: VII 139,9–16 K.

7sq. αἰσθητικὸν ἐδείξαμεν *ex* ἐδείξαμεν αἰσθητικὸν *corr.* P 9 ἐν *dubitanter add. Kalbfleisch, Zu Galenos, p. 691*

2sq. in – quam *bis scr. et verba iterata del.* B 4 quod] ut β tu] tñ (= tamen) γ: cum ε intelligat (-uat O) β in hoc] nichil β intellexerit (-ecxerit O) β fuerit β 5 perscruptatus C demonstratur ε complexionibus sunt] febribus sit C 7 *ante* Et *add.* Capitulum sextum de primo membro sensibili et uirtute eius et modo sui influxus et cui magis influit uel neruo uel carni. ε nos *om.* ε 12 quia] quod O ε ipso D 15 hec uirtus *post* expergitur *(lin. 16) trsp.* C hoc γ 16 expergitur ad] recipitur et spargitur ε 19 *ante* est *add. et del.* que B propter] per β 20 illius D 22 naturaliter *om.* B: naturalem ε 24 aqua *om.* E, *supra lin. add.* E[2] 25 curso O body is more sensitive than a colder one.

that the temperament of a *part* is a cold temperament and that in hot bodies there is greater sensation than in cold bodies, you ought to understand my meaning since you have understood well and examined well what I have shown; my meaning is that concerning these two temperaments my comments are the same as I made (about the dry and the wet).

6. We showed that the prime sensitive part (of the body), as earlier authorities agreed, was that in which the controlling part of the soul is situated: for from this there flows through the nerves to all parts of the body the power of sensation and of voluntary movement – as was said, it makes no difference whether one says "voluntary" or "deliberate" –. And this power on reaching each part, endows it with sensation. Hotter parts (of the body) accept more readily the change produced by this power and are thus more sensitive than the naturally colder.

2 This power, passing through the nerves as if through channels, renders also the nerves sensitive, but it does not make them more sensitive than any fleshy substance.

6. And this is what we showed, (namely,) that the prime sensitive part (of the body), according to the opinion of the ancients, is the part in which the controlling part of the parts of the soul is situated. And that there flows from this part through the nerves to the distant parts of the body the power of sensation and the power of voluntary movement. And since this power goes out to each part, it is made sensitive. And the receptivity of each particular body is hotter because of the change produced by this power. And so those parts are more sensitive than the parts which have a naturally cold temperament.

2 And the power that flows in the *members* is like water running in a channel and it provides the nerves with sensation. But it gives no more to the nerves than to flesh.

1 Orig.: νεῦρα (nerves)
26 Orig.: νεύρων (nerves)

et tu potes istud probare super quodcumque membrum animalis: ut discooperias neruos alicuius partis corporis et pungas cum aliquo corpore acuto uel cum acu, inuenies quod magis clamabit propter puncturam carnis quam propter puncturam nerui; plus enim recipit sensum doloris.

3 Νομίζεται δὲ ὑπὸ τῶν πολλῶν ἰατρῶν αἰσθητικώτερα τῶν σαρκῶν εἶναι τὰ νεῦρα διὰ τοὺς ἑπομένους κινδύνους ταῖς φλεγμοναῖς αὐτῶν, οὓς ἐπιφέρουσι, διότι τοῦ πρώτου τῶν αἰσθητικῶν μορίων ἀποβλαστήματά ἐστιν. ὡς εἴ γε διατέμοις ὅλον τὸ νεῦρον, οὐδεὶς κίνδυνος ἕπεται μηκέτι τῇ κατ' αὐτὸ φλεγμονῇ τῆς ἀρχῆς συμπασχούσης. καὶ μέντοι καὶ πολλοὶ τῶν ἰατρῶν φοβούμενοι τοὺς ἀκολουθοῦντας κινδύνους ταῖς φλεγμοναῖς τῶν νεύρων ὅλον ἐνίοτε διακόψαντες τὸ νενυγμένον νεῦρον καὶ φλεγμαῖνον ἔλαθον τὸν κάμνοντα μὴ δυνάμενοι λαθεῖν, ἐὰν σαρκῶδές
4 τι μόριον διακόψωσιν. οὕτω δὲ κἀν ταῖς φλεβοτομίαις ἄκοντες ἐνίοτε διακόψαντες νεῦρον τριχοειδὲς ἐπιτεταμένον τῇ τεμνομένῃ φλεβὶ κατὰ μὲν αὐτὴν τὴν το-

3 Et multi medicorum oppinati sunt quod nerui sunt magis sensibiles carne propter apostemata que accidunt membris elchatir. et hec apostemata nascuntur illis qui habent predictam infirmitatem, quia nerui sunt in cerebro sicut sunt rami in arbore. et quando mouetur membrum quod pungitur, non accidit ex apostemate quod accidit membro. et aliquando inciditur totus neruus qui est punctus, quem pupugerunt multi medicorum cum timuerunt de egritudine elchatir, que accidit ex apostemate nerui infirmi; non sentit incisionem, et si illa incisio facta fuisset in aliquo
4 membro carnoso sentiret infirmus. et secundum hoc exemplum inueni aliquos medicorum qui in hora fleubothomie inciderunt unam partem nerui subtilem ad modum capilli qui est in latere uene fleubothomate. et non accidit de hoc maior dolor ac si illa in-

7sq. διὰ – φλεγμοναῖς] *cf.* Gal. Meth. med. VI 2: X 391,4–12 K. 12 ὡς – 23] *cf.* Gal. De comp. med. per gen. III 2: XIII 607,11–609,18 K. 23–76,5 νεῦρον] *cf.* Gal. De anat. administr. III 9: p. 187,14–189,16 Garofalo = II 395,1–396,18 K.

9 ἐπιφέρει *(?)* P: *corr.* P^{2} 20 τόν ἐνιγμένον P: *corr. Helmreich* 22 δυνάμενος P: *corr. Helmreich*

1 tu *om.* β potest B illud β *post* probare *add.* fieri ε, *fort. recte* super *supra lin. inser.* E membrum *om.* C ut] *fort.* ut si *uel* si *scribendum est* discoperias C: discohoperias O: discooperias *e* scoop- *corr.* E: discooperiat D 3 sclamabit C carnis quam *in textu om., in marg. add.* B 3sq. propter puncturam *om.* B 5 *post* multi *add.* melioris B oppositi C 7 *ante* carne *add. et del.* carnes B 8 *ante* membris *add.* in O elchatit B: elchacir E, *qui in marg. ut interpretamentum* est egritudo que facit nasci apostemata que accidunt neruis, s. spasmus, uel punctura nerui spasmum inferens *scr.*: i. spasmus *in marg. ut interpretamentum scr.* B^{3} 14 *ante* membro *add.* in B membro] neruo ε 15 insciditur O 16 quem] quod β punxerunt β 17 elchacir E, spasmosa *ut interpretamentum supra lin.* E^{2}: spasmus *ut interpretamentum supra lin.* B^{3} 19 infirmi *om.* β: *fort.* infirmus *scribendum est* inscisionem O 20 inscisio γ fuisset facta β 21 sentiret *om.* C *post* infirmus *spatium 36 fere litt. in* C 23 qui] quod γ 24 insciderunt O: incidunt B 26 fleubothomathe E 27 dolor *om.* B., *in marg. add.* B^{2} inscisio O

And you can prove this on any part of an animal whenever you bare the nerves of one part of the body and prick them with a sharp object or with a needle, (for) you will find that it will complain more because of the pricking of the flesh than because of the pricking of the nerve; for the former has a greater sensitivity to pain.

It is thought by many doctors 3
that nerves are more sensitive than flesh because of the dangers that accompany inflammation of the nerves, which inflammation brings because they are offshoots of the most important of our sensory organs. Consequently, if you were to cut through the whole nerve, no danger would follow, since the source does not also suffer coincidentally through inflammation at this point. And indeed many doctors, afraid of the dangers consequent on inflammation of the nerves, have sometimes cut through the whole of the punctured and swollen nerve, without the patient realising this, which would not have been possible if they had cut through some fleshy
part. Similarly, during venesec- 4
tions they have sometimes unwittingly cut through a hairlike nerve which lies alongside the incised vein, by the same stroke

And many doctors have thought 3
that nerves are more sensitive than flesh through the swellings that happen to the *parts elchatir*. And these swellings arise in those with the aforesaid illness, because nerves are in the brain like branches in a tree. And when the *part* is moved that has been pricked, what happens to the *part* does not arise through the swelling. And sometimes the whole nerve is cut that has been pricked, which many doctors pricked when they were afraid of the disease *elchatir* which comes from a swelling of the patient's nerve; he does not feel the cut, although had that cut been made in a fleshy part, the patient would
feel it. And in this example I have 4
found some doctors who at the time for bleeding have cut a part of the thin hairlike nerve that lies beside the vein they have bled. And there did not arise from this any greater pain than if that cut had not been made. But at the end there follows *el-*

9 *parts*] Arabic transl.: nerves

9. 19 *elchatir*] Arabic transl.: *al-khaṭir* (the dangerous) or *al-khaṭar* (danger), orig.: κινδύνους (dangers)

13. 15 Arabic transl.: nerve

31 Arabic transl.: *al-khadir* (the numb) or *al-khadr* (numbness), orig.: ναρκώδους αἰσθήσεως, τὸ ναρκῶδες (numbness)

μὴν οὐδὲν μᾶλλον ὀδύνην εἰργάσαντο τῶν μὴ τεμνομένων· ὕστερον δὲ ναρκώδους αἰσθήσεως ἐπιγενομένης λογίζονται διηρηκέναι νεῦρον – τὸ δὲ ναρκῶδες ὀδύνης ἀμυδρᾶς ἐπὶ τῇ τῶν νεύ-
5 ρων φλεγμονῇ γνώρισμα –. καὶ
πολλοὶ μηδεμιᾶς ὀδύνης ἀξιολόγου κατὰ τὰς τῶν νεύρων φλεγμονὰς αἰσθανόμενοι μικρὸν ὕστερον ἐσπάσθησαν, ἐκ μὲν τοῦ σπασθῆναι δηλώσαντες οὐ μικρὰν εἶναι τὴν φλεγμονήν, ἐκ δὲ τοῦ μετρίως ἔμπροσθεν ὠδυνῆσθαι δηλοῦντες οὐκ εἶναι σφοδρὰν ὀδύνην ἐπὶ τῇ τῶν νεύρων φλεγμονῇ, διότι μηδ' ἰσχυρὰν αἴσθησιν.

cisio facta non esset. uerum in fine sequitur elchadir et propter hoc credunt medici quod neruus sit incisus – et manifestum est apud omnes homines quod elchadir est illa egritudo que facit nasci apostemata que accidunt neruis et sit similis isti speciei
5 doloris –. et accidit multis occasione
apostematum que accidunt neruis et sine sensu doloris perceptibili et post consumitur membrum, scilicet accidit illud quod accidit ex arefactione membri cum sint in eo multa apostemata. et significat paucitas doloris quod dolor qui accidit occasione apostematis existentis in neruo sit paruus, eo quod sensibilitas nerui non est multa.

6 et secundum quod oppinati sunt occasione elchatir que accidit ex apostemate nerui quod neruus sit magis sensibilis cum carne quam ⟨si⟩ sit in se, ita reprobauit Fisedis isto iudicio dicens neruum esse minime sensibilem. et si quis uult hoc perscrutari, inueniet neruum habere sensibilitatem; uerumptamen neruus non habet tantum de sensibilitate quantum habet membrum carnosum. et aliquando dicimus quod neruus sit magis sensibilis omnibus membris in infirmitate apostematum que accidit ipsis.

7. Et quia excusaui me non habere scientiam substantie anime que sit, et utrum sit mortalis aut immortalis, et uidetur michi possibile esse secundum

7–13 φλεγμονήν] *cf.* Gal. Meth. med. VI 3; XII 8: X 406,14–18; 872,9–11 K. Art. med. 31: I 388,11–17 K. 19 ita – 20] *cf.* Gal. De locis affectis II 8: VIII 90,8–10 K. 21 neruum – sensibilitatem] *cf.* Gal. De motu musc. I 2: IV 374,7sq. K. 25–26 immortalis] *cf. supra,* p. 60,3–6

4 λογίζονται *e* -ήζονται *corr.* P 5 νεῦρονο P 14 ὠδυνῆσθαι *ex* ὀδυνᾶσθαι *corr.* P

1 uerum] nam C: namque γ 2 elchidir B: elchatir D: elchacir E, spasmus *ut interpretamentum supra lin.* E[2] 3 inscisus γ 4 apud omnes *om.* C *spatio 20 fere litt. rel.* 5 alchadir O: elchacir E: elchatir D: alchidit B 6 aposteumata B 7 et *om.* C γ speciei isti C 11 *ante* membrum *add. et del.* neruus C scilicet] s. C O: et B ε 12 illud] idem B ε accidit *om.* B rarefactione C 13 cum] quod C B: que O 14 quod – 16 eo *bis scr.* C quod] et B 16 parui γ: parum C 18 sunt] fuerunt C O: fuerint B elchatis C B: alchacir E, i. spasmi *ut interpretamentum supra lin.* E[2] 19 *ante* magis *add.* et γ cum *om.* C γ si *add. Nickel* se *e* carne *corr.* E *ante* ita *add.* et C γ 20 fisodis B: fesedis D minime] inuerue O aliquis O 21 perscruptari C insensibilitatem B 21sq. uerumptamen – carnosum *om.* C 22 tantum de *om.* B sensibilitatem B 23 quod] quam O in *om.* γ 24 *ante* ipsis *add.* in C 25 *ante* Et *add.* Capitulum VII. de habitudine anime ad corpus et de natura corporis et spiritus. ε: ca[m] 4[m] *in marg. add.* B[4] quia] quamuis *malunt Kollesch et Nickel* non *om.* ε substantie *om.* C 26 aut immortalis *om.* C in mortalis O secundum *om.* C

creating no more pain than if the cut had not been made; but later on when numbness supervenes, they realise that they have sliced through the nerve – for numbness is an indication of slight pain at the inflammation of the nerves –.
5 And many have suffered spasms shortly after, although they have perceived no noticeable pain at the inflammation of their nerves, showing by their spasms that the inflammation was not minor, and revealing by their previously moderate pain that the pain involved in the inflammation of the nerves is not enormous, because the sensation of it is not great.

chadir, and from this the doctors believe that the nerve has been cut – and it is clear to everyone that *elchadir* is the disease which causes swellings to grow that happen to the nerves and that it is like that sort of pain –. 5
And it happens to many through the swellings that happen to the nerves and without any perceptible sense of pain and then the part is eaten away, to wit, there occurs what happens in the drying up of a part when there are many swellings in it. And the small amount of pain shows that the pain which arises on the occasion of a swelling existing on the nerve is small, for the reason that the sensitivity of a nerve is small.

And inasmuch as some have considered as a result of *elchatir* that arises from the inflammation of the nerve that a nerve has greater sensitivity with flesh than if it were by itself, *F i s e d i s* criticised this, saying that a nerve was hardly sensitive at all. If one wishes to pursue this matter, he will find that a nerve does possess sensation; but a nerve does not possess as much sensitivity as a fleshy part. Sometimes we say that a nerve is more sensitive than all (other) parts in the case of a condition of inflamed swellings that happens to them. 6

7. As I have refused all claim to knowledge of the substance of the soul, whatever it is, and whether it is mortal or immortal, and as it seems to me

3 Arabic transl.: *al-k͟hadir* (the numb) or *al-k͟hadr* (numbness), orig.: ναρκώδους αἰσθήσεως, τὸ ναρκῶδες (numbness)

19 Arabic transl.: *al-k͟haṭir* (the dangerous) or *al-k͟haṭar* (danger), orig.: κινδύνους (dangers)

21 Orig.: Ἀσκληπιάδης (Asclepiades)

hec duo dicta animam habitare in corpore, etsi sit immortalis et incorporea,
tamen uidetur michi conuenibile quod corpus, recipiens eam, rectum ab ea-
dem in dispositionibus suis in quibus conuenienter debet esse, sit sensibile; et
secundum quod dicimus oculum esse uidentem, aurem esse audientem et lin-
2 guam esse loquentem. et dico quod generatio corporis sit ex aliqua commixti-
one eadem commixtionibus elementorum; et si aduentus anime est cum aduen-
tu corporis, ergo generatio eius est ex quatuor elementis. impossibile autem
est quod aduentus anime sit ab uno et aduentus corporis sensibilis ab alio quia
substantia anime non est existens per se, sed inuenitur secundum speciem, di-
co autem formam corporis. intelligas a me cum dico secundum speciem quia
materia quam oppinantur sine qualitatibus aliquo modo sit materia.
3 Et egoipse monstraui quod hoc sit necessarium sine medio, cum non sci-
am substantiam anime. et hoc est quod anima quamuis sit immortalis et incor-
porea, tamen nos inuenimus eam manentem cum corpore, et possibile est quod
ipsa operetur mediantibus operationibus naturalibus. igitur oportet de hoc
quod corpus donec est custodiens complexionem sensibilem non moriatur. et
egoipse monstraui in prima dictione mei libri De regimento sanitatis quod
complexio corporis alteratur semper in frigiditatem et siccitatem quousque
desiccatur et infrigidatur in senii fine. et cum peruenit ad ultimitatem frigidi-
tatis et siccitatis, tunc non potest anima suas proprias operationes ⟨operari⟩,
sed ipsa etiam deficit prout deficit corpus; et uita post hoc extinguitur prop-
4 ter extinctionem suam. et sicut non refert apud medicum in medicando egritu-
dines utrum anima sit mortalis aut immortalis, ita etiam non refert utrum sub-
stantia sua sit incorporea prout uult aut sit corporea prout uult, cum iudicauit

3–5] *cf.* Gal. De instr. odor. 2,8: CMG Suppl. V, p. 38,13sq. 6–10] *cf.* Gal. Quod animi mores corp. temp. sequ. 3: Scr. min. II 37,16–38,4 Müller = IV 774,7–775,3 K. Arist. De anima II 1: 412 a 6–413 a 10 Metaph. Z 10; H 2: 1035 a 1–9; 1043 a 26–28 12–15] *cf. supra*, p. 76,25–78,3 Gal. In Plat. Tim. comm. III 2: CMG Suppl. I, p. 11,9–12, 21 17 in – sanitatis] *v.* Gal. De san. tuenda I 2,10sq.: CMG V 4,1, p. 5,8–15 22–80,1 spiritus] *cf.* Gal. In Hipp. Epid. VI comm. V 5: CMG V 10,2,2, p. 271,21–272,1

1 in mortalis O in corporea O 2 conuenibile *in textu om., in marg. add.* B eam *om.* β rectum] actum B ε *post* eadem *add.* dico C, dictio est O, dictio est *add. et del.* B 3 esse debet C et *om.* ε 4 diximus β aurem – audientem *om.* C 5 fit O ε 6 eadem] eodem modo C 7 est *supra lin. inser.* E inpossibile C: possibile ε 7sq. est autem ε 8 est *om.* γ anime] Nota opiniones de anima et de eius essenciis *in marg. add.* O^{2} sit *om.* β 10 autem] ante ε secundum speciem] speciei C 11 materia^{I}] materiam C opinatur β quantitatibus C 12 ego *e* go *corr.* C necessarium *e* ne/nec^{m} *corr.* C medio] me O E sciat C 13 et^{I}] ex γ quod] quia B quamuis anima ε 14 nos *om.* ε est *om.* O B, *supra lin. add.* B^{2} 16 complexionem] constructionem ε 17 libri mei ε De *om.* B, *supra lin. add.* B^{2} 18 complexio] constructio ε 19 senii] seni in O peruenerit ε 19sq. sic^{tis} et frigiditatis C 20 tunc *post* potest *trsp.* C *ante* suas *add.* in B^{2} *(supra lin.)* ε sua O operari *add. Kollesch et Nickel (cf. infra, p. 110,7)* 21 set O 22 meditando C 23 aut] uel C refertur C 23sq. substantia sua *scripsi*: scia sua C: scīa O: anima B ε 24 sit^{II} *om.* ε iudicauerit ε: iudicant C

possible, on these two points, for the soul to inhabit the body even if it were immortal and incorporeal, yet it seems probable that the body, on receiving it, should be endowed with sensation since it is controlled by it in the dispositions wherein it ought properly to be, just as we say that an eye sees, an ear
hears, and a tongue speaks. I also declare that the generation of the body de- 2
pends on a sort of mixture, identical with the mixtures of its elements; and if the soul arrives with the body, then it too is created from the four elements. But it is impossible that the soul should come from one thing and the sensible body from another, because the essence of the soul does not exist (independently) by itself but is found in conjunction with the appearance, I mean the form, of the body. You may understand from me when I say "in conjunction with the appearance", that the matter which they are considering is in some way matter without any qualities.

And I have shown that this is directly necessary, although I do not know 3
the essence of the soul. This is because although the soul is immortal and incorporeal, yet we find it co-existing with the body, and it is possible that it works through the medium of the natural activities (of the body). One should realise that so long as the body retains its sensible temperament it does not die. I have myself demonstrated in the first book of my work On the preservation of health that the constitution of the body is continually changing towards coldness and dryness until it dries up and is completely chilled in extreme old age. When it reaches the limit of cold and dryness, the soul can no longer perform its particular activities and itself grows weaker, just as the body does; and life is then extinguished through the extinction of the soul.
Just as it is irrelevant to the doctor in treating diseases whether the soul is 4
mortal or immortal, so it does not matter whether its substance is incorporeal, as this one wants, or corporeal, as that one wants, when he declared that the

quod substantia anime sit spiritus et non manifestauit, prout manifestauit Erasistratus, utrum spiritus anime contineatur in corporibus animalium in concauitatibus uel expandatur per omnia membra radicalia uel diuidatur in minutas partes prout uoluit Elumerephilis, dicens quod sit in unaquaque parte partium membri radicalis, ita quod nulla pars partium sit quod non sit in ipsa. et demonstraui in dictione per quam reprobaui dictionem libri Chrasis quod ipse in aliqua parte sui libri non declarauit hoc. ego autem non possum indagare prout dixi de substantia anime quid sit, sed secundum quod nomino corpus sensibile secundum corporis significationem quam dixi paulo ante, ita nomino spiritum animalem. et demonstraui in septima dictione libri De sententiis Ypocratis et Platonis et in aliis libris quod iste spiritus anime sit in uentriculis cerebri et quod sit primum instrumentorum anime rationalis; que anima habitat in corpore cerebri, non in uentriculis.

8. Sed multos medicorum et philosophorum inuenimus paratos ad multa iudicia per que iudicantur res secundum illos qui non credunt eis qui probant quod sol sit in ueritate maior tota terra. sed amatoris ueritatis non est uoluntas reprobare nec diligere inuentionem rei quod affirmet eam. uerumptamen cum audit aliquem affirmantem super aliquam rem, †audit† illam probationem post longum tempus; et postquam inuenit ueritatem uel ille expellit a se sen-

1 substantia – spiritus] *cf. infra,* p. 112,13–16 Gal. De simpl. med. temp. et fac. V 9: XI 730,2–731,17 K. De usu part. VII 8: I 394,6–9 Helmr. = III 542,2–5 K. 2 Erasistratus] *v. infra,* p. 161sq., comm. ad loc. 4 Elumerephilis] Heroph., T 145b v. Staden; *cf.* T 145a v. Staden 6 Chrasis] *v. infra,* p. 163, comm. ad loc. 7–8 sit] *cf. supra,* p. 60,3sq. 10sq. in – libris] *v.* Gal. De plac. Hipp. et Plat. VII 3,19–22: CMG V 4,1,2, p. 442,36–444,11 De respir. usu 5,1: p. 120,16–21 Furley-Wilkie = IV 501,13–502,2 K. De sympt. causis II 5: VII 191,9–16 K. De locis affectis III 9; IV 3: VIII 174,15–175,4; 233, 2–6 K. *cf.* Gal. De usu part. VIII 13: I 488,6–14; 489,5–7 Helmr. = III 673,2–9; 674,8–10 K. 12sq. que – cerebri] *cf.* Gal. De san. tuenda I 13,19: CMG V 4,2, p. 34,3sq. 16 quod – terra] *cf.* Gal. De cur. rat. per venae sect. 3: XI 256,2–15 K. De plac. Hipp. et Plat. VIII 1,20sq.: CMG V 4,1,2, p. 484,22–33 Arist. De anima III 3: 428 b 3sq. Aristarchi De magnit. et dist. solis et lunae, prop. 15sq.: p. 402,20–408,19 Heath Archim. Aren. 1,8; 2,1: p. 220,7–18; 232,27–234,11 Heiberg Posid., fr. 9 Edelstein-Kidd Pappi Coll. VI 72sq.: p. 558,5–560,10 Hultsch amatoris ueritatis] *cf.* Gal. De sympt. causis II 3: VII 165,5–7 K.

1 manifestauit[I]] manifestauerit ε prout manifestauit *om.* O B, *in marg. add.* B[2] 2 erasistrates C: archistrates O ε: architrastes B *ante* spiritus *add. et del.* con B *ante* in[II] *add.* aut O ε in[II] *om.* O 3 uel[II]] et B 4 minutas] multas β *post* prout *add.* ut E uoluit *om.* D elumpnerephilis C: elimerephilis ε: eliminerephilis B 5 parte *om.* β itaque E nulla] una O quod[II]] quoniam ε non *om.* ε in *om.* C 6 dictione] dictio O per – dictionem *om.* C ch`sis ε: charsis B: ebrasis O: ebrosis C 7 libri sui ε hoc *post* autem *trsp.* C autem ego γ 8 iudicare β 9 corporis] quod nomino corpus C *(cf. lin. 8sq.)*: quod corpus γ *post* ita *add.* et γ 11 et Platonis *om.* ε Platonis] pl`monis C anima C 12 uentribus O sit *om.* D principium ε que] quia B 13 anime O in[II] *om.* C *post* uentriculis *add.* rationalis C 14 *ante* Sed *add.* Capitulum octauum de moribus quorundam circa iudicia et de triplici principio in nobis secundum tres motus. ε 15 res *bis scr.* B eis] et α: *correxi* probunt B 16 ueritate] uirtute C amatores γ ueritatis] uirtutum β 17 quod] quoniam ε affirment B u[m]tn C 18 audit[I]] audit *ex* adit *corr.* C: audiuit ε rem aliquam ε audit[II]] *cruces posui*: agit *suspic. Kollesch et Nickel* 19 a se] asse O

substance of the soul is spirit and when he did not show clearly, as Erasistratus did, whether the soul's spirit is contained in bodies of living creatures in its cavities or whether it is spread out through all its fundamental parts, indeed distributes itself into minute parts, as *Elumerephilis* wanted when he declared that it is in every one of the particles of a fundamental part in such a way that there is no particle in which it is not. I also showed in my tract in which I criticised the exposition in the book of *Chrasis* that he himself never made this clear in any part of his book. As I have already said, I cannot make up my mind on what the substance of the soul is, but just as I call a body "sensitive" in the meaning of body I have given a little earlier, so I call the spirit "psychic". I showed in the seventh book of my work On the opinions of Hippocrates and Plato and in other treatises that this spirit of the soul exists in the ventricles of the brain and that it is the chief of the instruments of the rational soul; this soul inhabits the body of the brain, not its ventricles.

8. We have found many doctors and philosophers ready to accept several opinions by which matters are judged in accordance with those who do not believe those who prove that the sun is in truth larger than the whole earth. But the seeker after truth does not wish to criticise or approve the discovery of a thing because (someone) affirms it. But when he hears someone affirming something, he ... the proof then a long while; and when he discovers the truth, either he puts away from himself the false opinions which had been

4 Arabic transl.: *āl ʾīrufīlus* (the family of Herophilus) or *ahl ʾīrufīlus* (the followers of Herophilus), orig.: οἱ Ἡροφίλειοι (the Herophileans)

7 Orig.: Χρύσιππος (Chrysippus)

tentias falsas que erant formate in ipsam uel discooperit turpitudinem eorum contradicentium, et nullam sententiam reprobat multum, et si esset in turpitu-
2 dine. et propter hos uiros composui hunc meum librum ad exercitandum eos in probationibus quas posui super unamquamque sententiarum quas nominaui in hoc. et prohibeo eos de inuentione sillogismorum istarum propositionum, quia oportet in inuentionibus bonitatum anime quod debeat scire quod in nobis sunt tria principia per motus tres diuersos in genere; et oportet perscrutari hoc in curationibus egritudinum accidentium anime.

3 Et nos oportet scire quod principium istorum trium motuum sit in cerebro unius, alterius in corde, tertii in epate. et hoc demonstrauit Plato per operationem in libro suo, quod anima habet tres species, et omisit nominare locum corporis in quo habitat unaqueque istarum trium specierum. in libro autem suo qui nominatur Thimeus in quo locutus fuit de scientia naturali non sufficit ei iudicare quod anima sit tres species, sed quod sit in tribus locis,
4 quorum unus est in cerebro, alter in epate, tertius in corde. sed Chrosis et alii post ipsum narrauerunt membrum corporis in quo est pars regitiua partium anime, et omiserunt illud in quo est iuuamen illis qui uolunt addiscere philosophiam scientie et philosophiam pratice, prout omiserunt †mutant† illud quod prestat iuuamen scire dispositionem tonitrui et coruscationis et fulgoris

3 hunc meum librum] *immo* Gal. De demonstratione; *v. infra*, p. 166, comm. ad loc. 5 propositionum] *cf.* Gal. De plac. Hipp. et Plat. II 2,2sq.; 3,8–11: CMG V 4,1,2, p. 102,20–104,2; 110,15–112,2 9sq.] *v. supra*, p. 60,11sq. 10–12] *v.* Plat. Resp. IV: 439 d–441 a *cf.* Gal. De plac. Hipp. et Plat. II 7,19; V 7,1; IX 9,22: CMG V 4,1,2, p. 156,10sq.; 336,16–18; 602,18–21 12–15] *v.* Plat. Tim. 69 d–70 a. d–e *cf.* Gal. De plac. Hipp. et Plat. III 1,14: CMG V 4,1,2, p. 170,21–23 Galens Kommentar zu Platons Timaios, fr. 4: p. 50,2–8 Larrain Gal. In Plat. Tim. comm. III 2: CMG Suppl. I, p. 11,21–12,21 15sq. Chrosis – ipsum] Chrysippus, fr. 836–839; 843; 848; 879–881; 885; 887; 889–891; 893; 896–901; 910: SVF II, p. 227sq.; 229; 230; 235sq.; 238; 240; 241sq.; 244; 245–249; 258 Diog., fr. 29–30: SVF III, p. 215sq. *cf.* Gal. De plac. Hipp. et Plat. II 2,12; 3,3–7; III 2,1–9: CMG V 4,1,2, p. 106,7–14; 108,26–110,14; 174,25–176,30 18 prout – 84,3] *cf.* Gal. De animi cuiusl. pecc. dign. et cur. 3,7: CMG V 4,1,1, p. 47,12–21 In Hipp. Epid. VI comm. IV 20: CMG V 10,2,2, p. 229,22–231,3

1 que] secundum que B: secundum quod ε in ipsam uel] immanem uel O: uel immanem ε discohoperit C O 2 contrahentium B et^{II}] ac O D turpitudinis C 3 *ante* propter *in marg. add.* ca^{m} 5^{m} B^{4} propter] per C γ composui *om.* C librum meum γ meum *om.* ε excitandum C 4 sententiarum *e* sententiam *corr.* E: scientiarum B 5 de *bis scr.* B inuentione] denotatione E: denominatione D 6 in^{II} *om.* B 7 perscrubari C 8 hoc *om.* ε *post* hoc *add.* quod C 9 nos] non C istarum C 9sq. motuum – tertii *om.* C 10 unus, alter ... tertius β: *corr. Kollesch et Nickel* demostrauit O 11 *post* suo *uerba* de republica *desiderantur* habeat γ obmisit O: commisit C nōare B, *corr.* B^{2} 13 timeus B: tymeus O *ante* non *add.* et C γ 14 suffecit ε ei *om.* β indicare E sed] secundum γ D 15 est *om.* C set O crosis E 17 obmiserunt γ: commiserunt C iuuamentum ε: adiuuamen C addicere O E *ante* philosophiam *add.* scientiam uel ε 18 practice O ε obmiserunt γ: commiserunt C mutant] narrare ε: aliter narrare mutant O: multociens B, narrare *in marg.* B^{2}: *cruces posui; v. infra, p. 169, comm. ad loc.* illud] id B ε 19 prestant O iuuamentum ε fulgurationis β

formed on the subject or reveals the wickedness of those who contradict
(him), but he does not spend overmuch time on refutation, however wicked
the theory. It is for men like this that I have written the relevant book of 2
mine, in order to train them in the proofs which I have set out for each of the
opinions I have mentioned in it. I am also stopping them from discovering for-
mal arguments for propositions of this kind, since in trying to find the virtues
of the soul one has (only) to know that in man there are three principles for
three motions that are different in kind; and one should look out for this
when treating affections of the soul.

We should also know that of the principles of these three motions, one is 3
located in the brain, one in the heart, the third in the liver. Plato showed
this in fact in his book, that the soul has three forms, although he forgot to
name the organ of the body where each of these three forms has its seat.
However, in his book called the Timaeus, where he spoke about the theory of
nature, it was not enough for him to declare that the soul consists in three
forms, but (he stated) that it exists in three places, one in the brain, one in the
liver, and the third in the heart. *Chrosis* and his followers have specified 4
the part of the body where the controlling part of the soul is but they have
omitted that which helps men who wish to learn theoretical philosophy and
the philosophy of practical life, just as they have omitted ... whatever helps
(men) to know the make-up of thunder and lightning and thunderbolts, earth-

17 Orig.: Χρύσιππος (Chrysippus)

et terre motus et grandinis et niuis et yridis et signi quod apparet cum sole et cum luna aliquando mire diuisi et aliquando mire congregati et causas rerum que sunt in scientia metheororum. et hec omnia sunt necessaria illi perscrutari qui uult scire partem pratice philosophie tantum, et probaui in una dictione in qua reprobaui quendam philosophum de secta r e u b a c h. sed probaui medicis prodesse scire tria principia que sunt in nobis.

9. Et probaui etiam quod multum prodest scire illud quod multi medicorum neglexerunt, id est alterationem que accidit corpori. et hec in genere est duplex: una est unius qualitatis qualitatum actiuarum uel duarum qualitatum, id est caliditatis et frigiditatis et humiditatis et siccitatis; secunda est diuerso modo cum totalitate substantie actiue.

2 Ἐδείχθη ἔνια ἐν τοῖς Περὶ ⟨τῆς⟩ τῶν ἁπλῶν φαρμάκων δυνάμεως κατὰ τὸ θερμαίνειν ἢ ψύχειν ἢ ὑγραίνειν ἢ ξηραίνειν, ἔνια δὲ κατὰ συζυγίαν ἐνεργοῦντα τὸ θερμαίνειν ἅμα καὶ ὑγραίνειν ἢ τὸ ψύχειν ἅμα καὶ ξηραίνειν· ἕτερον δὲ γένος εἶναι φαρμάκων κατὰ τὴν ἰδιότητα τῆς ὅλης οὐσίας ἐνεργούντων. τοιαῦτα δ' ἐδείκνυον [ὄντα] τά τε καθαίροντα καὶ τὰ δηλητή-

2 Et ego demonstraui in libro meo De simplici medicina quia medicinarum que dicte sunt quedam alterant corpus uel caliditate uel frigiditate uel humiditate uel siccitate; et quedam alterant cum duabus qualitatibus uel cum caliditate et humiditate simul uel cum frigiditate et siccitate simul. et aliud genus istarum medicinarum alterant corpus proprietate totalitatis substantie sue, uerbi gratia sicut medicine laxatiue et medicine que nomi-

4 et – 5] *v. infra*, p. 170, comm. ad loc. 7–10] *cf.* Gal. In Hipp. De nat. hom. comm. I 7: CMG V 9,1, p. 22,26–28 9 qualitatum actiuarum] *cf.* Gal. De plac. Hipp. et Plat. VIII 4,20: CMG V 4,1,2, p. 502,17 De sem. II 5,24: CMG V 3,1, p. 184,10sq. 12 Ἐδείχθη – 21] *v.* Gal. De simpl. med. temp. et fac. V 1sq.: XI 705,11–706,17 K. 22 τοιαῦτα – 86,7] *cf.* Gal. De simpl. med. temp. et fac. V 18: XI 761,6–764,9 K. In Hipp. Epid. VI comm. VI 6: CMG V 10,2,2, p. 345,5–11 De temp. III 4: p. 101,1–15 Helmr. = I 670,6–671,3 K.

13 τῆς *add. Helmreich* 19 ἐστὶ Q 22 ὄντα *seclusi*

1 motus] maris C grandis C iridis B signum γ: sinnum D: finnum signum C: i. halonis *ut interpretamentum supra lin.* E^2 2 *post* luna *add.* et C mire$^{I\ et\ II}$] mirum γ diuisi – mire^{II} *supra lin. inser.* E causa C γ rerum *om.* ε 3 metherorum γ: metheorum ε: methauerorum C: *correxi* *ante* necessaria *add.* i. C illi necessaria ε 4 qui] quando B partem *om.* B, *in marg. add.* B^2 practice O ε 5 phy^m C: philosophorum ε *ante* medicis *add.* pro C 6 deesse B principia tria β 7 *ante* Et *add.* Capitulum nonum de modis qui de modis quibus alteratur corpus et de medicinis proportionaliter illis modis (illis modis *supra lin. inser.* E) alterantibus corpus et de diuisione operationum naturalium secundum hos modos. ε *ante* illud *add.* quod γ, quid C illud] id B ε 8 id est] .i. C B: in ε: .s. O alteratione ε: alterationi O qua O hoc B in genere *om.* C est^{II} *om.* γ 9 qualitatis unius ε: qualitatis unio γ qualitatum^{I} – duarum *om.* B actiuarum] actuarum C: primarum *ut interpretamentum supra lin.* D^2 E^2 10 id est] .i. C B D: .s. O E et^{II} *om.* C est diuerso] diuorso B: econuerso O ε B^2 *(in marg.)* 13 quia] quod ε 14 quedam] que C 16 uel siccitate *post* caliditate *(lin. 15) trsp.* E, *post* frigiditate *(lin. 15)* D 18 et] uel C 19 simul *om.* C 23 medicina ... nominatur β

quakes, hail, snow, rainbows, and of the phenomenon that appears with the sun and moon, sometimes wondrously separated (from them), and sometimes wondrously conjoined, and also the causes of things which are in the science of the heavens. All these must be investigated by the man who wishes to understand at least a part of practical philosophy, as I showed in one tract in which I criticised a philosopher of the sect *reubach*. I also proved that it is to the advantage of doctors to know the three principles within us.

9. I also declared that it was of great value to know what many doctors have neglected, i.e. the change that happens to the body. There are two kinds of change: one involves a change through one or two qualities being active, i.e. the hot, the cold, the wet and the dry; the other in a different way involves a change through the totality of the substance being active.

In my book On the properties 2
of simple drugs it was demonstrated that some (of them) act by heating or cooling or moistening or drying, and others by a joint action, by heating and moistening or by cooling and drying at the same time; but there is another group of drugs which work by the peculiar property of their entire substance. I showed that such (drugs) include the purgatives and the so-called de-

In my book On the simple 2
drug I demonstrated that some of medicines just mentioned alter the body by heat or cold or moistness or dryness; and others alter it by two qualities, by heat and moistness together or by cold and dryness together. And another group of these drugs alters the body through the peculiar property of the whole of its substance, e.g. like laxatives and those drugs called in Greek *gui-*

6 Orig.: οἱ Στωϊκοί (the Stoics)
24 Orig.: δηλητήρια (destructive drugs); cf. below, p. 172, the note ad loc.

ρια καλούμενα, διαφέροντα τῶν ἁπλῶς ϑανασίμων ὀνομαζομένων τῷ τὰ μὲν δηλητήρια μηδέποτ’ ὠφελεῖν ἡμᾶς, τὰ δὲ ϑανάσιμα φέρειν ὠφέλειαν ἔσϑ’ ὅτε βραχεῖαν λαμβανόμενα μετὰ μίξεως ἐνίοτε χρησίμων τινῶν. οὕτω γοῦν καὶ τῷ τῆς μήκωνος
3 ὀπῷ πολλάκις χρώμεϑα. τῶν δ’ ὠφελούντων ἡμᾶς φαρμάκων ἔνια μὲν κατὰ μίαν ἢ δύο ποιότητας ἐνεργοῦντα, τινὰ δὲ τῇ ὅλης τῆς οὐσίας ἰδιότητι. καὶ μέντοι καὶ τῶν τῆς φύσεως ἔργων ἔνια μὲν ὑπὸ μιᾶς ἢ δύο γίνεσϑαι ποιοτήτων, ἔνια δὲ καϑ’ ὅλην τὴν οὐσίαν, ὡς τὰς ἐν τῇ γαστρὶ πέψεις αἱματώσεις τε καϑ’ ἧπαρ ἔτι τε τὰς καϑ’ ἕκαστον μόριον αὐξήσεις τε καὶ ϑρέψεις, ὑπάρχειν τε τὰς ἐνεργείας ταύτας ἅπαντι μορίῳ τοῦ ζῴου. διοικεῖ⟨ν⟩ γὰρ ἕκαστον ἑαυτὸ κατὰ τὰς φυσικὰς ὀνομαζομένας δυνάμεις, ἃς κοινὰς ἔχει πρὸς τὰ φυτά, καϑάπερ τι ζῷον ἑαυτὸ διασῷζον, εἴ τὸ μὲν

nantur in Greca lingua guibentirie id est uenena. et differentia est inter istas et medicinas mortiferas quia de istis nullum habetur iuuamen; sed de medicinis mortiferis aliquando habetur iuuamen cum in parua quantitate sumitur cum commixtione aliarum medicinarum iuuantium. et hoc est quod utimur multotiens lac papaueris,
3 id est opium, et prodest. sed medicinarum que non prosunt quedam alterant corpus cum una qualitate uel cum duabus et quedam alterant cum proprietate totalitatis substantie sue. et demonstraui etiam quod operationes naturales diuiduntur per unam qualitatem uel per duas qualitates, et quedam adimplentur cum totalitate substantie, sicut digestio que fit in stomacho et generatio sanguinis que est in epate et nutritio uniuscuiusque membri animalium. et hoc est quod unumquodque membrorum †currit† uirtute naturali, in qua uirtute conueniunt plantis, quia etiam plante custodiunt substantiam earum et uiuunt sicut animalia, cum attrahunt illud quod

3 τὰ – 9] *cf.* Gal. De simpl. med. temp. et fac. V 19: XI 767,3–13 K. Apul. Apol. 32   7 οὕτω – 9] *cf.* Gal. De ther. ad Pis. 10: XIV 248,9–18 K. In Hipp. Epid. VI comm. II 5: CMG V 10,2,2, p. 64,1–3   23 διοικεῖν – 88,5] *cf.* Gal. De fac. nat. III 8sq.: Scr. min. III 229,14–230,4 Helmr. = II 177,6–178,3 K. De usu part. IV 7: I 201,14–202,13 Helmr. = III 275,3–276,8 K.

2 ἁπλῶς *ex* ἁπλῶν *corr.* P   3 *ante* τῷ *add.* ἐν Q   8 τῷ] νῶ P: *corr. Helmreich* τῆς] τοῦ P   9 ὀπῷ πολλάκις χρώμεϑα *scripsi*: πολλάκις ... (ὀπῶ *chartae detrimento euanuisse uidetur)* χρώμεϑα Q: ὀπῶ παρ.χρώμεϑα P   12sq. τῇ ὅλης] ὅλῃ τῇ P: *corr. Kollesch et Nickel*   13 ἰδιότητι] ποσότητι P^2 23 διοικεῖ P: *corr. Helmreich*   27 ἑαυτὸ *in* ἑαυτῶ *mut.* P   εἴη P: *corr. Helmreich*

1 lingua greca E   *post* lingua *add.* m^{e} (= medicine) C   guibentirie *scripsi*: quibentime O ε: quinbentime B: quebentime C   3 mortifferas C: *om.* O   4 ullum B iuuamentum C   set O   de *om.* C   5 medicis B: me^{is} O   *post* mortiferis *add. et del.* in C   7 sumuntur ε   9 quod] quando ε   hutimur C O   lacte ε   10 id est opium *om.* B   opio ε   sed] secundum C   14 totalitate proprietatis C   19 *post* substantie *add.* sue β   22 animalium membri O   23 unum O: unus B: unius C membrum *in* memborum *mut.* O   currit] *cruces posui*   24 *ante* uirtute^{I} *add.* cum E   25 plante etiam B ε: plante et O   26 substantiam] subiectum ε   27 attrahant ε: atrahant C: athrahant O   illud] id B ε

structive drugs, which differ from those simply called deadly in that destructive drugs never benefit us, unlike the deadly ones which are occasionally of some slight use when taken from time to time with an admixture of beneficial drugs. For example, we often make use of poppy juice in this way. Among be- 3
neficial drugs, some act through one or two qualities, others through the peculiarity of the whole of their substance. Similarly, natural processes are brought about sometimes by one or two qualities, sometimes by means of the whole substance, as with digestion in the stomach, bloodmaking in the liver, and growth and nutrition in each part (of the body); all these activities take place in every part of the animal. For each (of these) organises itself by means of what we call natural faculties, which it has in common with plants, preserving itself like any living being, if it at-

bentirie, i.e. poisons. The difference between these and the deadly drugs is that no help is gained from them; but help is occasionally gained from deadly drugs when they are taken in small amounts with an admixture of other drugs which are beneficial. This is why we often make use of poppy milk, i.e. opium, and it is of benefit. Some of the drugs 3
that do not benefit (us) alter the body with one or two qualities, and some alter it with the peculiarity of the whole of their substance. And I showed also that natural activities *are distributed to* one quality or *to* two qualities, and some are achieved by the totality of the substance, like digestion in the stomach, and bloodmaking in the liver and the nutrition of every part of animals. And this is because each of the parts ... with a natural faculty, in which faculty they share with plants, because plants too keep their substance and live like animals when

16 Orig.: ὑπὸ ... γίνεσθαι (are brought about by)

οἰκεῖον ἕλκει, τὸ δ' ἀλλότριον ἀποκρίνει μεταβάλλει τε καὶ ἀλλοιοῖ καὶ ἐξομοιοῖ πρὸς τὴν ἑαυτοῦ φύσιν ἕκαστον τῶν ἑλχθέντων.

10. Ἐπικουρίας δὲ αὐτὰ δεῖσθαι πρὸς τὸ διαμένειν ἐν τῷ κατὰ φύσιν ἥπατος μὲν ἐπιπέμποντός τε ἅμα τροφὴν ἐπιτήδειον αὐξάνοντός τε τὰς δυνάμεις, εἴ ποτε κάμνοιεν. εἶναι γὰρ οἷόν τινα ἑστίαν καὶ πηγὴν αὐτὸ τῶν φυσικῶν δυνάμεων, ὥσπερ ἐν τοῖς φυτοῖς τὸ μέρος, καθ' οὗ συμβάλλουσιν αἱ ῥίζαι τῷ πρέμνῳ. μέχρι γὰρ ἂν τοῦτο διασῴζῃ τὴν ἑαυτοῦ δύναμιν, ἂν καὶ τῶν ῥιζῶν τι καὶ τῶν κλάδων αὐανθῇ, σῴ-
2 ζεται τὸ φυτόν. οὐ μὴν ὁμοίως γε ταύτῃ τὴν ἐξ ἐγκεφάλου χορηγουμένην δύναμιν αἰσθήσεώς τε καὶ κινήσεως ἑκάστῳ τῶν μορίων ὑπάρχειν. ἐν γὰρ τῷ γίνεσθαι τὴν ὕπαρξιν ἔχειν ταύτην, οὐκ ἐν τῷ διαμένειν ἐπί τε τῶν ἀνθρωπίνων σωμάτων ὅσα τε τῶν ζῴων οὐ πόρρω τὴν φύσιν τῶν ἀνθρώπων.

est simile sibi et expellunt illud quod est contrarium et diuidunt unumquodque istorum quod attrahunt et alterant quousque unumquodque istorum assimiletur nature sue.

10. Et membra indigent ad hoc quod remaneant in natura eorum adiutorio epatis ut ipsis mittat nutrimentum simile ipsis. epar enim in uirtutibus naturalibus est tamquam radix plante. quia arbor, si radix eius conseruat uirtutem suam remanet magis intacta, licet desiccentur rami ipsius uel brance
2 diuise ipsius radicis. et dispositio uirtutis que uenit a cerebro et dat unicuique membro sensum et motum non est sicut dispositio istius uirtutis, quia de natura uirtutis fluentis a cerebro est currere si renouat se continue. ista uero est fixa in corpore humano permanens et in illis animalibus quorum natura non nutritur a natura hominis [et natura eorum non nutritur a natura eorum].

6 Ἐπικουρίας – 15] *cf.* Gal. De plac. Hipp. et Plat. VI 3,38–41; 4,1–3: CMG V 4,1,2, p. 382,14–28; 384,1–14 In Hipp. Epid. II comm. IV: CMG V 10,1, p. 313,20–31 18 οὐ – 90,6] *cf.* Gal. De plac. Hipp. et Plat. VII 1,4; 4,1–3: CMG V 4,1,2, p. 428,19–21; 448,4–24 In Hipp. Epid. VI comm. I 3: CMG V 10,2,2, p. 18,11–13

10 τε] δὲ P: *corr. Kalbfleisch, Zu Galenos, p. 692* 16 τὴν *e corr. in* P 17 αὐαν^{θ} P 21 ἑκάστω *e* -του *corr.* P 22 τῷ] τὸ P: *corr. Helmreich* 24 ἐπί τε] ἐπεί γε P: *corr. Kalbfleisch, Zu Galenos, p. 692* 26 τῶν ἀνθρώπων *coni. Kalbfleisch, Zu Galenos, p. 692*: τοῖς δ' ἂν P

1 est simile] assimilatur β et *supra lin. inser.* C expellat C illud] id B ε 2 diuidit C 3 attrahit C: atrahit O alterat C 4 unumquodque *om.* C γ 5 sue nature C 6 *ante* Et *add.* Capitulum decimum de utilitate epatis et uirtute eius et de comparatione dispositionis sue uirtutis ad dispositionem uirtutum cerebri et cordis et de errore male intelligentium corpus nostrum regi a tribus principiis. ε 6sq. ad hoc *om.* C γ 7 quod] ut D remaneat C 8 *post* ipsis *add.* et B 10 naturalibus *om.* C 11 tanquam γ 12 conseruet C 14 brancce O 15 diuisi α: *corr. Kollesch et Nickel* 18 ipsius D 19 *post* natura *add.* ipsius B 20 a] in B si] sed ε 21 ipsa C γ uero *om.* C γ 22 *ante* corpore *add. et del.* co. O permanens *post* fixa *trsp.* C 24 nutritur] mutatur ε hominis – 25 natura^{II} *om.* B hominis] eorum C 25 et – 26 eorum *seclusi* nutritur] mutatur ε 26 earum ε

tracts whatever is appropriate (for it), and rejects what is inappropriate, and changes, alters and assimilates to its own nature everything that has been attracted.

10. But to remain in their natural state, the parts (of our bodies) need the assistance, on the one hand, of the liver, which both delivers suitable nutriment and strengthens the powers whenever they weaken. It is, one might say, like a hearth and a source of these natural faculties, just as in plants that part where the roots come together with the stem. For as long as this retains its power, even if a root or a branch dries up, the plant is preserved. In a 2
somewhat different way the power of sense and motion is distributed from the brain to each part of the body. For this power exists in coming and going, not in remaining constant, both in human bodies and in animals that have a nature not greatly different from men's.

they attract what is like themselves and expel what is contrary and distribute each of what they attract and alter it until each of them is assimilated to their nature.

10. And in order to remain in their natural state the parts need the help of the liver to send them nutriment that is like themselves. For the liver is in the natural faculties like the root of a plant. For a tree, if its root keeps its power, remains more intact, even though its branches or the divided ramification of the root dry up. But the 2
disposition of the power which comes from the brain and gives each part sense and motion is not like the disposition of that power, for it is in the nature of the power flowing from the brain to be running if it renews itself continually. But that is fixed permanently in the human body and in those animals whose nature is not *nurtured* from that of man.

25 Orig.: πόρρω (different); cf. below, p. 175, the note ad loc.

3 Οὕτω δὲ καὶ τῆς τῶν ἀρτηριῶν κινήσεως τὴν δύναμιν ἐπιρρεῖν ἀπὸ τῆς καρδίας, οὐ μὴν διαμένειν γ' ἐν αὐταῖς, τὰς δὲ φυσικὰς ὀνομαζομένας δυνάμεις ἐμφύτους μένειν ἐν ταῖς οὐσίαις τῶν μορίων. εἰς δὲ τὸ διαμένειν τὴν εὐκρασίαν τῆς οὐσίας αὐτῶν οὐ σμικρὰ⟨ν⟩ γίνεσθαι βοήθειαν ἐκ τῶν σφυγμῶν, ὡς ἐν τῷ Περὶ χρείας σφυγμῶν δέδεικται γράμματι.

3 Et similiter uirtus mouens uenas pulsatiles transmittitur semper a corde et non est fixa in uenis. natura autem uirtutis naturalis est in substantia membrorum. uerumptamen ad hoc quod remaneat temperamentum complexionis substantie membri indiget adiutorio epatis et pulsus uenarum ⟨quod⟩ non est modicum secundum quod demonstraui in Iuuamento pulsuum.

4 Et errat in hoc loco ille qui non intelligit dictum ueraciter cum dico quod regimen nostrorum corporum compleatur tribus principiis, quia possibile est quod oppinatur quod uolui intelligere cum dixi principia a quibus est regimen animalium scilicet principia a quibus est generatio embrionis in matrice. ego autem scio secundum quod dixi quod regimen animalium postquam sunt generata completur a tribus principiis.

11. Et ego nescio que est illa uirtus inter ceteras uirtutes que format embrionem in matrice et que substantia sit. illud autem quod oppinor de hoc est quod hec uirtus sit illa que generat plantas et informat eas. et non figitur intentio mea in motu qui apparet in compositione cor-
2 poris nostri. et hoc declaraui in libro meo De iuuamento membrorum quia

νέος μὲν γὰρ ὢν εἱπόμην ἀνδράσιν ἀξιολόγοις ἡγουμένοις τὴν καρδίαν ἁπάντων πρώτην διαπλάττεσθαι· προϊὼν δὲ κατὰ τὴν ἡλικίαν ὑπώπτευσα τὸν λόγον

in iuuentute mea secutus sum multos antiquorum famosos qui oppinabantur quod informatio cordis precedit informationem aliorum membrorum et dixi secundum quod illi dicebant.

7 εἰς – 11] *v.* Gal. De usu puls. 3,3sq.; 8,1: p. 206; 226 Furley-Wilkie = V 160,17–161,17; 179,5–15 K. 16sq.] *cf. supra,* p. 60,11sq.; 82,9sq. 18sq.] *cf. supra,* p. 62,8–12 Gal. De foet. form. 6: IV 687,5–689,6; 696,8–702,4 K. 19sq.] *cf.* Gal. De sem. I 9,14–17: CMG V 3,1, p. 94,27–96,19 22 et – 92,3 certum] *haec verba citat* Gas: Pagel, Concordanciae, p. XLII et – 26 membrorum] *talia in* Gal. De usu part. *libris non inveniuntur* 23 νέος – 92,10] *cf.* Gal. De foet. form. 3: IV 660,8–13; 662,1–13; 663,11–664,9 K. De sem. I 8,2. 8; 9,4: CMG V 3,1, p. 90,12–14; 92,3–8. 25–27 23sq. ἀνδράσιν ἀξιολόγοις] *v. e.g.* Arist. De iuvent. 3: 468 b 28 De part. anim. III 4: 666 a 10sq. De generat. anim. II 4: 740 a 3sq. Chrys., fr. 761: SVF II, p. 214 Plin. Nat. hist. X 148; XI 181

8 σμικρὰ *e* μικρὰ *corr.* P: *corr. Helmreich* 10 τῷ *e* τὸ *corr.* P 23 εἱπόμην P: *corr. Helmreich*

1 similiter] sic est C B 3 corde *e* corpore *corr.* B et *om.* B 8 *ante* epatis *add. et del.* te B 9 quod *addidi* 12 erat C B D ueraciter *om.* C *spatio 19 fere litt. rel.* *post* dico *add.* in hoc loco C 14 uelim C est[II]] et D 15 scilicet *om.* ε ebrionis C 16 *ante* ego *add. et del.* co O 18 *ante* Et *add.* Capitulum undecimum de uirtute formatiua embrionis et plantarum et de ordine formationis membrorum et quid format membra. ε Et *om.* B 19 ebrionem C 19sq. illud – sit *om.* ε 21 ca[m] 6[m] *in marg. add.* B[4] que γ 23 mea *om.* ε sum *om.* γ 25 formatio *Gas* precedat C 26 formationem *Gas*

Finally, the faculty that 3
moves the arteries similarly flows from the heart, but it does not remain in them, whereas the so-called natural faculties remain innate in the substances of (bodily) parts. The pulses are also of no small assistance in maintaining a sound balance in their substance, as I showed in my work On the use of pulses.

And likewise the power that 3
moves the pulsatile veins is always being transmitted from the heart and is not fixed in the veins. But the nature of a natural faculty is in the substance of the parts. But for the temperament of the mixture of the substance of a part to remain requires the help of the liver and the pulse in those veins, which is not small as I showed in On the use of pulses.

In this connection the man is in error who does not understand the truth 4
of my statement here, that the organisation of our bodies is controlled by three principles, since it is possible that he thinks that I mean, of course, by the principles regulating the organisation of animals the principles which are responsible for the creation of the embryo in the womb. But I know according to my statements that the organisation of animals after birth is regulated by three principles.

11. On the other hand, I do not know what faculty above (all) others forms the embryo in the womb and what its substance is. My opinion is that this faculty is that which (also) produces plants and gives them their shape. My views on the movement which is clearly involved in the creation of our bodies
have also not been fixed. As I said in my book On the use of parts of the body, 2

For when I was young, I followed some weighty authorities in believing that the heart was formed first of all; but when I grew up, I suspected this argument was

in my youth I followed many famous among the ancients who thought that the formation of the heart preceded the formation of other parts, and I spoke as they spoke. And when I ὡς πιθανὸν μέν, οὐ μὴν ἀληθῆ· χωρὶς μὲν γὰρ αἵματος ἀδύνατόν ἐστι γεννηθῆναι τὸ σπλάγχνον τοῦτο. ⟨παρα⟩γίνεται δὲ αἷμα διὰ τῶν κατὰ τὴν μήτραν ἀγγείων, ἐξ οὗ τὴν γένεσιν ἔχει τὸ κυούμενον· ἀλλὰ τοῦτο τὸ αἷμα φαίνεται διὰ φλεβὸς ἐπὶ τὴν καρδίαν ἀφικνούμενον εἰς ἧπαρ πρότερον ἐμφυομένης.

et cum perueni ad perfectam etatem ego percepi quod istud dictum est uerisimile, non tamen certum. impossibile enim est quod istud membrum sit generatum sine sanguine. et sanguis peruenit ad embrionem per uenas continuatas cum matrice, et ex ipso est generatio embrionis. et uideo quod iste sanguis in primis uenit per uenas continuatas cum epate, licet ueniat a matrice sua ad cor per uenas pulsatiles — spiritus tantum aut spi-
3 ritus et sanguis agitur —. uia sua est longior satis uenarum non pulsatilium, quia uene pulsatiles que ueniunt ad cor embrionis a matrice sua, cum transierint diafragma, reuoluuntur circa uesicam et componuntur in primis super os positum in extremitate radicis, id est in cauda, spine. et postea coniunguntur cum uena pulsatili expansa super dorsum et postea transit secundum longitudinem spine usque infra duas spatulas in directo pectoris quousque reuertitur usque ad uentrem sinistrum duorum uentrum cordis. et ministrat ei illam substantiam quam recepit a matre embrionis — uel est spiritus tantum uel cum eo aliquid sangui-
4 nis —. et non dicitur ueraciter quod cor sit prius generatum diafragmate et uenis pulsatilibus que ministrant ei spiritum et sanguinem, quos recipiunt a muliere.

οὐ μὴν οὐδὲ τοῦ ἥπατος εἰκὸς αὐτὴν διαπλάττεσθαι προτέραν φαινομένης γε σαφῶς τῆς ἐκ τῶν κατὰ τὸ χόριον ἁπασῶν φλεβῶν γενομένης φλεβὸς εἰς τὸ ἧπαρ ἀφι-

et non est uerisimile quod generatio cordis sit prior generatione epatis, eo quod nos uidemus uenam generatam ex congregatione uenarum que sunt in diafragmate uenire

12–18] *cf.* Gal. De foet. form. 3: IV 661,10–662,1 K. De plac. Hipp. et Plat. VI 6,49–52: CMG V 4,1,2, p. 404,12–20 De usu part. XV 4: II 349,16–351,25 Helmr. = IV 227,18–231,2 K. De ven. arter. dissect. 10: II 824,3–11 K. 15 radicis ... spine] *cf.* Simon, Gal. Anat. II, p. 18,17. 35 Gal. De usu part. XIII 1: II 233,14 Helmr. = IV 72,7 K. 20sq.] *cf.* Gal. De foet. form. 5: IV 682,9–18 K.

4 παραγίνεται *dubitanter coni. Kalbfleisch, Zu Galenos, p. 692*: ... γίνεται P

1 predictam γ: dictam ε: perfectam *Gas* 2 istud] id B ε: illud O *Gas* 4 est enim β 7 matrice – 10 cum *om.* C 9 uenit *om.* γ 11 *post* licet *addiderim* et ad cor *om.* C γ pulsatiles – 12 agitur] pulsatiles tantum. quia uene pulsatiles quibus spiritus aut sanguis agitur ε: pulsatiles tantum. spiritus autem ipse agitur B: pulsatiles. spiritus aut spiritus aut sanguis agitur O 12 longinquior C 13 transiuerint E dyafragma O: dyoflama C 14 uexicam C componuntur/tur C 15 radicis] matricis C et – 16 dorsum *post* pectoris *(lin. 17) colloc.* α: *trsp. Kollesch et Nickel* et *om.* β coniungitur C γ 16 expressa ε transeunt ε 17 in directo] et C: et de γ reuertantur ε 18 ministrant ε ei *ex* enim *corr.* C quam] suam quam ε: suam C γ: *correxi* 19 recipiunt ε matrice C *ante* uel^{I} *add.* que ε cum eo *om.* C γ aliquid] substantia C 20 ueraciter – 22 non *om.* D quod] quia C dyafragmate O: dyafl`ate C 21 ei] illi C quos] que C B a *ex* ea *corr.* B 23 primo generatione γ: ante generationem C 25 ex] et C congregationem C: agregatione B 26 dyafragmate O D: dyafl`ate C

plausible rather than true: for this organ cannot be created without blood. Besides, it is through the vessels in the womb that there arrives the blood from which the foetus has its genesis; but this blood clearly reaches the heart through a vein which has been first implanted in the liver.

reached adulthood, I saw that that statement is plausible, but not certain. For it is impossible that that part is generated without blood. And blood reaches the embryo through veins linked with the womb, and the generation of the embryo comes from this. And I see that that blood first comes through veins linked with the liver

although it may reach the heart from the womb through pulsatile veins –
pneuma alone or pneuma and blood are carried –. Their path is somewhat 3
longer than that of the non-pulsatile veins, because the pulsatile veins that go to the heart of the embryo from the womb, after passing through the *diafragma*, are curled round the bladder and (then) are first brought together above the bone that is at the end of the root, i.e. the tail, of the spine. They then join the pulsatile vein which spreads out over the back, and they then proceed along the length of the spine straight to the chest to just below the two shoulder blades and then it returns to the left chamber of the two chambers of the heart. There it delivers the substance it has received from the embryo's mother – it
is either pneuma by itself or with a certain amount of blood as well –. So it is 4
wrong to say that the heart is created before the *diafragma* and the pulsatile veins that distribute to it the pneuma and blood they receive from the woman.

And it is equally unlikely that it is formed before the liver, since we can see clearly that a vein produced from all the veins coming together in the chorion comes to

And it is not probable that the generation of the heart is before the generation of the liver, from the fact that we see a vein generated from the coming together of veins

13 Orig.: ὀμφαλός (umbilicus)
21 Orig.: χόριον (chorion)

κυουμένης πρότερον ἤπερ εἰς τὴν καρδίαν.

Ἔτι δὲ ἀτοπώτερος ὁ λόγος εἶναί μοι φαίνεται τῶν οἰομένων ὑπὸ τῆς καρδίας διαπλάττεσθαι τὰ κυούμενα μόρια. τὸ γὰρ αὐτήν τε τὴν καρδίαν διαπλάσαν, ἔτι δὲ πρὸ αὐτῆς τάς τε ἀρτηρίας καὶ τὰς φλέβας εὔλογόν ἐστιν, ὥσπερ ταῦτα καὶ σὺν αὐτοῖς τὸ ἧπαρ, οὕτω καὶ τἄλλα διαπλάττειν, ὅπερ ἔνιοι μὲν ἡγοῦνται τὸ καταβαλλόμενον εἰς τὰς μήτρας εἶναι σπέρμα, τινὲς δὲ τοῦτο μὲν ὄργανον, ἕτερον δέ τι θειότερον ὑπάρχειν τὸ διαπλάττον τὰ κυούμενα νομίζουσιν.

prius ad epar, et postmodum extenditur ad cor.

Et turpe est dicere quod a corde generantur omnia membra et quod prius debet esse generans cor et uenas pulsatiles et epar similiter cum ipsis quam illud prout creat omnia alia membra. et quidam dicunt quod ille qui est faciens hoc est sperma quod proicitur in matrice, et quidam dicunt quod sperma est loco instrumenti et quod formator embrionis in matrice sit aliquid nobilius spermate; et propinquius est dicere quod sit deus omnipotens.

12. Sed compositiones que sunt sanguis, fleuma, colera citrina ego demonstraui sententiam meam de ipsis in commento meo quod feci super librum Ypocratis De humana natura et in libro meo De elementis secundum sententiam Ypocratis. et monstraui quod ipse uideat quod quatuor compositiones generantur in omnibus corporibus sanis uel non sanis. et quidam uident quod sanguis tantum sit similis nature ⟨et⟩ appropriatus ei, sed generatio om-

3 Ἔτι – 17] *cf.* Gal. De foet. form. 6: IV 687,5–702,4 K. 12 ὅπερ – 14 σπέρμα] *cf.* Arist. De generat. anim. I 2. 20; II 3: 716 a 4–7; 729 a 9–14; 736 a 24–27 Gal. De sem. I 3,1–8: CMG V 3,1, p. 68,3–26 *(de Peripateticis)* De fac. nat. II 3: Scr. min. III 159, 26–163,7 Helmr. = II 81,9–85,16 K. *(de Erasistrato)* De foet. form. 6: IV 699,13–700,2 K. *(de Chrysippo)* 14 τινὲς – 17] *cf. e.g.* Gal. De foet. form. 6: IV 687,12–688,2; 700,2–701,10 K. De plac. Hipp. et Plat. IX 8,22–27: CMG V 4,1,2, p. 596,5–29 15 τι θειότερον] *cf.* Gal. De plac. Hipp. et Plat. IX 9,1–3: CMG V 4,1,2, p. 596,30–598,11 De foet. form. 6: IV 687,16 K. 19 in – 21] *v.* Gal. In Hipp. De nat. hom. comm. I 26: CMG V 9,1, p. 35,18–36,12 De elem. ex Hipp. sent. 8,11–14; 10,2–7: CMG V 1,2, p. 126,1–16; 138,15–140,14 22–96,1] *cf.* Gal. In Hipp. De nat. hom. comm. I 4sq.: CMG V 9,1, p. 19, 13–20,19 De elem. ex Hipp. sent. 3,52–64: CMG V 1,2, p. 82,14–86,10

1 εἴπερ P: *corr. Helmreich* 7 δὲ] τε *malunt Kollesch et Nickel coll. CMG V 8,1, p. 84,3* 12 ἅπερ P: „Legendum ὅπερ" *Helmreich* 14 τινὲς] τὸν ἐς P: *corr. Kalbfleisch, Zu Galenos, p. 692*

4 generentur γ 6 et[1] *om.* C E 7 quam] quod C illud] id ε: cor *ut interpretamentum supra lin.* D[2] E[2] 9sq. ille – quod *om.* B, qui facit hoc *in marg. add.* B[2] 10 *fort.* matricem *scribendum est* 11 dicunt quidam O 12 *ante* est *add.* non O ε loco instrumenti] istud ε *ante* quod *add.* et quidam dicunt B[2], *del.* B[3] formatio C 13 *ante* embrionis *add. et del.* e O ebrionis C 13sq. aliud nobilius O: anobili C 18 *ante* Sed *add.* Capitulum duodecimum de humoribus et habitudine medicinarum (melaxatiuarum *add. et del.* E) laxatiuarum ad eos. ε compōnes C B fl'a C: flegma O E: *om.* B colera citrina *post* sanguis *trsp.* O ε *post* citrina *add.* et melancolia ε: *fort.* colera <nigra, colera> citrina *scribendum est* 19 quod] quem O ε 21 uiderat C 22 in] ex D 23 sit tantum C et *addidi* appropriatis ε

the liver before it goes to the heart.

Still more curious, in my opinion, seems to be the argument of those who think that the foetal limbs are moulded by the heart. For it is logical that whatever moulded the heart itself, and before that the arteries and veins, and the liver also with them, should also mould the rest: some people think that this is the seed which has been projected into the womb, others believe that the seed is a (mere) instrument and that what moulds the embryos is something else more divine.

in the *diafragma* come first to the liver, and then it extends to the heart.

And it is bad to say that every part is generated by the heart and that what produces the heart and arteries and liver similarly with them must be before it, just as it creates all other parts. And some say that what does this is seed which is projected into the womb, and some say that seed acts like an instrument and that the moulder of the embryo in the womb is something more noble than seed; and it is more appropriate to say that it is almighty God.

12. I have given my opinion about the compositions, blood, phlegm, yellow bile, in my commentary on Hippocrates' book On the nature of man and in my book On elements according to Hippocrates. I also demonstrated that he believed that these four compositions are generated in all bodies, healthy or unhealthy. Some, however, believe that only blood is similar to nature and appropriate to it and that all other admixtures are produced unnatu-

1 Orig.: χόριον (chorion)

nium aliarum commixtionum extra naturam. et hoc est sententia uerisimilis,
uerum sententia Ypocratis est uerior. et probatio huius procedit ab una
2 sententiarum quas monstraui in alio libro quam in isto libro. et hoc est quod
unaqueque medicinarum laxatiuarum et uomicarum attrahit unam de commix-
tionibus. et quedam earum attrahunt cum commixtione sibi simili aliquid de
aliis duabus commixtionibus uel de una tantum. et quidam uident quod natura
medicine non solum attrahit unum humorum corporis, sed attrahit omnes hu-
mores a uenis equaliter et postea conuertit eos in naturam aut in ipsam. et ego
locutus sum super hiis non bis, sed pluries; et scripsi post hoc unam dictionem
De medicinis purgatiuis et monstraui quod unaqueque istarum medicinarum
purgatiuarum habet uirtutem per quam attrahit aliquem humorem.
3 Et qui uult quod secum consentiam quod medicina purgatiua in hora at-
tractionis humoris alterat illud quod attrahit alteratione debili, non redarguo
ipsum in hoc. sed quod manifestius est, illa alteratio fit debilis propter cole-
ram quam attrahit in ipsa illud quod attrahit inter omnes. et probaui quod
plus magis proprius et magis similis inter omnes humores animalibus habenti-
bus sanguinem sit sanguis solum, et unumquodque genus aliorum animalium
non habentium sanguinem habent humorem similem nature eorum in loco san-
4 guinis. igitur demonstratum est demonstratione manifesta quod unumquemque
humorum existentium intra uenas attrahit natura istarum medicinarum purga-
tiuarum, uerbi gratia, si patienti stillea detur medicina euacuatiua que euacuet
magnam quantitatem aquose humiditatis erit diminutio inflationis secundum
quod euacuatur de ipsa aqua. et si detur patienti iarcan ⟨...⟩, erit diminutio

2sq. una sententiarum] *v.* Hipp. De nat. hom. 5,3: CMG I 1,3, p. 176,10–178,6 3 quas – libro[I]] *v.* Gal. In Hipp. De nat. hom. comm. I 28: CMG V 9,1, p. 38,1–22 De elem. ex Hipp. sent. 13,1–10: CMG V 1,2, p. 148,15–150,19 3–11. 19–98,4] *cf.* Gal. De purg. med. fac. 1–3: XI 324,3–335,18 K. In Hipp. De nat. hom. comm. I 28. 32: CMG V 9,1, p. 38,23–39,18; 42,16–18 De elem. ex Hipp. sent. 13,11–23: CMG V 1,2, p. 150,20–154,10 De atra bile 6,9–12; 8,1–10: CMG V 4,1,1, p. 83,24–84,18; 92,4–93,28 Adv. Iul. 1,11; 8, 1–16: CMG V 10,3, p. 35,22–36,3; 62,16–67,22 De fac. nat. I 13: Scr. min. III 130,10–131, 13 Helmr. = II 40,12–42,2 K. In Hipp. Aphor. comm. IV 2: XVII B 657,16–658,15 K. 15 probaui] *v.* Gal. De elem. ex Hipp. sent. 13,23: CMG V 1,2, p. 154,9sq. De temp. II 3: p. 59,20sq. Helmr. = I 603,7sq. K.

1 *ante* extra *add.* est C: *post* extra *supra lin. add.* sit D[2] E[2] hec ε est *om.* C 2 hius B: hec C: minus O 3 quam – libro[II] *om.* D in[II] *om.* C γ et *om.* C 5 et *om.* C γ quedam – 6 commixtionibus *in textu om., in marg. add.* B eorum γ 7 attrahit[I]] atrahit O: atrahunt C unum *in textu om., in marg. add.* B humorum] humorem ε 8 et[I] *om.* B et[II] *om.* B, *supra lin. add.* B[2] 10 purguatiuis O istarum *om.* ε 12 consensiam O 13 humoris *om.* C illud] id β 14 sed] sit O fit] sit C B 15 ipso ε *ante* inter *addiderim* coleram 15sq. et – omnes *om.* B, *in marg. add.* B[2] 16 magis[I] *om.* ε 18 habentibus C habet ε in *om.* C 18sq. igitur sanguis B: igitur sanguinis O 19 unumquodque C γ 20 humorum *om.* C existentium *om.* ε natura] medicina γ: medicinas C purgatiuarum *om.* E, *supra lin. add.* E[2] 21 si *om.* B squilla O: squinanciam B: squinantiam ε: al-istisqā' *Arabice* que *om.* C euat/ad C 22 mangnam C *ante* erit *add.* et C γ infl\`ationis C 23 datur α: *correxi* iarcan] raicham β: .i. ictericiam *ut interpretamentum supra lin.* D[2] E[2] *lac. indic. Kollesch et Nickel; supple fere* medicina purgatiua colere 23sq. erit – infirmitatis *in textu om., in marg. add.* E: *om.* C γ

rally. And this is a plausible belief, but Hippocrates' view is more truthful. The proof of this starts from one of (his) arguments I put forward in another work than this. This is that each purgative and emetic drug attracts one 2
of these admixtures. And some of them attract, in addition to the admixture that resembles them, something from the two other admixtures or only from one. Some people observe that the nature of the drug not only attracts one bodily humour but attracts all humours alike from the veins and then turns them either into its own nature or into the drug itself. I have spoken about this not twice but several times; and I have written later one treatise On purgatives, and showed that each purgative drug has a property by which it attracts a humour.

As for the man who wants me to agree with him that a purgative at the 3
moment of attracting the humour alters slightly what it attracts, I see no reason to refute him on this point. But what is certainly clearer is that such an alteration is slight because of the bile which of itself is attracted by whatever attracts +bile+[1] among all (the humours). Indeed, I also proved that to sanguineous animals the far more appropriate and similar of all the humours is blood alone, and that every type of non-sanguineous animal has a humour similar to its nature instead of blood. So it has been clearly demonstrated that the na- 4
ture of these purgatives has a particular attraction for one of the humours existing in the veins, e.g. if *a sufferer from stillea* is given a purgative to remove a large amount of watery humour, there will be a lessening of the swelling inasmuch as water is removed therefrom. And if +a purgative drug that removes bile+[2] be given to *a sufferer from iarcan*, the infirmity will become

21 Orig.: e.g. ὁ ὑδεριῶν (sufferer from dropsy)
24 Orig.: e.g. ὁ ἰκτεριῶν (sufferer from jaundice)

1 +bile+: see the app. crit.
2 +a – bile+: see the app. crit.

infirmitatis secundum euacuationem colere citrine; et si contrario modo, per contrarium, ut si detur medicina purgatiua aque patienti iarcan et patienti listilia medicina ⟨...⟩ de humore simili sibi, in magna quantitate cum magna uiolentia, et ⟨in⟩ illa euacuatione iuuamentum est.

5 Et demonstrauit Y p o c r a s in libro De humana natura quod illud quod generatur in corpore existente in infirmitate sua, non solum est sanguis, sed fleuma et colera citrina et colera nigra. et est causa in corpore que ex necessitate generat sanguinem. et merito si diuersificatur cum dictum sit quod solum sanguis approprietur corpori et assimiletur, et sit uerisimile quod si iste sanguis esset similis corpori uel esset fortior humoribus in similitudine, igitur sufficeret nobis euacuare superhabundantiam duarum colerarum et fleumatis et inquirere regimentum conseruans sanitatem non utendo cibariis fleumaticis et generantibus coleram ne superhabundent isti humores in corpore. 6 et non nocet in speculatione operis medicine quod nos debeamus accipere quamcumque duarum rationum uolumus, id est quod nos dicamus quod quatuor humores generantur in corpore secundum prius et sunt in loco quatuor elementorum, et quod omnium aliorum humorum generatio sequitur generationem suam necessario.

ὅτι γὰρ χρὴ τό γε περιττὸν τῶν χολῶν καὶ τοῦ φλέγματος ἐκκρίνεσθαι προνοεῖσθαι κατὰ τὴν ὑγιεινὴν δίαιταν, ὅπως μὴ πλεονάσαντες ἐν φλεγματικοῖς ἢ χολοποιοῖς ἐδέσμασιν αὐξήσωμέν τινα τῶν χυμῶν τούτων, εὔδηλόν ἐστι.
6 τοῦτο οὖν ὁμολογούμενον ἔχοντες οὐδὲν εἰς τὰ τῆς τέχνης ἔργα βλαβησόμεθα κατ' οὐδετέραν δόξαν, ἐάν τε στοιχειώδεις τοὺς τέσσαρας χυμοὺς λέγωμεν ἐάν τε τὸ μὲν αἷμα μόνον ὑπὸ τῆς φύσεως γίνεσθαι κατὰ πρῶτον λόγον, ἕπεσθαι δ' ἐξ ἀνάγκης αὐτοῦ τῇ γενέσει τοὺς ἄλλους τρεῖς χυμούς.

7 Et dico etiam quod si apparet calor in ipsis spleneticis uel sit in ipso splene eruptio uel aliqua alia dispositio mala declinans in corruptionem suam,

5 Ypocras – natura] Hipp. De nat. hom. 4: CMG I 1,3, p. 172,13–174,10 8–10 similitudine] *cf.* Gal. In Hipp. De nat. hom. comm. I 31: CMG V 9,1, p. 41,26–29 De temp. II 3: p. 59,20sq. Helmr. = I 603,7sq. K. 8 cum – sit] *cf. supra,* p. 94,22–96,1 18 τοῦτο – 26] *cf.* Gal. De elem. ex Hipp. sent. 11,1–3: CMG V 1,2, p. 140,15–142,1

2 ut *om.* C γ aqua C γ iarcha B: raicham O: artheticam ε lintissia γ: leutissimam ε: .i. yposarcam *ut interpretamentum supra lin.* D^2 E^2 *(cf. supra, p. 96,21)* 3 *lac. indic. Kollesch et Nickel* humore] hisore B: hysore O: ysore ε: .i. busbo *ut interpretamentum in marg.* E^2: .i. ... ouo .. a *ut interpretamentum supra lin.* D^2, *sed litterae paene deletae* 4 et – euacuatione] et euacuatione illa γ: et illa euõe C: euomere illa ε: *corr. Kollesch et Nickel* est *om.* C O B, *supra lin. add.* B^2: *fort. post* euacuatione *addendum est* non est 5 illud] id B ε 6 in^{II} *om.* C γ non] sed O solus E set O 7 $colera^{II}$ *om.* C causa *om.* β que] quod B ε 8 medico β si *om.* ε 9 solus ε approprietur *om.* E, *supra lin. add.* E^2 fit ε quod] quia C O 11 superhabundantiam – 13 inquirere *om.* B, *in marg. add.* B^2 12 duorum B colerum O E: $coler^{m}$ C: co. B 13 et^{II} *om.* γ regim̄ C 15 fl`aticis C: fl`is B: $fl`ati^{c}$ O 17 nocet *scripsi*: decet C γ E: dicet D 19 debemus D quamque B D 20 duorum canonum C 24sq. et – humorum] scilicet omnes alii (-os C) tres humores C γ 26 suam] sanguinis ε 27 etiam *om.* B ε color C in ipsis *om.* C illis O: alīs (= aliquibus) B 28 eruptatio γ: erutuatio C declinas C corruptione sua C γ

less in proportion to the evacuation of yellow bile; and if the opposite is done, the result will be the opposite, just as if a hydragogue were given to *a sufferer from iarcan* and *a sufferer from listilia* were given a drug ... of a humour like itself in large quantity and with great violence, and there is benefit in that evacuation.

Hippocrates in his tract On the nature of man showed that during illness not only blood is produced within the body but (also) phlegm and yellow and black bile. And a cause exists in the body that necessarily produces blood. And rightly so, if (blood) is particularly special, since it is stated that only blood is appropriate and assimilated to the body, and that it is probable that if blood alone were like the body or were far more like the body than the (other) humours, 5

Clearly we should have to seek to remove the excess of the biles and of phlegm in accordance with a healthy regimen, in order to prevent an increase in any of these humours by using an excess of phlegm- or bile-producing foods. If we are agreed on this, we shall 6 suffer no disaster in our medical practice for either opinion, whether we declare that the four humours are elemental or that only blood is produced naturally in the first place, and that the other three humours are necessarily consequent on its production.

it would then suffice for us to remove the superabundance of the two biles and phlegm and look for a regimen that preserves health by not using phlegmatic foods and those that produce bile, lest these humours abound to excess in the body. And 6 there is no harm in speculation on the practice of medicine that we should accept whichever of the two arguments we want, i.e. that we say that the four humours are produced primarily in the body and take the place of the four elements, and that the production of all other humours follows of necessity on its production.

I also declare that when heat affects sufferers from the spleen or there 7 is some eruption in the spleen itself or some other unhealthy condition that

2–3 Orig.: e.g. ὁ ἰκτεριῶν (sufferer from jaundice)
3 Orig.: e.g. ὁ ὑδεριῶν (sufferer from dropsy)

non nocet in opere medicine quod dicamus quod attrahat humorem nigrum,
sed non dicimus quod sit generatus in ipso. et hoc est quod demonstraui in li-
bro meo De colera nigra, quod oportet manifestare uerum de duobus dictis
cum manifestum sit. et demonstraui etiam in hoc libro omnem rem quam opor-
8 tet querere necessario de ista colera. ⟨...⟩ sed quod peius est quod hunc debe-
at inquirere reprobationem sillogismi probatione et dimittit reprobare propo-
sitiones sillogismi ex quibus contexitur sillogismus. et quidam sunt qui num-
quam prouident in hoc, et si prouident, numquam prouident nisi raro, et in
hoc nolunt continuare studium. et multi etiam sunt qui desiderant intelligere
sillogismum, et maxime quoniam reperiuntur in eo aliqua conuenientia in ho-
mine, sicut in significatione humoris melancholici – quia de sanguine intelli-
guntur duo, non sicut intelligitur de significatione colere nigre una res –, item
quia humor generatur in epate antequam fiat colera nigra. sed possibile est
quod fiet si diu permanet in uenis aut superat in corpore animalium mala
9 complexio calida et sicca. et colera nigra nominatur secundum quod nomina-
tur colera nigra humor niger; et erit illud quod significa[n]t hec [dicitur] no-
minatio, hoc est humor niger, conturbatio sanguinis [ypostasma] que est sicut
fex in uino et in oleo. et istud etiam denominatur humor niger, eo quod natura
sua est ut conuertatur in purum nigrum modica occasione. et secundum istam
significationem dicimus de aliquibus potibus quod sint fleumatici et de aliqui-
bus quod sint melancolici.
10 Et demonstraui in libro meo De uirtutibus naturalibus et in alio meo li-
bro De medicinis purgantibus quod uene que tribuunt cibum per totum corpus

2sq. in^{II} – nigra] *v.* Gal. De atra bile: CMG V 4,1,1, p. 71–93 15–18] *cf.* Gal. De atra bile 3,5sq.; 6,6: CMG V 4,1,1, p. 75,6–16; 83,13sq. De purg. med. fac. 3: XI 335,16–18 K. In Hipp. Progn. comm. III 32: CMG V 9,2, p. 356,4–7 Meth. med. XIV 9: X 973, 12–14; 974,14–975,6 K. In Hipp. Epid. VI comm. VI: CMG V 10,2,2, p. 384,34–38
22sq. in^{I} – purgantibus] *cf.* Gal. De fac. nat. II 9: Scr. min. III 200,6–9 Helmr. = II 136,11–15 K. De purg. med. fac. 1: XI 326,3–7 K.

1 medicine *om.* ε atrahat C: *correxi*: attrahit B: atrahit O: contrahit ε 2 *ante* sed *supra lin. add.* et B^2 non *om.* C γ *fort.* dicamus *scribendum est* 3 uerum] unum C 4 etiam *om.* O quam] suam C γ 5 inquirere *in textu,* aliter querere *in marg.* O ipsa D *lac. indicavi (v. infra, p. 189sq., comm. ad loc.)* 6 sill'i C: sil'i γ: simili ε probationi ε: probationis C γ: *correxi* dimittit quia B ε: dimititque O: dittet in C: *correxi* probare B propositiones] probationes C B 7 sillogismi] sill'i C: sil'i γ: illius ε contentetur B: continetur O: continue ε 8 in hoc] in hos O: in os C: mos B numquam prouident *om.* C raro] ratio O: *om.* C B 9 hoc] hos O: l/os C: mos B etiam *om.* ε *ante* intelligere *add.* quod C 10 reperientur γ nomine ε 12 non] nam O intellingitur C item] roȝ (= rationem) C 13 generatus C γ fiat *om.* B, *supra lin. add.* B^2 14 *fort.* fiat *scribendum est* aut] u^t C 15 et^I *om.* C γ sic B et^{II} *om.* C γ nigra] rubee C: *om.* B nominatur^I – 16 colera *in textu om., in marg. add.* B *ante* secundum *add.* et C γ 16 colera *bis scr.* C et – 17 niger *om.* β significant C: *correxi* dicitur *seclusi* 17 a^d turbatio C B: aliud turbatio O *post* sanguinis *add.* et fex C ypostasma *secl. Kollesch et Nickel, nisi alia exciderunt* que] quod C 18 et^I *om.* O B, *supra lin. add.* B^2 etiam *om.* β 19 uomica actione C 20 de^I *om.* C sint – 21 quod *om.* B sunt O fl'atici C: fl'ici O et *om.* B, *supra lin. add.* B^2 22 et *om.* B, *supra lin. add.* B^2 aliquo C

leads to its corruption, our practice of medicine is not affected if we say that
it attracts the black humour but not that it is being produced there. This is
what I showed in my work On black bile, because one should make clear
which of two statements is true when it becomes clear. I also showed in this
book all that is necessary to look for in connection with that bile. ... What is 8
worse is that this man should look for the refutation of a syllogism by a proof
and yet refuses to refute the premisses of the syllogism from which the syllo-
gism is constructed. Some men never bother themselves with this, or if they
do so, do so only rarely, and they do not wish to prolong their study to its
end. But there are also many who want to understand a syllogism, especially
since there are found some things relating to man, as in the term "melancholic
humour" – for there are two possible meanings of "blood", but only one
meaning of "black bile" is readily understood –, and also the fact that the hu-
mour is produced in the liver before becoming black bile. But it is possible
that it would become so if it were to remain for a long time in the veins or if
an unhealthy hot and dry mixture were to predominate in the bodies of living
beings. It is called black bile inasmuch as black bile is called a black humour; 9
and what this name signifies, i.e. black humour, is going to be a disturbance in
the blood like the dregs of wine and oil. This is also called a black humour,
because it can be naturally and very easily be turned into pure blackness. It is
in this sense of the word that we say that some drinks promote phlegm, and
others black bile.

I have shown in my book On the natural faculties and in another book of 10
mine, On purgatives, that the veins which distribute food throughout the body

⟨...⟩ in illis currit colera nigra et aliquando sanguis. ergo festinauit in iudicio dicens quod impossibile est quod uena que extenditur usque ad splenem attrahat de uena que est in epate, que uocatur portanaria, sanguinem nigrum, et nutriatur inde splen. sed et fortasse oppinaberis quod non sit impossibile quod unumquodque medicamentum purgatiuum attrahat humorem sibi similem, et non sit possibile secundum unamquamque uenarum que nutriuntur ex ipso; et certe res ita non se habet. sed et fortasse oppinaris quod humor similis omnibus membris sit unus humor, et quod ille est sanguis, sicut oppinati fuerunt antequam ratiocinati fuerunt quod multa animalia ⟨sint⟩ sine sanguine et quod de animalibus que sunt sine sanguine [quod] nutrimentum eorum sit ex humore simili qui est proportionatus sanguini; uerumptamen habeant caliditatem naturalem in loco caliditatis innate que est in epate et in unoquoque membro corporis.

13. Sed propter hoc dico de corde quod est loco illius quod accendit caliditatem que est in corporibus animalium. et in plantis est aliud genus caliditatis in quo communicat corpus nostrum et secundum hunc modum communicant cum eo in uirtute que nominatur naturalis. et secundum hoc tu potes nominare uirtutem que est in epate uirtutem naturalem, et potes eam nominare
2 animam sicut nominauerunt eam Plato et Aristotiles. sed dico quod epar est principium caloris naturalis et est in animalibus loco rei similis radici plantarum, et quod calor qui portatur a corde in totum corpus et dat sensum [sentis corpus] calidum tactu [qui] est alter a calore isto; et accidit a paucitate

1–4] *cf.* Gal. De usu part. IV 4. 15: I 198,19–199,9; 232,14–233,13 Helmr. = III 271, 7–272,3; 316,13–318,1 K. De atra bile 7,21: CMG V 4,1,1, p. 89,9–18 De fac. nat. II 9: Scr. min. III 201,13–22 Helmr. = II 138,7–15 K. 14sq.] *cf. supra*, p. 62,1sq. Gal. De usu part. VI 7: I 318,15–19 Helmr. = III 436,3–7 K. Meth. med. IX 10: X 635,15–18 K. 15–19] *cf.* Gal. De plac. Hipp. et Plat. VI 3,7: CMG V 4,1,2, p. 374,9–17 In Hipp. Epid. III comm. I 17: CMG V 10,2,1, p. 46,10–15 In Hipp. Epid. VI comm. I 3; V 5: CMG V 10,2,2, p. 18,12sq.; 272,25–273,19 19 Plato et Aristotiles] *cf. supra*, p. 62,12–14 Gal. De foet. form. 3: IV 665,10–15 K. De usu part. IV 13: I 226,18–21 Helmr. = III 308,17–309,3 K. 19–20 naturalis] *cf.* Gal. In Hipp. Epid. VI comm. V 5: CMG V 10,2,2, p. 274,3–7 20sq. et – plantarum] *cf.* Gal. De plac. Hipp. et Plat. VI 3,39sq.; 5,20: CMG V 4,1,2, p. 382,17–23; 392,1–5

1 *lac. indic. Kollesch et Nickel* festinaui C 3 ue/uena B uocatur *om.* γ: est ε B^{2} *(supra lin.)* portonaria C: portat O 4 inde] in C O 5 attrahit B ε: atrahat O 6 secundum] sed sunt γ: sed sibi C unaqueque C γ 7 se non E non *om.* D 8 membris *om.* B unius O 8sq. antequam – fuerunt *om.* D 9 fuerint γ E animalia] alia γ: a^{a} (= alia) C sint *add. Kollesch et Nickel* 9sq. et – sanguine *om.* ε 10 quod *seclusi* 11 similiter B qui] quod C γ proportionatum C *post* sanguini *iter.* est B habeat β 12 in^{III} *om.* β 14 *ante* Sed *add.* Capitulum tredecimum quod cor est fons caloris animalium; et de comparatione dicti caloris ad calorem naturalem inuentum in plantis et nobis. et de diuersitate platonis super animam, scilicet quibus communicatur corporibus, et de differentia inter animalia et plantas. ε *post* Sed *add.* et C quod^{I} *om.* C γ *ante* loco *add.* in ε quod^{II}] qui β 15 que – animalium *om.* D 16 communicant] communicat C ε 18 *ante* potes *add.* tu O 19 nominauit ε Plato et *om.* ε, Plato *om.* γ quod] etiam B 20 locis res γ 22 sentis corpus *seclusi* setis C: sentit ε B^{2} *(supra lin.)* tactu] motu β qui *seclusi* est *om.* C altum C

... in them there runs black bile and occasionally blood. And so he was hasty in his explanation, saying that it is impossible that the vein extending to the spleen attracts black blood from the vein in the liver which is called the portal vein, and that the spleen receives its nutriment from there. But perhaps you may also think that it is not impossible that each purgative drug should attract a humour similar to itself, but that this is impossible for each of the veins that are nourished by it; certainly this is not so. But perhaps you also think that the humour which resembles all parts of the body is a single humour and that this is blood, as men thought before they considered that many animals lack blood and that in these bloodless animals their nutriment comes from a similar humour that corresponds to blood; but they may have a natural heat in place of the innate heat which is in the liver and in every part of the body.

13. For this reason my opinion on the heart is that it is the thing which produces heat in the bodies of animals. In plants there is another sort of heat, in which our body shares, and in this way (plants) share with us in (the possession of) a so-called natural faculty. On this basis you can call the faculty present in the liver a natural faculty and you can also follow Plato and Aristotle in referring to it as "soul". But I say that the liver is the source 2
of natural heat and is in animals that thing which is similar to the root in plants, and that the heat which is carried from the heart throughout the body and gives a feeling of heat to the touch is different from the natural heat: it

caloris naturalis quod non percipiatur sensu. et propter hoc idem dicimus in plantis in comparatione ad corpora animalium quod ibi non sit caliditas.

IV 757 K. 3 Καί τις ἴσως δόξει διαφωνίαν ἀξιόλογον εἶναι ἡμῶν λεγόντων θερμὰ μὲν εἶναι τὰ ζῷα, ψυχρὰ δὲ τὰ φυτὰ μὴ γινώσκων, ὡς, ὅταν μὲν ἀκριβέστερόν τις ἐπεξέρχηται πᾶν τὸ ἀκόλουθον ζητῶν, ἄχρι ⟨τῆς βεβαίας γνώσεως ἥκειν χρή⟩, ὅταν δὲ περί τινος ἄλλου πράγματος σκοπούμενος ἐν παρέργῳ περὶ τούτων ἀποφαίνηται, τὸ πρὸς τὴν πρόχειρον αἴσθησιν θερμὸν ἢ ψυχρὸν λέγων ἀρκεῖται.

3 Et propter hoc oppinatur quod sit diuersitas inter antiquos medicos et philosophos cum dixerunt quod animal sit calidum et planta sit frigida. et nescit quod debet inquirere res quousque deueniat ad firmam notitiam ipsarum; et cum inquisierit aliqua de hiis et uoluerit iudicare de hiis, sufficiet dicere calidum et frigidum secundum sensum manifestum et hoc sufficit ei.

4 Πλάτων γοῦν αὐτὸς ἔμψυχα μὲν ἀεὶ λέγει τὰ ζῷα, τοὺς
758 λίθους δὲ καὶ τὰς πόας καὶ | τὰ ξύλα καὶ καθόλου φάναι τὰ φυτὰ πάντα τῶν ἀψύχων σωμάτων εἶναί φησιν. ἀλλ' ὅταν ἐν Τιμαίῳ τὴν φυσικὴν θεωρίαν ὀλιγίστοις ἀκροαταῖς κατακολουθεῖν ἐπιστημονικοῖς λόγοις δυναμένοις ἀποχωρίσας τῶν τοῖς πολλοῖς δοκούντων εἰς ὅλον τὸν κόσμον ἐκτετάσθαι λέγῃ τὴν ψυχὴν αὐτοῦ, διαφωνίαν οὐ χρὴ

4 Et hoc est quod inuenies Platonem dicentem in omni loco de animalibus quod sint animata, et dicit de lapidibus et lignis et omnibus plantis quod sint corpora non habentia animam. uerumptamen cum in libro suo Thimeo de scientia naturali ad opus aliquorum qui sunt potentes ad intelligendum uera dicta dissentiebat in illis in quibus multi conueniebant, et dixit quod anima mundi expansa est per totum mundum, [et] non est iustum quod dicatur quod sermo-

15 Πλάτων – 20] *cf.* Gal. In Plat. Tim. comm. III 2: CMG Suppl. I, p. 11,11sq. 20–27 αὐτοῦ] *cf.* Plat. Tim. 34 b; 36 e; 41 d; 43 a Galens Kommentar zu Platons Timaios, fr. 21: p. 140,1–4 Larrain Gal. Compend. Tim. Plat. 4 a/b: p. 42–44 Kraus-Walzer De foet. form. 6: IV 700,17sq. K. 27 διαφωνίαν – 106,6 ἑταίροις] Theophr., fr. 42 Fortenbaugh 27sq. διαφωνίαν – εἶναι] *cf.* Gal. De foet. form. 6: IV 699,15–700,2 K.

3 διαφωνίας *edd.* 4 ἡμῶν] τῶν A: *corr. Kollesch et Nickel* 7 ἀκριβέστερόν τις] ἀκριβ... ις A *spatio 6 litt. rel.: in marg. suppl.* A^2 8 *post* ἀκόλουθον *Gallicus quidam in exemplari editionis Basileensis nunc Cantabrigiae conservato* λέγει *vel* λέγῃ *deesse putat* ζητούμενον A: *corr. Nickel* 8sq. ἄχρι ... ὅταν A *spatio 20 fere litt. rel.*: τῆς βεβαίας γνώσεως ἥκειν χρή *sec. versionem Latinam addidi*: τῆς ἐσχάτης ἐπιστήμης *add. edd., post* ἐπιστήμης *deesse e. g.* ἐπεξέρχεται *suspic. in adn. Goulst.* 13 θερμὸν ἢ ψυχρὸν] θε... ρὸν A: *in marg. suppl.* A^2 18 καθόλου φάναι *deleverit Goulst.*^{Bas} 24 ἀποχωρήσας A: *corr. Nickel* 26 λέγει A: *corr. Kühn*

1 percipietur C: percipitur B: participatur ε propter *om.* ε idem *om.* C 2 corpus C 5 dix̄ C: dixit O: dicit B 7 sit *om.* C 8 deueniant C 9 ipsorum β 10 inquisieris C 15 quod *in marg. add.* B^2 inueniens C 16 in omni loco *post* animalibus *(lin. 17) trsp.* C de *om.* C 18 *ante* omnibus *add.* de β 19 sunt D 20 ca^m 7^m *in marg. add.* B^4 cum *om.* ε 21 *post* suo *add.* de ε thymeo C: timeo B: tymeo O 23 dicentiebat C 26 mundum *om.* C γ et *secl. Kollesch et Nickel*

derives from a deficiency of natural heat that it is imperceptible to the senses. That is why we say that in plants there is no heat by comparison with the bodies of animals.

3 Possibly someone will believe that there is a significant disagreement when we say that animals are warm and plants cold, not realising that when one attacks (a problem) with greater precision, investigating all its consequences, one must reach a firm understanding; on the other hand, if one is investigating some other problem and commenting on this in passing, it is enough to say that a thing is hot or cold as far as the immediate sensation is concerned.

4 Plato himself always describes animals as endowed with a soul, and considers that stones, grasses, pieces of wood, and, generally speaking, plants are all bodies without souls. Yet when in the Timaeus to suit a very small audience who can follow his scientific arguments he separates his theory of nature from the common opinion and states that the world soul stretches throughout the whole world, one should not consider this to be a contradiction on the part of a

3 And for this reason one thinks that there is a divergence between ancient doctors and philosophers when they said that an animal is warm and a plant cold. And one does not know that one should investigate things until one has reached a firm understanding of them; and when one has investigated some of them and wishes to pronounce on them, it will be enough to talk of hot and cold in accordance with manifest sensation, and this is enough for him.

4 And this is because you will find Plato always saying about animals that they are animate, and he says about stones and pieces of wood and all plants that they are bodies not having a soul. But when in his book Timaeus on natural science for the use of some who are capable of understanding the truth when it is uttered he dissented in matters on which most people agreed, and said that the soul of the world is spread through all the world, it is not fair to say that his words are inconsistent one with another and that he gives each statement a

τοῦτο νομίζειν εἶναι τἀνδρὸς ἑαυτῷ τἀναντία λέγοντος, ὥσπερ οὐδ' Ἀριστοτέλους ἢ Θεοφράστου, τὰ μὲν τοῖς πολλοῖς γεγραφότων, τὰς δὲ ἀκροάσεις τοῖς ἑταίροις. ὅταν γάρ τι τῶν ἐκφευγόντων ἅπασαν αἴσθησιν δόγμα πολλῶν λόγων δεόμενον εἰς ἀπόδειξιν ἀκαίρως λέγηται, προσκρούει τοῖς
5 ἀκούουσιν. οὔκουν χρὴ περὶ τῶν τοιούτων ἀποφαίνεσθαι πρὶν τοῦ κατὰ βραχὺ διὰ μακρᾶς ἀποδείξεως ἐπὶ τὸ συμπέρασμα τοῦ λόγου παντὸς ἀφικέσθαι, οὐδὲ διὰ τῶν λίθων καὶ τῶν ὀστράκων καὶ τῆς ψάμμου καὶ τῶν κατακαιομένων ἢ σηπομένων νεκρῶν ζῴων τὴν τοῦ κόσμου διήκειν ψυχήν. εἰ γὰρ ἁπλῶς οὕτως ἀναφανδὸν ἀκουόντων τῶν πολλῶν ὁ Πλάτων εἶπέ τι τοιοῦτον, κατεγίνωσκον ἂν οἱ παρ-
759 6 όντες αὐτοῦ πάντες. | ἐγὼ δ' οὖν, ἀφ' ὧν μὲν κινούμενος ἐπὶ τὴν δόξαν ταύτην ἀφίκετο, δι' ἑτέρων ὑπομνημάτων ἐδήλωσα μὴ συναποφηνάμενος αὐτῷ ἢ διατεινόμενος – οὐδὲ γὰρ αὐτὸς ἐκεῖνος

nes sui non conueniunt adinuicem et quod unumquodque dicat contrarium secundum quod sermones Aristotilis et Theopha contradicunt eis adinuicem qui composuerunt libros ad opus multorum in aliquibus rebus et libros ad opus discipulorum suorum. eo quod sententie que exeunt extra diffinitionem illius rei que percipitur sensibus indigent in eis multis sermonibus ad earum probationem, et si nar⟨r⟩atur in aliis locis quam in propriis, nar⟨r⟩atio eorum arguat au-
5 dientes. igitur non conuenit quod iudicetur in similibus sine probatione paulatiua quousque colligitur inde sillogismus totius sermonis, et non debet dici quod anima mundi sit in lapidibus et in testis et in arenis et in cadaueribus combustis uel putrefactis. et hoc est quod si Plato dixisset hunc sermonem, admirarentur omnes
6 et dicerent quod esset insanus. sed ego demonstraui in aliis libris quid coegit Platonem dicere hunc sermonem, et non quod ego iudicarem cum eodem in hiis in quibus iudicauit. et non sum ausus dicere super hoc iudicium, quia Plato non ponit

3sq. Ἀριστοτέλους ἢ Θεοφράστου] Theophr., fr. 37; 498 Fortenbaugh 16 οὐδὲ – 20] *cf.* Gal. De foet. form. 6: IV 700,18–701,6 K. 26sq. δι' – ἐδήλωσα] *cf. supra,* p. 62,3–17 29 οὐδὲ – 108,4 φησιν] *cf.* Plat. Tim. 29 c–d; 72 d Gal. De plac. Hipp. et Plat. IX 9,3–7. 12: CMG V 4,1,2, p. 598,7–28; 600,21–25

15 τοῦ *bis scr. et primum del.* A

2 unumquodque – 3 quod *om.* ε contrarium] arteriam C γ: *corr. Kollesch et Nickel* 3 Aristotiles α: *correxi* 4 Theopha] thempha O: tempha B: sententie ε contradicant C ei γ: eĩ C 5 inuicem β qui] tamen C 6 quibus C: aliquos β: *correxi* 8 eo quod] et C 9 rei *om.* C recipitur C 10 sensibus] sorisibus C: *correxi*: cum fortibus β indiget C γ D 11 eorum α: *correxi* 12 et – 15 probatione *om.* β naratur C quam] quod C: *correxi* 13 naratio C 16 paulatiuam β collegitur C: *correxi*: confirmetur ε: consil'r γ 17 *post* sermonis *add.* ad eorum probationem *(cf. lin. 11)* B 19 testis] intestinis B harenis B in^{III} *om.* C B 20 adustis B uel] et B 21 *ante* quod *supra lin. add.* uerum D^2 E^2 *ante* Plato *add. et del.* co. B 22 admirentur B, *corr.* B^2 23 dicent E 24 libris *om.* β 24sq. quod cohegit O 25 coegit – 27 hiis *(verba* dicere – 26 non *omissis) bis scr.* B 26 et *om.* ε quod] quam B 27 iudicaui C γ 29 hunc β ponit] po^t C: posuit ε

man who is uttering inconsistencies, nor on the part of Aristotle and Theophrastus when they wrote some things for general circulation as well as lectures for their pupils. For the listeners are greatly struck when a theory that goes beyond universal perception and requires a great deal of argument for its proof is expounded inopportunely. So one must not pronounce 5
about such matters without first progressing gradually through a long demonstration to the conclusion of the whole argument, nor that the world soul stretches through stones and pots and sand and bodies of dead animals that are being burnt or rotting away. Now if Plato had said something like this bluntly and so openly to a general audience, all those who were there would have censured him. However, I 6
have shown in other writings how he was moved to reach this belief, neither supporting him nor pressing the point – for he

contrary, just as the comments of Aristotle and *Theopha* are inconsistent one with another when they wrote books on some topics for the use of many people and books for the use of their students. The reason is that those opinions which go beyond the definition of that which is perceived need in them many arguments for their proof, and if it is reported in other than appropriate places, their reporting points at the listeners. Thus 5
it is not fitting for a pronouncement to be made in such matters without a gradual demonstration until the syllogism of the whole argument is put together, and it ought not to be said that the soul of the world exists in stones, and in pots and in sand and in burnt or putrefied corpses. And this is because if Plato had made this speech, all would be astounded and say that he was insane. But I have shown in 6
other books what made Plato make this speech, and not that I would agree with him in these matters on which he pronounced. And I did not dare to pronounce on this judgment because Plato does not put down as

2 Orig.: Θεοφράστου (Theophrastus)

οὕτως ἀποφαίνεται τὰ τῆς φυσικῆς θεωρίας, ἀλλ' ἄχρι τοῦ πιθανοῦ καὶ εἰκότος αὐτὴν προέρχεσθαί φησιν –, ὅτι μέντοι τὰ φυτὰ κινήσεως ἀρχὴν ἐν αὑτοῖς ἔχει καὶ τὴν τῶν οἰκείων τε καὶ ἀλλοτρίων αἴσθησιν, ἀληθὲς εἶναι νομίζω, λέγειν δὲ ἀκαίρως τὰ τοιαῦτα φυλάττομαι μᾶλλον ἢ αὐτὸς ἐκεῖνος.

7 Ἀλλ' ἐὰν ἔρηταί μέ τις, τί πλεονεκτεῖ τῶν φυτῶν τὰ ζῷα, τήν τε αἴσθησιν λέγω καὶ τὴν καθ' ὁρμὴν κίνησιν, καὶ τὰς [τε] δυνάμεις, ἃς εἶπον ἄρτι, τήν τε ἑλκτικὴν καὶ τὴν ἀποκριτικὴν καὶ τὴν καθεκτικήν τε καὶ ἀλλοιωτικήν, οὐ ψυχικάς, ἀλλὰ φυσικὰς ὀνομάζω[ν] μηδὲν ἐκ τούτου μήτε τὴν ἰατρικὴν τέχνην μήτε τὴν ἠθικὴν φιλοσοφίαν βλαπτομένην ὁρῶν. ὅταν δὲ τῆς ἠθικῆς φιλοσοφίας τὸ φυσικὸν μέρος, ὁποῖόν τι Πλάτων ἡγεῖται, λέγειν ἀναγκαῖόν μοι γένηται, τινὰ μὲν ἄντικρυς ἐπαινῶ καὶ συναποφαίνομαι τἀνδρί· περὶ τι-
760 νῶν δὲ ἄχρι τοῦ πιθανοῦ προέρ|χομαι, καθάπερ ἐπ' ἐνίων ἀπορῶ[ν]

iudicium suum hoc quod dicit de scientia naturali. immo dicit quod finis istius scientie ducit hominem ad sufficientiam. et quod dictum est quod in plantis sit principium motus et sensus in hiis que assimilantur et sunt contraria eis, uidetur michi quod sit uerum. sed ego timeo hec narrare non in proprio suo loco plus quam timuit Plato.

7 Sed si fuero interrogatus quid sit illud in quo differant animalia plantis, dicam quod est motus uoluntarius; et nominabo uirtutem quam paulo ante narraui, scilicet uirtutem appetitiuam, expulsiuam, retentiuam et digestiuam, uirtutem †tristiuam†, non animalem, et ego non uideo quod hoc noceat arti medicine et parti philosophie moralis. et cum erit michi necessarium quod narrem sententiam Platonis in parte naturali philosophie, ego laudabo partem dicti sui et iudicabo secum prout ipse iudicauit; et dicam quod in parte est sufficiens

4 ὅτι – 7 νομίζω] *cf. supra*, p. 62,3sq. Gal. In Plat. Tim. comm. III 2: CMG Suppl. I, p. 11,9–20 De fac. nat. I 1: Scr. min. III 101,1–15 Helmr. = II 1,3–2,5 K. 11 Ἀλλ' – 21] *cf.* Gal. De plac. Hipp. et Plat. IX 9,9: CMG V 4,1,2, p. 600,10–19 In Plat. Tim. comm. III 2: CMG Suppl. I, p. 12,18–21

2 ἀλλὰ χρὴ A: *corr. Ald.* 5 αὐτοῖς A: *corr. Kühn* 11 ἔρηταί – πλεονεκτεῖ *in marg. rescr.* A^2 13 τὴν καθ' ὁρμὴν *in marg. rescr.* A^2 14 τε *incertum esse putat Schröder, in: CMG Suppl. I, p. 41 comm. ad p. 11,14sq.: seclusi* 18 ὀνομάζων A: *correxi* μηδὲν – τούτου *in marg. rescr.* A^2 20 βλαπτομένην *in marg. rescr.* A^2 22 τὸ – ὁποῖον *in marg. rescr.* A^2 24 τινὰ – ἄντικρυς *in marg. rescr.* A^2 27 ἀπορῶν A: *corr. Ald.*

2 immo dixit B: y^o dicit C: ymmo dicit D: ymo dicit E: i modicit O 3 ficientiam D 4 $quod^{II}$ *om.* O 5 fit γ initium β motus *supra lin. add.* E^2 5sq. sensus et motus γ 6 in *om.* B 7 *post* eis *add.* sed ε 8 *post* sed *add.* quod γ hic ε: hoc O narare C 9 non] si γ 11 set O 12 quid] quod γ est C γ, *fort. recte* frigidant B: fr`ant C 12sq. animalia differant ε 13 *ante* plantis *add.* a ε 14 uolomptarius C 15 naraui C: nominaui D 16 scilicet *scripsi*: sicut ε: sic C γ 18 tristiuam β: cresciteuam C: *cruces posui* 19 uideor B: uidear O 21 philophie E: phĩe B D: $phy^e$ C 22 nararem C 23 sciam (= scientiam) C 24 $phy^e$ nat` C naturalis D laudo C 25 et *om.* B, *supra lin. add.* B^2 26 dicam *e* dixi *corr.* E

himself is not declaring in this way the details of physical theory, but, as he says, he is merely proceeding to a plausible and probable conclusion –, but I think that it is true that plants have a source of motion within them and some sense of what is suitable and unsuitable for them, but I am even more careful than he not to relate this inopportunely.

But if I am asked why animals are superior to plants, I say that it is in their possession of sensation and voluntary motion and I call the faculties I mentioned earlier, the attractive, the expulsive, the retentive and the transformative, natural, not psychical, being well aware that neither medical art nor moral philosophy is ruined by this statement. But whenever I have to describe Plato's view of the natural part of moral philosophy, I praise some (of his doctrines) outright and agree with him; but there are others that I accept only as plausible, just as I refuse to make up my mind at all on some oth- 7

his judgment what he says here about natural science. No, rather he says that the end of that knowledge leads man to plausibility. And what is said that in plants there is a source of motion and sense about these things that are like them and are contrary to them, seems to me that it is true. But I am afraid to talk of these things not in their proper place more than Plato was.

But if I am asked in what animals differ from plants, I will say that it is voluntary motion, and I will call the faculty I mentioned a little earlier, to wit, the appetitive faculty, the expulsive, the retentive and the digestive, a ... faculty, not psychical, and I do not see that it harms the art of medicine and the part of moral philosophy. And when it is necessary for me to report the opinion of Plato in the natural part of philosophy, I will praise part of his comment and pronounce with him as he himself pronounced; and I will say that in part it is plausible and 7

18 ...] Orig.: φυσικὰς (natural)

παντάπασιν οὐδεμίαν ἔχων ῥοπὴν ἐπὶ τῶν διαφωνουμένων, ὡς εἴη τὸ ἕτερον αὐτῶν πιθανώτερον.

14. ⟨...⟩ ὥσπερ ὅτι ψυχὴν ἔχομεν, ἐπίστανται πάντες οἱ ἄνθρωποι θεώμενοι μὲν ἐναργῶς τὰ διὰ τοῦ σώματος ἐνεργούμενα βαδιζόντων καὶ τρεχόντων καὶ παλαιόντων αἰσθανομένων τε πολυειδῶς, ἐννοοῦντες δὲ καὶ τῶν ἔργων τούτων αἰτίας τινὰς ὑπάρχειν ἔκ τινος ἀξιώματος πιστοῦ φύσει πᾶσιν ἡμῖν, καθ' ὃ μηδὲν ἀναιτίως γίνεσθαι νοοῦμεν, ἀλλὰ καὶ διὰ τὸ μὴ γινώσκειν, ἥτις ἐστὶν ἡ αἰτία τῶν ἔργων τούτων, ὄνομα θέμενοι ἀπὸ τοῦ δύνασθαι ποιεῖν, ἃ ποιεῖ, δύναμιν [εἶναι] τῶν γινομένων ἑκάστου ποιητικήν. οὕτω γοῦν καὶ τὴν σκαμμωνίαν ἅπαντές φασι δύναμιν ἔχειν καθαρτικήν, ὥσπερ τὸ μέ-
2 σπιλον ἐφεκτικὴν γαστρός. οἱ δὲ τὴν φυσικὴν ὀνομαζομένην

et in hiis in quibus cadit diuersitas est magis sufficiens.

14. De substantia autem uirtutum sentio prout alii senserunt scilicet quod habeant animam, eo quod uident manifeste operationes quas operatur corpus in dispositione eundi et redeundi et in dispositione surgendi et luctandi et in sensu nostro diuersarum rerum. ergo sentiunt quod in istis operationibus sint certe occasiones et nichil de hiis accidit sine occasione. uerumptamen nesciunt occasionem operatiuam istarum operationum et nominauerunt secundum quod dicunt quod homo est potens ad faciendum, hoc est quod in ipso est potentia unaqueque actiua istarum operationum. et tu inuenies omnes dicentes quod in scamonea sit potentia laxatiua et in zarolis
2 sit potentia constipatiua. sed illos qui sunt exercitati in scientia naturali inuenio diuersos, et unusquisque dicit secundum mensuram sue potentie: qui-

4–9 παλαιόντων] *cf.* Gal. De plac. Hipp. et Plat. VIII 1,1sq.: CMG V 4,1,2, p. 480,7–13   10 ἐννοοῦντες – 20 ποιητικήν] *cf.* Gal. De fac. nat. I 4: Scr. min. III 107,14–20 Helmr. = II 9,13–10,1 K.   21 τὴν σκαμμωνίαν – 23 καθαρτικήν] *cf.* Gal. De ther. ad Pis. 3: XIV 223,2sq. K. De fac. nat. I 13: Scr. min. III 132,3–8 Helmr. = II 42,15–43,3 K. 23 τὸ μέσπιλον – 24] *cf.* Gal. De simpl. med. temp. et fac. VII 10; 12: XII 41,17sq.; 72,4sq. K.

1 ἔχων *ex* ἔχον *corr.* A   4 Γαληνοῦ περὶ τῆς οὐσίας τῶν φυσικῶν δυνάμεων *velut titulum add.* L A   *lac. indicavi*   5 οἱ *om.* A   7 *ante* τὰ *add.* καὶ L   8 *post* τρεχόντων *add.* ἔσθ' ὅτε A   11 καὶ *om.* L   12 αἰτίαν τινὰ L *Nic.* (causam aliquam) 13sq. πιστοῦ – ἡμῖν] φυσικοῦ πᾶσιν ἡμῖν πιστοῦται A   15 ἀλλὰ] ita *Nic.*   καὶ *om.* A   16 ἡ *om.* A   18 θεμένων L A: *in marg. corr. Goulst.*: imposuerunt *Nic.*: ἔθεντο *sec. Nic. coni. Corn.*   19 ἃ ποιεῖ *om.* A   εἶναι *secl. De Lacy per litt.*: dicentes *Nic.*: *post* εἶναι *add.* λέγομεν *Goulst.*[Bas]   20 ἑκάστων L   21 σκαμωνίαν L

4 *ante* De *add.* Capitulum quartumdecimum de substantia uirtutum et de opinionibus circa substantiam anime. ε   5 senserunt] sentiunt C: sentierunt γ   9 et[I] *om.* B   in *om.* C   et[II] *om.* β   12 occasiones] .i. cause *ut interpretamentum supra lin.* D[2] E[2] 15 nominauerunt *scripsi*: diuinauerunt α   18sq. actiua unaqueque C   19 actiua] accidentia B   20 scamo[a] γ   21 fit B: est C   zarolis] .i. sorbis *ut interpretamentum supra lin.* D[2] E[2]   22 set O   23 exercitati *bis scr.* C   25 secundum *e* quod *corr.* B

er (issues), having no inclination to declare on such disputed questions that one answer is any more plausible.

14. ... just as all men know that we have a soul, because they see clearly activities that are performed through the body – walking, running, wrestling, and a variety of ways of sensation – and because, working from a principle that is naturally trusted by all of us, inasmuch as we believe that nothing happens without a cause, they consider that there exist some causes of these actions, and, since they do not know what the cause of these actions is, they have given it a name from its being able to do what it does, i.e. a faculty which brings about each of the things that take place. So, for instance, all are agreed that scammony has a cathartic faculty, and the medlar a property that binds
the stomach. But experts in so- 2

that on those matters where there is disagreement it is more plausible.

14. But on the substance of the faculties I feel as others have felt, to wit, that they have a soul, in that they see clearly activities which the body performs in its disposition of coming and going and in its disposition of getting up and wrestling and in our sensation of various things. Thus they feel that in those activities there are certain causes and none of them happens without a cause. But they do not know the cause productive of those activities and they have given it a name according to the fact that they say that a man is capable of acting, this is that in him is each active faculty for those activities. And you will find everyone saying that in scammony there is a laxative faculty, and in
medlars a constipative faculty. But 2
those who are trained in natural science I find in disagreement and each one speaks according to the measure

ἐκπονήσαντες ϑεωρίαν, ἄλλος ἄλλο πείσαντες ἑαυτούς, οἱ μὲν ἀσωμάτους τινὰς ἀπεφήναντο δυνάμεις ἐνοικεῖν ταῖς αἰσϑηταῖς οὐσίαις, οἱ δὲ αὐτὰς ἐνεργεῖν τὰς οὐσίας κατ' ἰδίαν ἑκάστης φύσιν, ἤτοι γε ἐκ τῆς τῶν τεττάρων στοιχείων κράσεως
761 γενομένην ἢ ποιᾶς | συνϑέσεως
τῶν πρώτων σωμάτων, ἃ τινὲς μὲν ἄτομα, τινὲς δὲ ἄναρμα, τινὲς δὲ ἀμερῆ, τινὲς δὲ ὁμοιομερῆ
3 φασιν εἶναι. καὶ γάρ τοι καὶ
τὴν ψυχὴν ἡμῶν αὐτὴν οἱ μὲν ἀσώματόν τινα νομίζουσιν οὐσίαν εἶναι, τινὲς δὲ πνεῦμα, καϑάπερ ἄλλοι μηδὲ εἶναί τινα ὕπαρξιν αὐτῆς ἰδίαν, ἀλλὰ τὴν ἰδιότητα τῆς τοῦ σώματος οὐσίας, ὧν ποιεῖν πέφυκε, τούτων ἔχειν λέγεσϑαι δυνάμεις, οὐκ οὐσ⟨ι⟩ῶν τινων ἐκείνων ἰδίαν

dam iudicauerunt quod in substantiis sensibilibus sint uirtutes incorporee, et quidam eorum iudicauerunt quod unaqueque substantiarum id quod operatur non operatur nisi per naturam propriam generatam in ipsa ex commixtione quatuor elementorum aut ex compositione primorum, de quibus uident aliqui quod sint indiuisibilia; et quidam uident quod possint continuari; et quidam uident quod non possint diuidi, et quidam uident quod non pos-
3 sint similium partium esse. et dixerunt
etiam de anima dictum simile huic. et hoc est quod aliqui uident quod sit substantia incorporea, et quidam uident quod sit spiritus, et quidam alii dicunt quod anima non sit ens existens per se et diuisum ab alio; sed de proprietate corporis dicitur quod habeat operari ea que sibi pertinent operari et non quod habeat eam naturam ap-

10 τῶν – 13] *cf.* Gal. De san. tuenda I 5,11: CMG V 4,2, p. 9,11sq. De elem. ex Hipp. sent. 2,9: CMG V 1,2, p. 60,2sq. De causis content. 9,4: CMG Suppl. Or. II, p. 69, 22–26 = p. 140,17–20 14 τὴν – 16 εἶναι] *cf.* Plat. Tim. 69 c Gal. De plac. Hipp. et Plat. VII 3,19; 7,25: CMG V 4,1,2, p. 442,37sq.; 474,25sq. Galens Kommentar zu Platons Timaios, fr. 6. 9: p. 67; 86 Larrain [Gal.] Hist. philos. 24 (9): Diels, Doxographi Graeci, p. 613,12sq. = XIX 254,13sq. K. 16 τινὲς – 19 οὐσίας] *cf.* Gal. Quod animi mores corp. temp. sequ. 4: Scr. min. II 45,5sq. Müller = IV 783,10sq. K. In Hipp. Epid. VI comm. V 5: CMG V 10,2,2, p. 270,26; 272,20–22 De simpl. med. temp. et fac. V 9: XI 731,3sq. K. [Gal.] Hist. philos. 24 (9): Diels, Doxographi Graeci, p. 613,14 = XIX 254,15sq. K.

1 ϑεωρίαν *post* ὀνομαζομένην *(p. 110,25) trsp.* A 1sq. ἄλλος – πείσαντες] ἄλλως ἄλλοι πάντες A 2 *ante* ἑαυτούς *add.* τε L αὐτοὺς A 3 ἀσωμάτους] ἀσωκρα^τ A τινὰς *om.* A *spatio 5 litt. rel.* 4 δύναμιν A ἐνοικεῖν ταῖς *om.* A *spatio 10 fere litt. rel.* αἰσϑητικαῖς A 6 ἑκάστην L A *Nic.* (unamquamque): *in marg. corr. Goulst.* 7 γε *om.* L *Ald.* 8 τεττάρων] δ' A κράσιν L 9 γεναμένην A συνϑ' L 12 τινὲς δὲ ὁμοιομερῆ *om.* A 14 αὐτην ἡμῶν A 15 ὀνομάζουσιν L 17 μηδὲ *om.* L *Nic.* τινα] τὴν L 18 ἰδίαν αὐτῆς A 22 οὐσων L A *Nic.* (existentibus): *corr. ignotus in exemplari editionis Basileensis nunc Cantabrigiae conservato*

1 *post* substantiis *add. et del.* meris B 4 substantiam *in* substantiarum *supra lin. corr.* O: substantia scientiarum C id] illud C 6 ex *om.* B 7 ex *om.* β 8 commixtione C 9 indiuisibilia] scil. corpora athomalia *in marg. add.* B², *supra lin.* D² E² 10 quidam *om.* B *post* uident *add.* alii β *ante* possint *fort.* non *addendum est* possunt C γ 11 uident *om.* ε possunt C γ 12 possunt C γ 14 simile *e* similem *corr.* O 15 est *om.* O 18 ens *om.* β 19 de *om.* β 21 pertinet O imparari C 22 quod non B habeant γ

called theory of nature have proposed various contrary explanations: some have declared that incorporeal faculties inhabit sensible substances, others that the substances themselves act according to their own particular nature, which derives either from a mixture of the four elements or from some conjunction of primary bodies, which some say to be atoms, others unlinked, indivisible, or homogeneous particles. Indeed, some think that 3
our soul itself is some incorporeal substance, others spirit, others that it has no independent existence of its own, but that the individuality of the body's substance is said to include the faculties of doing what it is born to do; they do not have the specific nature

of his power: some have declared that there are incorporeal virtues in sensible substances, and some of them have declared that each of the substances does not do what it does except through its particular nature produced in itself either out of a mixture of four elements or of a conjunction of primary bodies; with regard to these, some see that they are indivisible; and some see that they can be linked together; and some see that they cannot be divided; and some see that they
cannot be of similar parts. And they 3
have even stated of the soul a statement like this. And this is because some see that it is an incorporeal substance, and some see that it is spirit, and some others say that the soul is not an entity existing of itself and apart from something else; but of the propriety of the body it is said that it

φύσιν ἐχουσῶν, ἀλλὰ τῆς ἐνεργούσης οὐσίας κατ' αὐτὴν πρὸς τὰ γινόμενα δι' αὐτῆς τε καὶ ὑπ' αὐτῆς δυνάμεις ἔχειν λεγομένης, ὧν πέφυκε δρᾶν.

4 Ἐγὼ τοίνυν ἐν τούτοις ⟨εἰς⟩ μέσην τινὰ τάξιν ἐμαυτὸν ἔταξα. περὶ γὰρ ἄλλων δογμάτων ἀποφαινόμενος ἁπλῶς, τῶν μὲν ὡς εἰδείην τὴν ἐν αὐτοῖς ἀλήθειαν, τῶν δὲ ὡς οὐδὲν αὐτῆς εἰδείην, ἐν οἷς ἄρτι διῆλθον, ἄχρι τοῦ πιθανοῦ προέρχομαι βέλτιον μὲν εἶναι νομίζων, εἴπερ ἐγνώκειν οὕτω περὶ αὐτῶν ὡς ἀποφαίνεσθαι καθάπερ ἐπ' ἄλλων, οὐ μὴν ἀναπείθων ἐμαυτόν, ὥσπερ ἕτεροι, βεβαίαν ἔχειν γνῶσιν ὧν οὐκ ἔσχον ἀπόδειξιν βεβαί-
762 5 αν. εἰπεῖν οὖν | βούλομαι καὶ περὶ τῶν τοιούτων ἁπάντων, ὅσα τὴν μὲν γνῶσιν οὐκ ἀναγκαίαν ἔχει πρὸς ὑγείαν σώματος ἢ τὰς τῆς ψυχῆς ἠθικὰς ἀρετάς, ἐπεκόσμησε δ' ἄν, εἴπερ ἐγνώσθη βεβαίως, τὰ διὰ τῶν γιγνωσκομένων ἀκριβῶς ἀποτελούμενα κατὰ ἰατρικήν τε καὶ τὴν ἠθικὴν φιλοσοφίαν, ἣν ἐγώ φημι χρησίμην τε ἅμα καὶ δυνατὴν εἶναι πᾶσι τοῖς βουλομένοις ἀσκῆ-

propriatam ei †ratione respectum†. uerumptamen substantia operatiua est dicta rerum procedentium ab ipsa et mediante ipsa, quod habeat uirtutes quibus illud quod pertinet ei operatur.

4 Et de hiis sententiis est gradus mediocris. et hoc est quod iudicaui in aliquibus sententiis iudicio naturali quod sentio de certitudine ipsarum et in aliquibus ex ipsis quod non habeo aliquam notitiam. sed de hiis que ante narraui habeo notitiam secundum modum sufficientie. et mee expositiones essent nobiliores si scirem eas firmiter et iudicarem de hiis prout iudicaui de aliis. uerumptamen anima mea non sentit scire ea ueraciter, eo quod sunt res in quibus non inuenitur uera probatio secundum quod alii senserunt.
5 et ego monstrabo ea quorum notitia non est necessaria ad sanitatem corporis neque ad nobilitatem anime; si darentur cum uera notitia esset additio in hiis quorum notitia est in medicina et in morali philosophia quod iuuat et est possibile scire omnibus uolentibus hoc. et ego compilaui de hiis duas dicti-

12 ἄχρι – 19] *cf. supra*, p. 108,25–110,3 *infra*, p. 124,12sq. Gal. In Hipp. Epid. VI comm. V 5: CMG V 10,2,2, p. 271,12–19

2 κατ' αὐτὴν] κατά τι A 4 δύναμιν A 6 εἰς *add. Kollesch et Nickel* 7 ἐμαυτὸν *ante* μέσην *trsp.* A 9 τῶν] τὴν A εἰδείην – 11 αὐτῆς *om.* L 11 ὡς] ἄλλως A: *corr. Ald.* 13 νομίζω A 15 ὡς *fort. delendum est*: *post* ὡς *add.* ἔοικεν *Goulst.*^{Bas} 18 οὐδ' L ἔχον A 21 ἔχει *ex* -ειν *corr.* L 22 ὑγίειαν *Chart.* 23 ἐπεσκόσμησε A 24 τὰ *om.* L 26sq. τε – ἠθικὴν *om.* L 29 βουληθεῖσιν A

1 eis γ ratione respectus ε: *cruces posui* 2 u^{m}tn C 3 *ante* et *add. et del.* quod B 4 mediante *e* medicante *corr.* E ipsa] hoc *supra lin.* D^2 E^2 uirtutem C 5 quibus] qua C γ illud] id O operari C γ 6 Et *om.* C 9 sentiens C: senciens γ ipsorum C γ 10 et *om.* ε 11 habeo *post* notitiam *trsp.* β *supra* notitiam *add.* certam D^2 E^2 sed] se O 14 me B, mee *supra lin.* B^2 15 si] sed γ eam C γ *post* firmiter *iter.* et – scirem *(lin. 14sq.)* C 17 mea *om.* β non *bis scr.* O 20 secundum] set O 21sq. ea – est] modo ea non esse C 22 *post* est *add. et del.* et B 23 nec B anime] que ε 24 cum uera] cura C 25 esset – notitia *in textu om., in marg. add.* E addatio C: adicio B: additione E in hiis] unius E quod E 27 *ante* quod *add.* eius ε quia B

of various substances, rather the substance, acting according to its individuality with regard to what is done through and by itself, is said to have the faculties of doing what it has been created to do.

In this debate, I take a middle 4
course. For I simply declare about other topics that I recognise the truth of some of them, and know nothing of it in others; in what I have just described, I admit (only) a plausible conclusion, considering that it would be better if I had understood them, so as to pronounce about them as I did about others, but not persuading myself, as others have done, that I have a sure knowledge of things of which I have no sure proof. So I should 5
like to speak (here) also of all those things of which knowledge is not essential for the health of the body or the moral wellbeing of the soul, but which, if they were known for certain, would be an additional adornment to those things that are achieved through careful understanding in medicine and moral philosophy, which I believe both useful and attainable by all

can do what pertains to it to do and not that it has this nature appropriate to it ... But the operative substance of those things that proceed from it and through its mediation is said to have faculties by which it performs what is appropriate for it.

And in these opinions there is 4
a middle way. And this is because I have declared about some opinions with a natural judgment that I am aware of their certainty and in some of them that I have no knowledge whatsoever. But of what I have said earlier I have knowledge (only) of plausibility. And my expositions would be better if I knew them firmly and could judge about them as I have judged about others. But my soul does not feel it knows them truly, in that they are things in which no true proof has been found as others have felt. And I will show 5
those things, knowledge of which is not necessary for the health of the body or the well-being of the soul; if they were made available with a true knowledge, there would be an increase in those things of which knowledge exists in medicine and in moral philosophy, which is of use and possible for all who want it to

σαι. καὶ γέγραπταί μοι περὶ τούτου δύο βιβλία, νυνὶ δέ, ὅπερ ὑπεσχόμην, προσάξω τὴν ἀρχὴν ἐνθένδε ποιησάμενος.

15. Ὅτι μὲν ἐκ τῆς τῶν δ' στοιχείων κράσεως ἅπαντα τὰ παρ' ἡμῖν σώματα γίγνεται, βεβαίως γιγνώσκειν φημί, καὶ προσέτι δι' ὅλων αὐτῶν κεραννυμένων, οὐχ ὡς ὁ Ἐμπεδοκλῆς ἡγεῖτο, κατὰ σμικρὰ μόρια καταθραυομένων. εἴτε δὲ τῶν σωματικῶν οὐσιῶν ὅλων δι' ἀλλήλων ἰουσῶν εἴτε τῶν ποιοτήτων μόνων, οὔτ' ἀναγκαῖον εἶναί φημι γιγνώσκειν οὔτε ἀποφαίνομαι. πιθανώτερον δὲ εἶναι νομίζω κατὰ τὰς ποιότητας γίγνεσθαι τὰς κράσεις.
2 τήν γε μὴν ψυχήν, εἰ μὲν ἀθάνατος οὖσα ταῖς σωματικαῖς οὐσίαις κεραννυμένη τὰ ζῷα διοικεῖ, γιγνώσκειν βεβαίως οὐκ ἐπ-
763 αγγέλλομαι, καθάπερ | οὐδὲ εἰ μηδεμία καθ' ἑαυτὴν ἔστιν οὐσία ψυχῆς. ἐκεῖνο μέντοι φαίνεταί μοι σαφῶς, ὅτι, κἂν εἰσοικί-

ones. sed in hoc tempore nostro narrabo illud quod promisi dicere, faciens principium huius ab hoc loco.

15. Igitur dico quod sum sciens uera notitia quod generatio omnium istorum corporum existentium ante nos que narrauimus sit ex commixtione quatuor elementorum. et ego scio etiam quod commixtio quatuor elementorum in generatione istorum corporum sit cum sua totalitate, non secundum quod oppinatus fuit Empedocles, qui ea diuisit in minimas particulas. sed utrum hoc sit quod substantie corporee incorporent se adinuicem, uel hoc non accidit nisi in earum qualitatibus tantum, igitur dico quod scientia istarum rerum non est necessaria et non habeo iudicium de ipsa. sed ego uideo quod magis conueniens est sumere dictum dicentis quod
2 commixtio sit in qualitatibus. sed de anima utrum sit immortalis eo quod ipsa regit animalia commixtione sua cum substantiis corporeis ego non sum certus de hac scientia, nec utrum sit

5 Ὅτι – 8 φημί] *cf.* Gal. De elem. ex Hipp. sent.: CMG V 1,2, p. 56–158 10 Ἐμπεδοκλῆς] *cf.* Empedocl., A 43: I, p. 291,15–26 D.-K. Gal. In Hipp. De nat. hom. comm. I 3; 13: CMG V 9,1, p. 19,7–12; 27,24–27 De constit. artis med. 7,9: CMG V 1,3, p. 76,4–7 [Gal.] Hist. philos. 29 (10): Diels, Doxographi Graeci, p. 616,12sq. = XIX 258,12sq. K. 12 εἴτε – 17] *cf.* Gal. De elem. ex Hipp. sent. 9,33: CMG V 1,2, p. 136,15–18

1 *fort.* τούτων *scribendum est; cf. vers. Lat.* (hiis) 2 νῦν A 3 πράξω A ἐνθένδεν A 10 ὁ *om.* A 11 μόρια *om.* L 12 καταθραυμένων L 13 τῶν *om.* L οὐσῶν L *Nic.* (existentibus) 16 γινώσκων A 21 οὐσίαις *om.* A *spatio 4 litt. rel.* 22 κεραννῦν ψυχῆς L διοικῆ A 23 ἀπαγγέλλομαι L 25 μὴ δὲ μία L *ante* οὐσία *add.* ἡ A 27 εἰσοικίζεται A

1 set O 2 illud] id B ε 3 huius] haberi β 5 *ante* Igitur *add.* Capitulum quintumdecimum de hiis quorum habetur certa noticia in medicina et de hiis quorum non. et de quibus est cura. ε: cap^m octauum *in marg. add.* B^4 sum sentiens C: scio sane ε 6 quia C 6sq. horum corporum omnium C 8 sint C: sicut γ 9sq. quatuor – commixtio *om.* β 11 in] et O 12 sunt C γ: *correxi*: *om.* ε 14 qui] quia C: quod γ eas γ minimas *e* menimas *corr.* B: mimas O 15 utrum] u^t C 17 uel *scripsi*: sed α eius C O: eis B: eorum ε, sc. elementorum *ut interpretamentum* D^2 E^2: *correxi* 19 scientia *coni. Kollesch et Nickel*: $\overline{sba}$ C γ: substantia ε non *om.* ε 19sq. necessaria est ε 23 comixtio O: mixtio ε 24 mortalis ε

who wish to exercise it. I have written two treatises on this theme, but for the moment I shall say (only) what I have promised to say, starting from the following point.

15. I declare that I know for certain that all our bodies come from a mixing together of the four elements, and besides through their complete mixture, not, as Empedocles believed, through being broken up into small particles. But whether (this happens) because the corporeal substances interpenetrate thoroughly one another or only the qualities I neither consider it necessary to know, nor do I make any definite pronouncement (about it). I think it more likely, however, that the mixture occurs
in the qualities. Neither do I claim 2
to know for certain whether the soul is immortal and governs animals by being mixed with the substances of the body, or whether the substance of the soul has no existence per se. However, it seems clear to me that even if the

know. And I wrote on this two treatises. But at this moment of ours I shall expound what I promised to say, making a beginning of it from here.

15. Thus I say that I know with a true knowledge that the generation of all these bodies existing before us that we have mentioned derives from a mixture of the four elements. And I also know that the mixture of the four elements in the generation of those bodies takes place in its totality, not as Empedocles believed, who divided them up into very small particles. But whether this is because the corporeal substances incorporate themselves or this does not happen except only in their qualities, so I say that the knowledge of these things is not necessary and I have no opinion on it. But I see that it is more plausible to accept the statement of him who says that the mixture is of
the qualities. But as to the soul 2
whether it is immortal, by the fact that it governs animals by its mixture with the substances of the body I am not sure of this knowledge, nor

ζηται τοῖς σώμασι, δουλεύει ταῖς φύσεσιν αὐτῶν, αἵπερ εἰσίν, ὡς ἔφην, ἐκ τῆς τῶν δ' στοιχείων ποιᾶς κράσεως γιγνόμεναι. καὶ κατά γε τοῦτο πρὸς τὴν ἰατρικὴν τέχνην οὐδὲν ἡγοῦμαι βλαβήσεσθαί τινα διὰ τὴν ἄγνοιαν τῆς καλουμένης ἐμψυχώσεώς τε καὶ μετεμψυχώσε-
3 ως. ἐπιτήδειόν τε γὰρ εἶναι χρὴ τὸ σῶμα τὸ δεξόμενον τὴν ψυχὴν ἀλλοιωθέντος τε αὐτοῦ μεγάλην ἀλλοίωσιν ἐν τῇ κράσει παραχρῆμα τὴν ψυχὴν ἐξιέναι, ψυχομένου μέντοι σφοδρῶς ἐν ταῖς κενώσεσι τοῦ αἵματος καὶ ἐν ταῖς πόσεσι τῶν ψυχόντων φαρμάκων ὅταν τε σφοδρῶς ᾖ τὸ περιέχον ψυχρόν, ἀμέτρως τε θερμαινομένου κατά τε τοὺς πυρετοὺς καὶ τὰς εἰσπνοὰς τῆς φλογὸς ἢ τῶν ὑπερθερμαινόντων φαρμάκων πόσεις.

4 Οὐ μόνον δὲ οὕτως ἀλλοιωθείσης τῆς κράσεως τοῦ σώματος τὴν ψυχὴν ὁρῶμεν αὐτοῦ χωριζομένην, ἀλλὰ κἀπειδὰν τῆς ἀναπνοῆς στερηθῇ πάντως κἀνταῦθά τινος γινομένης ἀλλοιώσεως κατὰ τὸ σῶμα. τη-

substantia existens per se. uerumptamen illud quidem manifestum est nobis quod cum sit disposita in corporibus, nos inuenimus naturas que sunt generate secundum quod dixi ex commixtione quatuor elementorum. et ego non uideo quod alicui noceat in arte medicine nescire modum quo currit
3 dispositio uite. et nos scimus quod conuenit quod corpus quod est preparatum ad recipiendum animam sit conueniens ad receptionem eius. quod quando alteratur in complexione sua uehementi alteratione anima dimittit illud. et alteratio eius est uel frigiditate secundum quod accidit quando euacuatur multum a sanguine et quando repletur medicinis et quando aer continens nos est multum frigidus; sed per caliditatem secundum quod accidit in febribus et secundum quod accidit in attractione flamme ignis et in potione medicinarum calidarum in ultimitate.

4 Et non solum propter istam causam recedit anima a corpore, sed propter defectum hanelitus. et impossibile est quod anima recedat a corpore quousque corpus consistit in sua complexione na-

1 δουλεύει – 5] *cf.* Gal. Quod animi mores corp. temp. sequ. 3: Scr. min. II 41,15–18 Müller = IV 779,11–13 K. 3 ὡς ἔφην] *v. supra,* p. 62,19

3 ὡς ἔφην *om.* A δ' *om.* L στοιχείων *om.* A 7 διὰ *om.* L 9 τε – μετεμψυχώσεως *om.* A 10 γὰρ *om.* A 10sq. τὸ σῶμα χρὴ L 16 τοῦ αἵματος *ante* ἐν *(lin. 15) trsp.* A 17 ἐν *om.* L 20 τε[I]] γε L: *corr. Ald.*: δὲ A 23 πόσις A 26 ὁρῶμεν *om.* A 27 τῆς *om.* A στερηθείη L

2 illud] id B ε quidem] quod C γ 3 quod] et B dispositio α: *correxi* 4 *post* nos *add.* non β naturas] materias ε B^3 *in marg.* 5 generate secundum *scripsi*: generatio eius α ex] in B, *fort. recte* 10 uenit O 13 quando] uero ε 15 illud] id B ε: eum C frigiditate] stante C γ 16 *ante* secundum *add.* uel β 18 medicinis] materiis ε 19 per] propter C 20 secundum *om.* O 22 potatione C 23 ul/ultimitate *in* ultimitate *corr.* B 26 defectum *e* defectam *corr.* C anhelitus D*(?)*E: anelitus C 27 recedit B 28 *ante* corpus *add.* etiam O, et B

soul (merely) takes up residence in bodies, it is subservient to their natures, which are, as I have said, derived from some mixture of the four elements. And, as far as this goes, I think that no one is going to suffer in his medical art from his ignorance of so-called empsychosis and metempsychosis. For 3
the body has to be suitable for receiving the soul and if it suffers some grave alteration in its mixture the soul must depart from it immediately, for example, when the body is greatly chilled through the evacuation of blood and through drinking chilling drugs, and when the surrounding atmosphere is very cold, and when the body is heated to excess by fevers and by breathing in a flame or by drinking superheating drugs.

It is not only when the mixture 4
of the body undergoes such a change that we see the soul depart from it but also when it is totally deprived of breath, because here, too, a change takes place in the

whether it is a substance existing by itself. But what is clear to us is that when it is disposed in bodies, we find natures which are generated, as I have mentioned, from a mixture of the four elements. And I do not see that it harms anyone in the art of medicine not to know the way in which the disposition of life runs.
And we know that it is appropriate 3
that the body which is prepared to receive the soul should be fit for its reception. When it is altered in its temperament by a great change, the soul leaves it. And its alteration is either through cold when it happens that much blood is removed and when it is filled with drugs and when the air surrounding us is very cold; but by heat as happens in fevers and as happens in the taking in of a flame of fire and in drinking extremely hot drugs.

And not only for this reason 4
does the soul depart from the body but from a deficiency of breath. And it is impossible that the soul should leave the body as long as the body remains in its own natural

ρουμένης οὖν τῆς φυσικῆς εὐκρασίας
764 ἐν τῷ σώματι τὴν | ψυχὴν αὐτοῦ χωρισϑῆναι δοκῶ μοι γιγνώσκειν ἀδύ-
5 νατον εἶναι. καὶ διὰ τοῦτο τὴν οὐσίαν αὐτῆς, ἥτις ἐστίν, οὐκ ἀναγκαῖον οὔτε εἰς τὰς ἰάσεις τῶν νοσημάτων οὔτε εἰς τὴν φυλακὴν τῆς ὑγείας ἐπίστασϑαι, καϑάπερ οὐδὲ εἰς τὴν ἠϑικὴν φιλοσοφίαν, πρακτικήν τε καὶ πολιτικήν – ὀνομαζέτω γὰρ αὐτὴν ἕκαστος, ὡς ἂν ἐϑέλῃ, χωρίζων τῆς ϑεωρητικῆς. ἐπὶ πλέον δὲ περὶ τούτων ἐν ἑτέροις ὑπομνήμασι γέγρα-
6 πταί μοι. τῶν δὲ φυσικῶν δυνάμεων ἐπιδεδειγμένων, ὁπόσαι τέ εἰσι καὶ ὁποῖαι, ζήτησίς τις γίνεται κατὰ ἀκολουϑίαν, ὅπως φαμὲν αὐτὰς ἕλκειν μὲν τὸ οἰκεῖον, ἀποκρίνειν δὲ τὸ ἀλλότριον. ἀδύνατον γὰρ εἶναι φαίνεται πρὶν γνωρίσαι σαφῶς, ὁποῖον μέν τι τὸ οἰκεῖόν ἐστιν, ὁποῖον δέ τι τὸ ἀλλότριον, ἢ τὴν ὁλκὴν τῶν οἰκείων ἢ τὴν ἀπόκρισιν τῶν ἀλλοτρίων ποιεῖσϑαι. τὸ δὲ γνωρίζειν αἰσϑητικῆς δυνάμεως ἔργον εἶναι φαίνεται.

5 turali. et propter hoc non est necessarium scire quid sit substantia anime in curatione morborum neque in conseruatione sanitatis neque in aptatione morum. et si placet nominare hanc particulam moralem siue consuetudine siue quia docet bene operari, hoc est licitum unicuique nominare eam sicut uult, dummodo ponat differentiam inter ipsam et opus pratice. et ego locutus sum in aliis libris euidentius quam modo lo-
6 quor. et cum demonstratum sit quot sint uirtutes naturales et quid sint, modo restat perscrutari quot modis dicitur quod uirtus attractiua attrahat illud quod est conueniens sibi, expulsiua expellat illud quod est contrarium sibi. et impossibile est quod una istarum attrahat rem conuenientem sibi et ⟨...⟩ rem contrariam sibi naturaliter. et notitia non est nisi a uirtute sensitiua.

4 καὶ – 10 πολιτικήν] *cf. supra,* p. 108,18–21 Gal. In Hipp. Epid. VI comm. V 5: CMG V 10,2,2, p. 271,19–272,1 De plac. Hipp. et Plat. IX 7,9–12: CMG V 4,1,2, p. 588, 7–22 13 ἐν ἑτέροις ὑπομνήμασι] *v. e.g.* Gal. Quod animi mores corp. temp. sequ.; De plac. Hipp. et Plat.; In Plat. Tim. comm. 15sq. ὁπόσαι – ὁποῖαι] *cf. supra,* p. 108,14–18

2 ἐν τῷ σώματι] τοῦ σώματος A 5 ἀναγκαῖα A 7 τὴν *om.* L ὑγιείας *Chart.* 8–10 ἠϑικήν τε καὶ πρακτικὴν καὶ πολιτικὴν φιλοσοφίαν A 11 ἂν ἐϑέλῃ] βούλεται A 15 εἰσι *post* ὁποῖαι *(lin. 16) trsp.* L 18 μὲν *om.* L δὲ] τὸ *in* τε *mut.* L 19 εἶναι γὰρ A 20 πρὶν γνωρίσαι] προγνωρίσαι L *Nic.* (precognoscere): πρὶν *in marg.*, „πρὶν γν.] Ita Adelph. Ms. excus." *in adn. Goulst.* 21 μέν τι] μέντοι L: *corr. Kühn*: μὲν A: quidem nimirum *Nic.* τι^{II} *om.* A 24 τὸ δὲ γνωρίζειν *bis scr.* L

2 scire *om.* β quod α: *correxi* 3 morborum *e* uerborum *corr.* E 4sq. nec ... nec B 7 siue consuetudine *bis scr.* B: siue consuetudine *e* consuetudine siue consuetudine *corr.* E 8 quia] qua C *ante* hoc *add.* quia C γ 9 unicuique *om.* ε 11 opus] oȝ (= oportet) γ practice ε 12 ego *om.* ε 12sq. locutus – euidentius *post* modo *iter.* B 15 quod α: *correxi* 16 quid] quot ε perscruptari C: perscruti B 17 atractiua O: attractia C 18 atrahat C: attrahit D illud] id B ε 19sq. sibi – contrarium *om.* β 23 *lac. indicavi; fort.* altera expellat *addendum est*

body. I think that I know that the soul cannot leave the body as long as the natural balanced mixture in
it is maintained. For this reason it is 5
not necessary to understand what is the substance of the soul either in treating diseases or in maintaining health or in moral philosophy, both practical and political – you can give it whatever name you like, provided that you separate it from theoretical philosophy. I have written at greater length on this in oth-
er works. Since I have (already) 6
shown how many and of what kind are the natural faculties, the next question to ask is what we meant by saying that they attract what was appropriate and reject what was inappropriate. For it seems impossible that they can secure the attraction of the appropriate and the rejection of the inappropriate without first recognising clearly what sort of thing is appropriate and what inappropriate. Thus recognition seems to be the work of some sensory faculty.

temperament. And for this reason it 5
is not necessary to know what the substance of the soul is in the treatment of diseases nor in the conservation of health nor in the improvement of morals. And if one prefers to call this part moral either by custom or because it teaches how to work well, this is permitted for anyone to call it what one wants, provided that one makes a distinction between this and the work of practice. And I spoke (about this) in other books more clearly than I
speak now. And since it has been 6
shown how many the natural faculties are and what they are, it just remains to investigate in what ways it is said that the attractive faculty attracts what is appropriate for itself, the expulsive (faculty) expels what is opposed to itself. And it is impossible that one of them attracts something appropriate to itself and +the other expels+[1] something opposed to itself naturally. And there is no knowledge except from a sensory faculty.

1 +the other expels+: see the app. crit.

7 Διὰ τοῦτο οὖν ἐν τῷ λόγῳ τούτῳ παρακοή τίς ἐστι καίτοι σαφῶς εἰρηκότος τοῦ Πλάτωνος ἕτερον εἶναι γένος αἰσθήσεως ἐν τοῖς φυτοῖς οἰομένων τῶν ἀκουόντων εἶναί τινα γνωριστικὴν δύναμιν ἐν αὐτοῖς τῶν
765 οἰκείων | τε καὶ ἀλλοτρίων. τούτων γὰρ μόνων ἐστὶν ἡ διάγνωσις αὐτοῖς, ἥ τε καθ' ἡδονὴν ἥ τε κατ' ἀνίαν ἥ τε κατά τινα παραπλήσια τούτοις ἢ ἀνάλογα παθήματα γιγνομένη, τῶν ἄλλων αἰσθητικῶν διαγνώσεων οὐ μετεχούσης τῆς φυτικῆς ψυχῆς. οὔτε γὰρ τῶν ὁρατῶν οὔτε τῶν ἀκουστῶν οὔτε τῶν ὀσφραντῶν οὔτε τῶν γευστῶν οὔτε τῶν ἁπτῶν ποιοτήτων ἔχει διάγνωσιν, ἀλλὰ μόνον τῶν τρέφειν αὐτὴν ἢ μὴ τρέφειν δυναμένων. τὰ μὲν γὰρ τρέφειν δυνάμενα πρὸς ἑαυτὴν ἕλκουσα καὶ κατέχουσα καὶ πέττουσα καὶ μεταβάλ-

7 Et propter hoc accidit de hoc quod dico error cum Plato dixerit manifeste quod in plantis est aliud genus sensus propter quod ⟨...⟩

[Arist.] De pomo: ⟨...⟩ magnum gradum, que trahit hominem ab obscuritate ignorantie et a tenebris stultitie ad lucem scientie et claritatem intellectus. respondit Aristotiles: qui uult intelligere philosophiam et uult esse sapiens legat et discat VIII primos libros quos agregaui quousque perueniat ad librum De anima. et dum cognoscet et intelliget, ubi in corpore est sedes anime sue et naturam suam et si est in ipso incarcerata aut si est antiqua aut creata cum corpore aut si requiescit in eo et si surget et suscita-

3 Πλάτωνος] *v.* Plat. Tim. 77 a *cf.* Gal. In Plat. Tim. comm. III 2: CMG Suppl. I, p. 10,4–11,20 6 magnum – 124,12 docentes] [Arist.] De pomo: p. 58,4–59,2 Plezia 11 qui – 124,9 gradus] *haec verba citat* Gas: Pagel, Concordanciae, p. XLII

2 τίς *om.* A *spatio 3 litt. rel.* ἔσται A 3 τοῦ *om.* A *post* Πλάτωνος *add. et del.* ὡς *Goulst.*^{Bas}: ὡς *in marg. add. Goulst.* ἐστι L 7 ἀλλοτρίων τε καὶ οἰκείων A *post* τούτων *supra lin. add.* τε A 8 μόν͡ A 9sq. εἴτε ... εἴτε ... εἴτε A 9 ἥ τε κατ' ἀνίαν *supra lin. inser.* L 10 παραπλησίαν L A: *correxi* 11 ἀνάλογα παθήματα] ἀνάλογα τὰ παθήματα L: *correxi*: ἀνάλογον ὄντα A γιγνομένων L 13 φυσικῆς A 14sq. τῆς ὁρατῆς ... τῆς ἀκουστῆς ... τῆς ὀσφραντῆς L 15sq. οὔτε τῶν γευστῶν *om.* A 17 ἔχει *om.* A μόνων L A *Nic.*^{chik} (solorum): solum *Nic.*^{bj}: *corr. Ald.* 18 αὐτὴν *om.* L εἰ A 21 πέπτουσα *Ald.*

1 accidit de hoc *om.* B, *in marg. add.* B^2 2 dixerit] dixit O: dicit B ε 4 aliud] a^d C γ: aliquid ε *post* aliud *supra lin. add.* de uirtute sensitiua D^2 E^2 genus *scripsi*: igitur α 4sq. propterea quid ε 5 *post* quod *spatium 16 fere litt. in* C *hic finem tractatus Galeni in hac versione servati primus statuit Einarson, p. 258sq.; incipit fragmentum libri [Arist.] De pomo, p. 58,4–59,2 Plezia* 6 *lac. indicavi* 6sq. magnum – que *om.* O magnum gradum] magnum est ε: mag. B: manifeste B^4 7 que] quod ε: *om.* B extrahit ε: atrahit O ab] in C γ 8 obscuritatem C: oscuritate E ingnorantie C 10 claritate C intellecti O B, *corr.* B^4: intelligit C respondit *om.* β: ait *post* Aristotiles *(lin. 11) supra lin. add.* D^2 E^2 12 philosophiam] sapientiam *Gas* *ante* et *add. et del.* d C 13 leguat O et discat *om. Gas* disat B VIII primos libros] VIII° librorum megategni *Gas* VIII *om.* ε libros *om.* C 14 aggregaui ε 15 dum] tunc ε *Gas*: de ipso *Arist.* 16 cognoscet et *om. Gas* 16sq. in corpore *om. Gas* 17 sue *om. Gas* 18 est – 19 si *om.* O est in ipso] ipsa est *Arist.* in ipso *om. Gas* incarceratio B E: incarceratus D 19 antequam *Arist.* 20 si *om.* β quiescit O ε *Gas*: quiescat B 21 et^1] aut *Arist.*

For this reason there is (possible) misunderstanding in this argument although Plato clearly stated that there is a different sort of perception in plants, (a misunderstanding) if his audience understood him to mean that there is in plants a cognitive faculty of what is appropriate or inappropriate. For plants have the capacity to distinguish between these things alone, and it is brought about by feelings of pleasure and pain or affections similar or akin to them, while the vegetable soul shares in no other kinds of sensory diagnostic. It cannot distinguish things by how their qualities appear to sight, sound, smell, taste or touch, but only by whether they can nurture it or not. It attracts the things that can nurture it, retains them, digests them 7

And for this reason there occurs an error in what I say although Plato clearly stated that in plants there is a different sort of perception, (an error) insofar as ... 7

[Arist.], De pomo: ... large step (of philosophy) which draws men out of the darkness of ignorance and from the shadows of folly into the light of knowledge and the brilliance of understanding. Aristotle declared: Whosoever wishes to understand philosophy and wishes to be wise, let him read and learn the first 8 books I have put together until he reaches the book On the soul. And whenever he knows and understands where in the body is the seat of his soul and what its nature is, and if it is imprisoned within it or is of old or created with the body or if it dies with it or if it is

λουσα πρὸς τὰς οἰκείας τοῖς τρεφο-
μένοις οὐσίας, τὰ δὲ μὴ δυνάμενα
τρέφειν οὐ προσίεται, ὥστε μοι
Πλάτων ὀρθῶς δοκεῖ λέγειν αἴ-
σθησιν ἔχειν τὰ φυτά, τῶν οἰκείων
τε καὶ ἀλλοτρίων δηλονότι, καὶ κα-
τὰ τοῦτο ζῷα προσηκόντως ἂν λε-
χθῆναι μετὰ τοῦ μηδὲ τῆς ἐξ ἑαυτῶν
8 κινήσεως ἐστερῆσθαι. ἀλλὰ μηδὲ τῆς
τοιαύτης γνώσεως ἀναγκαίας οὔσης
εἰς τὴν ἰατρικὴν φιλοσοφίαν ἀρκοῦ-
μαι διὰ τὴν ἀκολουθίαν μόνον ἄχρι
τοῦ πιθανοῦ προερχόμενος ἐπαινεῖν
766 τὸν Πλάτωνα | καὶ ζῷα καλοῦντα τὰ φυτὰ καὶ μετέχειν αἰσθήσεως μό-
νης φάσκοντα τῆς τῶν οἰκείων τε καὶ ἀλλοτρίων διαγνωστικῆς, ἥτις, ἂν
ἀκριβῶς σκοπῇς, τοῦ γένους τῶν ἡδέων τε καὶ οὐχ ἡδέων οὖσα φανεῖται.
δι' οὐδὲν γὰρ ἄλλο δυνατὸν εἰπεῖν ἕλκειν αὐτὰ τὸ οἰκεῖον ἢ ἐξομοιοῦν ἑαυ-
9 τοῖς ἢ διὰ τὴν ἀπόλαυσίν τε καὶ τὴν ἐγγινομένην αὐτοῖς ἡδονήν. ἀλλ', ὡς
ἔφην, ἀρκεῖ πρὸς ἰατρικὴν ἐπίστασθαι τοῦτο μόνον, ὡς ἕλκει μὲν τὸ οἰκεῖ-
ον, ᾧπερ καὶ τρέφεται, ἀποκρίνει δὲ τὸ ἀλλότριον. ἔτι δὲ μᾶλλον εἰς φιλο-
σοφίαν ἠθικὴν ἄχρηστος ἡ τῶν τοιούτων ἀκριβὴς γνῶσις, ὅθεν οὐδὲ ὁ
Πλάτων αὐτῆς ἐμνημόνευσεν.

bitur aut quia ⟨celatur⟩ oculis omnium animalium postquam exierit a corpore ⟨aut finietur⟩ cum eo, et cum respiciet in hiis euentibus, tunc cognoscit creatorem suum et ibit in uiam recti, non declinabit ad dexteram siue ad sinistram. et hic maximus gradus et altior gradus. et ego iam declaraui uobis uiam ueritatis ⟨et non⟩ exiui a semita recta quia docentes ⟨...⟩

18sq. ὡς ἔφην] *cf. supra*, p. 108,14–21

1 τὸ οἰκεῖον A τῆς τρεφομένης *Caius (sec. Ad.), Corn., Goulst.*[Bas]*, Chart.* 2 οὐσίας *om.* A 5 ἔχειν *e* σχειν *corr.* A 7 τοῦτο] τὰ A *post* λεχθῆναι *add. et del.* πρ L 8 μήτε L αὐτῶν L 9 ἐστερεῖσθαι L 12 μόνην L A: *correxi* 14 μόνης *om.* A 15 εἴ τις A 16 τε σκοπῇ A 17 ἑαυτῆς L 19 ἀρκεῖν A ἕλκειν A 20 ὥσπερ καὶ τὸ τρέφεσθαι πέφυκεν ἀποκρίνειν A ἔτι δὲ] „ἔστι δὲ] Ita Adelph. excus. ἔτι δὲ" *in adn. Goulst.* 21 ὁ *om.* A 22 „f. αὐτοῦ" *in adn. Goulst.* τέλος περὶ τῶν ἑαυτῷ δοκούντων A: τέλος τοῦ περὶ τῶν φυσικῶν δυνάμεων L

1 aut – 5 cognoscit *om. Gas* aut quia *ex* atque *corr.* B: ante ε celatur *sec. Arist. addidi*: *lac. 11 fere litt. in* C occulis O: oculos ε 2 exierit *om.* O B, recesserit, ueniet *post* corpore *in marg. add.* B[4]: *lac. 20 fere litt. in* C: recedet *Arist.* 3 aut finietur *sec. Arist. addidi*: *lac. 18 fere litt. in* C 4 cum respiciet] c...... t B, *corr.* B[4] recipiet O in – 5 cognoscit *om.* β *post* euentibus *add.* anime *Arist.* 5 cognoscet *Arist.* 6 uia C recta C: rectam *Arist. Gas* 7 declinabitur O ε *Gas* B, *corr.* B[4] dextram C ε siue] uel *Arist.*: nec *Gas* 8 *post* hic *add.* est *Arist. Gas* gradus *om. Gas* 9 et[I] – gradus *om.* B: quo non est altior *Arist.* et[I] *om.* C 10sq. et non exiui *sec. Arist. scripsi*: ex uia α 11 semita *e* -itta *corr.* E: secuta B quia] que B: queque ε 12 dicentes β *lac. indicavi*: et dantes doctrinam non debent mentiri nec falsificare sermones meos. *Arist.* Explicit liber Galieni de sententiis medicorum B: Explicit liber de sententiis G. O: explicit liber sententiarum G. id est de sententiis medicorum C: explicit liber Galieni de sentenciis ε

and turns them into substances appropriate to what are being nurtured, and it does not take up the things that cannot nurture it; so Plato seems to me to be right when he says that plants have perception, namely of what is appropriate and what is inappropriate, and for this reason they could be properly called living beings, as well as because they are not deprived of motion in themselves. But since this sort of knowledge is not essential for medical philosophy, because of consistency (of the argument) I am content to reach only plausibility and to praise Plato for calling plants living beings and for saying that they have a sense that can distinguish only between things appropriate and things inappropriate (to them), which, if you look closely, will be obviously one that distinguishes between pleasant and unpleasant. Indeed, one might say that they attract what is appropriate and assimilate it to themselves for no other reason than the enjoyment and pleasure that they derive therefrom. But, as I said (before), it is enough for 9
medicine to know only that they attract what is appropriate, from which they obtain nutriment, and that they reject what is inappropriate. But a detailed knowledge of such matters is even less useful for moral philosophy, which is why Plato made no mention of it.

to rise and be raised up or that it is hidden from the eyes of all living creatures after it departs from the body or has done with it, and when he will look back at these events (of the soul), then he will know his creator and will walk in the way of righteousness, and will stray neither to the right nor to the left. This is the greatest and higher step. And I have declared to you the way
8 of truth, and I have not departed from the right way because teachers ...

COMMENTARY

P. 54,2: For a possible Platonising parallel to the title, see below, p. 131, comm. to p. 56,7–10.

P. 54,5–18: The text opens with an elaborate preface, characteristic of Galen in that a past incident provides justification for the writing of the present treatise.[1] De venae sectione adversus Erasistrateos Romae degentes begins with a case-history (1: XI 187,3–194,14 K.), De anatomicis administrationibus with a survey of Galen's education and early writings in anatomy (I 1: pp. 1, 1–5,10 Garofalo = II 215,5–218,15 K.), Quod optimus medicus sit etiam philosophus and De praecognitione with ornate descriptions of the dreadful conditions of contemporary society (1: Scr. min. II 1,1–2,20 Müller = I 53,3–55,9 K.; 1: CMG V 8,1, pp. 68,1–74,11). Other treatises open with a claim that there has been a dispute, over treatment or the meaning of words, which Galen will subsequently resolve, e.g. De partibus artis medicativae (1: CMG Suppl. Or. II, pp. 24,2–26,8 = pp. 119,3–120,6) and De atra bile (1,1–3: CMG V 4,1,1, p. 71, 2–20). The closest parallel to the preface of On my own opinions is provided by the opening of De libris propriis (Scr. min. II 91,1–93,16 Müller = XIX 8, 3–11,11 K.), in which Galen describes how he came across in Rome two men disputing the authenticity of a tract that was being sold under his name. One was convinced it was genuine, but the other, who had enjoyed a proper education in rhetoric and grammar, could determine by reading only a few lines that the book was not by Galen. But, Galen goes on to argue, such talents are now increasingly rare, and in order to assist those who might unwittingly be led astray by these fraudulent imitations, he has decided to write a tract that will help to authenticate the works of his in circulation.

But the preface to On my own opinions differs in one important respect from all the rest: Galen is neither himself a participant nor concerned about the specific point at issue in the debate. Instead, by a nice rhetorical conceit he takes a story about Parthenius the poet in order to distinguish between two, at first sight similar, situations: he contrasts the living poet among friends with the living author accessible only through his books and his scientific methods.

Galen then adds a further individual twist. Whereas, in De libris propriis, he had listed the books he had written under their various subjects by title

[1] For a survey of Galen's prefaces, see L. Alexander, The preface to St. Luke's Gospel. Literary convention and social context in Luke 1:1–4 and Acts 1:1, Cambridge, 1993, and, from a different perspective, Mansfeld, Prolegomena, pp. 116–131.

and, as with some of his works on anatomy, also by summarising their contents, here, by contrast, he refers to relatively few books, and excludes almost entirely his non-medical writings. Instead, he summarises the main doctrines that, he declares, have been with him throughout his life, with one exception. Any treatise passing under his name and containing ideas at variance with what is given here is henceforth to be rejected as spurious.[1]

Such a zeal for authenticity goes far beyond the familiar literary concern for the survival of one's own writings, and involves criteria that would have been foreign to most, if not all, of the writers of the second century. Galen applies to his own books techniques which he had deployed, if not in large part himself developed, in dealing with the multitude of writings that constitute the Hippocratic Corpus. There, faced with a series of competing claims to convey the ideas of the historical Hippocrates, he had used a variety of tests, notably language and consistency of doctrine, to determine how a particular book represented what Hippocrates had taught.[2] Here, in De libris propriis, and in De ordine librorum suorum, he goes out of his way to suggest methods of interpretation that will minimise any possible misunderstanding and misrepresentation of the authentic voice of Galen. He is determined to ensure that his books are read properly, and that spurious writings are not allowed to disseminate error and falsehood to his detriment.[3] He did not succeed entirely, for works like the Introductio sive medicus circulated even in his lifetime alongside genuine material.

P. 54,5 Ait Galienus: Many mediaeval medical texts, and especially translations taken from the Arabic, begin with the phrase, "so-and-so says", which also serves to ensure the identity of the author should the title of the treatise be lost, as was not uncommon in manuscripts. Openings with "inquit" are more frequent than those with "ait", see the lists in: L. Thorndike and P. Kibre, A catalogue of Incipits of mediaeval scientific writings in Latin, 2nd ed., London, 1963, cols. 72 and 746–751, which is a reason for preferring the less familiar "ait" of the β-group.

Parthenius of Nicaea was a Greek poet whose learned complexity found many admirers among the intellectual coteries of Rome in the last years of the Republic, c. 70–30 B.C. Papyri from Roman Egypt show that his works

1 Cf. also W. Speyer, Die literarische Fälschung im heidnischen und christlichen Altertum. Ein Versuch ihrer Deutung, Munich, 1971 (Handb. d. Altertumswiss. 1,2), pp. 55; 93; 128, for similar attempts to defy forgery and misrepresentation.

2 See W. D. Smith, pp. 61–176; F. Kudlien, Hippokrates-Rezeption im Hellenismus, in: Die hippokratischen Epidemien. Theorie – Praxis – Tradition. Verhandlungen des Ve Colloque international hippocratique, veranstaltet von der Berliner Gesellschaft für Geschichte der Medizin in Verbindung mit dem Institut für Geschichte der Medizin der Freien Universität Berlin, 10. – 15. 9. 1984, ed. G. Baader and R. Winau, Stuttgart, 1989 (Sudhoffs Archiv, Beih. 27), pp. 355–376; Lloyd, Galen on Hellenistics and Hippocrateans, in: Lloyd, Methods and problems, pp. 398–416, and in: Galen und das hellenistische Erbe, pp. 125–143; D. Manetti and A. Roselli, Galeno commentatore di Ippocrate, in: ANRW II 37,2, Berlin and New York, 1994, pp. 1529–1635.

3 Mansfeld, Prolegomena, passim, shows how discussions of questions of authenticity came to form part of the standard introductory material within the tradition of commentary, even if codification into a fixed order of approaches may have post-dated Galen.

long continued to be copied and read, but little of his writing survives today, except for some short prose Fabulae amatoriae dedicated to the Latin poet, Cornelius Gallus.[1] The nature of his elegiac poems can be discerned from the fact that he joined Callimachus and Euphorion as a favourite author of the emperor Tiberius (Suet., Tib. 70), an association confirmed in an epigram by Pollianus, Anth. Pal. XI 130.[2] Galen's contemporary, Artemidorus, in his Onirocritica (IV 63: p. 287,9–12 Pack), commenting on the many "strange and unusual stories" in his poetry, likens him in style and content to such deliberately obscure poets as Lycophron in his Alexandra. The examples Artemidorus gives of the myths and legends used by these poets, as well as the rare words that make up the bulk of his surviving fragments, show how the elucidation of his choice and allusive vocabulary would have been an appropriate task for a schoolmaster.[3] Nevertheless, there is no reason to trust too much in the historicity of this incident, for the tale of the obscure poet having to step in to confirm his own meaning might have been applied to any of the many learned writers of the Hellenistic and Roman periods.[4] It also exemplified what Galen, and many others in a variety of disciplines, believed about the priority of the "living voice" in determining the doctrine of a particular master, cf. Gal., De comp. med. sec. loc. VI 1: XII 894,1–6 K.; De alim. fac. I 1,47: CMG V 4,2, p. 216,19–27; Gell., Noctes Att. XIV 2,1; Euseb., Hist. eccl. V 10, 4: p. 452,2–5 Schwartz.

P. 54,7 inuenit – 8 uersuum: One of the main tasks of the *grammaticus* was the exposition of the meaning (and etymology) of the words of a chosen text.[5] This was usually taken from Homer or the tragedians, but Statius's father, who taught Greek at Naples around 40 A.D., also commented on such unusual authors as Lycophron, Sophron, and Corinna (Statius, Silvae V 3). Galen's story implies that even contemporary authors might be selected. Since schoolmasters frequently held their classes in the open-air or in a public colonnade, there was nothing to stop passers-by from interfering or joining the debate, see St. F. Bonner, Education in ancient Rome. From the elder Cato to the younger Pliny, Berkeley and Los Angeles, 1977, pp. 116–117; 227–249. A

1 R. A. Pack, The Greek literary texts from Greco-Roman Egypt, 2nd ed., Ann Arbor, 1967, nos. 1337–1338, cf. also nos. 1754; 1783; H. Lloyd-Jones and P. Parsons, Supplementum Hellenisticum, Berlin and New York, 1983 (Texte und Kommentare 11), nos. 605–666.

2 Line six of this epigram may include an example of Parthenius' choice wording.

3 See R. Pfeiffer, A fragment of Parthenios' Arete, Classical Quarterly 37, 1943, pp. 29–32 (repr. in: R. Pfeiffer, Ausgewählte Schriften. Aufsätze und Vorträge zur griechischen Dichtung und zum Humanismus, ed. W. Bühler, Munich, 1960, pp. 142–147). Parthenius' choice vocabulary would have appealed to Galen, a connoisseur of linguistic peculiarities, and may account for his appearance in Galen's preface.

4 In this it resembles the story of the meeting of Erasistratus and the painter reported by an Arab source, but from a possible Greek intermediary, see F. Rosenthal, Four essays on art and literature, Leiden, 1971, p. 4. The story is not given in: Erasistrati fragmenta, ed. I. Garofalo, Pisa, 1988.

5 D. M. Schenkeveld, Scholarship and grammar, in: La philologie grecque à l'époque hellénistique et romaine, ed. F. Montanari, Geneva, 1994 (Entretiens sur l'antiquité classique 40), pp. 263–301.

similar story of an outsider's intervention in a dispute, this time between philosophers, is imagined by Galen at De animi cuiusl. pecc. dign. et cur. 7,2–6: CMG V 4,1,1, pp. 66,1–67,1.

P. 54,19–56,1: Galen's complaint that contemporary doctors rejected both philosophy and proper medicine is a commonplace in his writings, see the passages cited in the testimonia ad loc. But his point here is more fundamental. Grammar is, for him, one of the basics of any education, an honourable art (Protr. 14,4: CMG V 1,1, p. 150,12–14). It is on these grounds that Galen justifies his own substantial studies of the meanings of words, both medical and non-medical, and explains to his audience the necessity for precision of terms and meaning.[1] But one might well doubt how far this perception was shared by other practitioners, or their patients.

P. 56,1 et – complementum: Although Galen throughout his writings aims to instruct the "complete" or "accomplished" physician, at De opt. med. cogn. 11,7: CMG Suppl. Or. IV, p. 123,7–9, he allows that even a physician without total mastery of all medical knowledge might still prove useful and effective. Soranus, Gyn. I 4,2: CMG IV, p. 5,8–10, interestingly defines the "accomplished" midwife as one who just achieves her medical aims, whereas the "best" practitioner will always add something more. The Greek word τέλειος and its cognates, which lie behind the Latin here, are frequently found on inscriptions honouring physicians for their services, see D. Gourevitch, Un thérapeute accompli. Note sur l'adjectif τέλειος, Revue philologique 61, 1987, pp. 95–99.

P. 56,2 potuerunt: The manuscripts are here divided between the perfect (C) and the future tense (β). Since Galen is referring to those who are already practising medicine and doing it badly, the perfect, referring to their past education, is preferable to a reading that would imply that, even if they were, at some future date, to find Galen's works, they would be unable to profit from them. Galen frequently comments on the inability of others to read and understand his writings, and there is no reason to suppose that he envisaged such a situation as still in the future.

P. 56,4 qui – 5 antiqui: In De optimo medico cognoscendo Galen lays down his requirements for the ideal practitioner and advises a potential patient on how to choose a physician when the normal method of personal experience and recommendation is not available.[2] His first criterion is book learning (5,1–3: CMG Suppl. Or. IV, p. 69,1–20). The patient should ask questions that will reveal how well the doctor knows the writings of the ancients, whom Galen defines as Hippocrates, followed, at some distance, by Diocles, Pleistonicus, Phylotimus, Praxagoras, Dieuches, Herophilus, and Erasistratus (all of whom lived and wrote between 350 and 250 B.C.) and by Asclepiades

[1] See M. S. Silk, LSJ and the problem of poetic archaism: from meanings to iconyms, Classical Quarterly, n. s. 33, 1983, pp. 308–309. Galen wrote a tract specifically on medical nomenclature, De nominibus medicis: Galen, Über die medizinischen Namen, ed. and transl. M. Meyerhof and J. Schacht.

[2] See V. Nutton, The patient's choice: a new treatise by Galen, Classical Quarterly, n. s. 40, 1990, pp. 236–257.

(fl. 92 B.C.). The absence of writers from the Empiricist, Pneumatist, or Methodist traditions is instructive. Given that, by 200 A.D., copies of the writings of any of these ancients would have been hard to find, it is likely that information on their doctrines and divergencies would have been most easily located in doxographical handbooks. Surviving fragments of such works, and other (non-Galenic) lists of distinguished physicians in the Hippocratic or 'dogmatist' tradition (e.g. Introd. s. med. 4: XIV 683,6–11 K.), confirm, at least in part, Galen's selection of the good and great, and imply, more generally, that the basis for such doxographies was laid in third-century Alexandria[1], and that relatively few names were later added to the list.

P. 56,6 sed – 10: What did Galen call to witness on his behalf? The manuscript tradition is divided over what Galen mentioned alongside the catalogues of his own books as a guarantee of authenticity, and this dilemma is not helped by Galen's own immediate admission that his somewhat oracular statement requires exemplification to be fully intelligible. But although an exact text and translation of the Latin are impossible to determine, Galen's original meaning has not been entirely lost, and can be reconstructed from parallel passages elsewhere.

At the end of the treatise (pp. 108,25–110,3; 114,8–19 / 108,26–110,2; 114,9–20), Galen makes a triple distinction between the epistemological status of the topics under discussion. Upon some of them he can pronounce with certainty; others he believes have been shown to be plausible, likely to be true, and hence to be provisionally adopted[2]; on others he can reach no decision in any way. Behind the confusion here one can glimpse this same triple division. A comparison with the later passages, where the original Greek survives, shows that "secundum uiam sufficientie" represents some form of πιθανός. "de scientia uirtuosa" would then be a good translation of an Arabic circumlocution for an original Greek adverb or adverbial phrase (βεβαίως). The manuscripts place a full stop after "sufficientie", but "non habeo notitiam" corresponds exactly to an original Greek ἀγνοῶ or ἀπορῶ, and "illud" (line 9) thus depends on "conuoco" as the third type of knowledge. But difficulties still remain. The phrase "de hoc quod probaui", if right, looks backwards either to "composui" or to "sciui", but in neither instance does it give great sense. The best solution is to delete "de", to make this the second type of knowledge, again dependent on "conuoco".[3] Finally, "quod est in ipso" is vague, if not entirely meaningless. Unless the translator misunderstood his source, or corruption had already occurred within the Arabic, we expect some reference to matters that are equivocal or obscure and some linkage to what follows, perhaps "in obscuro ⟨de quo⟩", but I have preferred to obelise. Nonetheless, even if the exact wording of the Latin translation may be be-

1 For the creation of medical doxographies, see J. Kollesch, Untersuchungen zu den pseudogalenischen Definitiones medicae, Berlin, 1973 (Schriften zur Geschichte und Kultur der Antike 7), pp. 78–88; Mansfeld, Doxography, pp. 3058–3060; 3099–3108.

2 See A. Debru, Expérience, plausibilité et certitude chez Galien, in: Galeno: obra, pensamiento e influencia, pp. 31–40.

3 C has unfortunately lost some of the sentence through switching from one "probaui" to the next, and cannot be brought to support any interpretation of this crux.

yond recovery, Galen's overall meaning can still be ascertained, thanks to the parallel passages surviving in Greek.

P. 56,7 quod composui de meis libris: This reference to De libris propriis (Scr. min. II 91–124 Müller = XIX 8–48 K.) and to De ordine librorum suorum (Scr. min. II 80–90 Müller = XIX 49–61 K.) not only helps to establish the authenticity of the present treatise but also explains why it is not mentioned in any of Galen's bibliographical writings: it was written at the very end of Galen's life.

P. 56,7 et probaui – 10: Galen's title and his argument at the end of this section find a close parallel in the life of Plato by Diogenes Laertius, who is generally assumed to have been a contemporary of Galen. At De clar. philos. vitis III 51–52, Diogenes, in answer to the question whether Plato was a dogmatic or a sceptic, states that he was both: "Plato both explains what his opinions are and thoroughly refutes falsehoods: and about doubtful matters he suspends judgment; for what he believes in (περὶ τῶν αὐτῷ δοκούντων), he uses four characters, Socrates, Timaeus, the Athenian Stranger, and the Eleatic Stranger . . ." This triple division becomes even more interesting if Mansfeld (Prolegomena, p. 76) is right to argue that there are links between the lists of Plato's writings drawn up by Diogenes and those by Galen's Platonist teacher, Albinus. But the parallel is at best suggestive, and there is no conclusive reason to believe that Galen deliberately adopted the title and the threefold division directly from a book or in order to allude to a Platonist characterisation of one of his heroes.

P. 56,12–20: Galen's agnosticism (non habeo scientiam), as P. Moraux has amply demonstrated, is based on a sound appreciation of the limitations of experience and logical argument.[1] It is not that he is unwilling ever to make up his mind, or that he regards all the problems to which he refers as incapable of resolution because of their irrelevance to medicine (although his practical bias leads him to underestimate the views of those more theoretically inclined) – to Galen when talking and writing as a philosopher such questions would be highly appropriate.[2] Rather, they cannot be solved either by experiment (De plac. Hipp. et Plat. IX 6,21: CMG V 4,1,2, pp. 576,27–578,1) or by logical demonstration, but are merely rhetorical testpieces (De animi cuiusl. pecc. dign. et cur. 7,11: CMG V 4,1,1, p. 68,2–4). Assent to any conclusion in such an insoluble question is thus the sign of slavish adherence to the doctrines of a sect, not the mark of an independent thinker.

1 Moraux, Der Aristotelismus, vol. II, pp. 785–791. Cf. for a similar appreciation, R. J. Hankinson, Galen's philosophical eclecticism, in: ANRW II 36,5, Berlin and New York, 1992, pp. 3505–3522.

2 Indeed, at De locis affectis III 5: VIII 157,17–159,9 K., Galen takes an apparently more favourable view of these questions: one can choose from among these alternatives in the domain of physics without necessarily contradicting one's own opinion on the seat of the regent part of the soul (on which, as we shall see, Galen did hold a firm view). But Galen in this context is making no claims for the truth or falsity of any position on these disputed question, but using them in order to make the general point that all the dogmata of one sect are not shaken if a single one is refuted; various topics are neither logically consistent nor inconsistent.

Not all have been so generous to Galen. P. L. Donini in his general survey of Galen's philosophy, rightly, if somewhat harshly, remarks that this critical independence is neither particularly profound nor philosophically fruitful if it consists largely in saying "no" to the standard solutions while at the same time accepting, for practical purposes, the conceptual structures just denied. Galen's refusal to commit himself, although at times understandable and praiseworthy, is also bought at a price: an inability to appreciate the problems involved or the subtleties and intellectual weight of the interlocutors in the debate. By concentrating on narrow questions of functional logic, Galen paradoxically comes close to separating one's activities as a human being from the ideas that might sustain them.[1]

Galen's agnosticism, as the testimonia show, was familiar to later philosophers in the Islamic world, and they openly chided him for it. At the very least it proved that he was no philosopher, unworthy to be given the highest title of "sage".[2]

The topics singled out here and elsewhere in this treatise as incapable of resolution one way or the other would have been familiar to any one who had had a minimum of instruction in philosophy. The positions taken up by leading thinkers and by the various philosophical sects had been discussed for centuries, at least since the time of Aristotle, and were recorded in widely read doxographies, like the pseudo-Galenic Historia philosopha (Diels, Doxographi Graeci, pp. 597–648 = XIX 222–345 K.); see Mansfeld, Doxography, who shows brilliantly how pervasive the influence of this doxographical tradition was.

P. 56,12 non habeo – 13 generatus: Galen more than once remarks on the impossibility of coming to any conclusion about whether the world was created or not (see the testimonia). His agnosticism is shared by his contemporary Lucian, who likewise describes the dispute over the creation or non-creation of the world as the best example of a useless, but highly popular, argument (Icaromenippus 8).[3] For a variety of views on the creation of the world, see Diels, Doxographi Graeci, pp. 330,13–332,17; 468,6–469,10; 485,17–491,18; 609,11–610,6; W. Wieland, Die Ewigkeit der Welt, in: Die Gegenwart der Griechen im neueren Denken, Festschrift für Hans-Georg Gadamer zum 60. Geburtstag, ed. D. Henrich, W. Schulz, K.-H. Volkmann-Schluck, Tübingen, 1960, pp. 291–316.

Galen's agnosticism, however, did not prevent him from intervening in the debate in a variety of ways. Firstly, he insisted that there was no logical link between creation and mortality or between immortality and uncreatedness: that was a plausible supposition, but one that was far from proven, De marcore 2: VII 671,12–672,2 K.

1 P. L. Donini, Galeno e la filosofia, in: ANRW II 36,5, Berlin and New York, 1992, pp. 3502–3504.

2 See the version of this condemnation reported by as-Sijistānī, lines 83–87 Dunlop. In general, see also Temkin, pp. 71–94.

3 And, one might add, historically long-lived; cf. Arist., Top. I 11. 14: 104 b 8; 105 b 24–25.

Secondly, in interpreting Plato's Timaeus, the most influential of all ancient books on creation, he emphasised that Plato had believed that the world was created in time. Galen did this both by stressing the active role of the Demiourgos and, if the Arabic text of Compend. Tim. Plat. 17 a: pp. 72–73 Kraus-Walzer is accurate, by making more explicit Plato's own formulations; cf. also ibid. 2 b/c; 8 b: pp. 38–39; 57 Kraus-Walzer. He was thus opposing a tendency, which became even stronger in Porphyry and later Neoplatonism, cf. Ioann. Philop., De aet. mundi VI 2: p. 126,13–18 Rabe, to believe in a world without beginning in time and eternal. In particular, he was taking up a position directly opposed to that of his teacher Albinus (see Procl., In Plat. Tim. comm. II: I 219,2–3 Diehl) who denied there was ever a time when there was no world (see Alcinous [or Albinus], Didasc. 14: p. 32,32–34 Whittaker), as well as that of his contemporaries Calvenus (or Calvisius) Taurus (see Ioann. Philop., De aet. mundi VI 8: p. 145,1–12 Rabe) and Apuleius (see Apul., De Plat. et eius dogm. I 8: p. 97,8–13 Moreschini). For a valuable survey of ancient interpretations of Plato's views on the creation of the world, see M. Baltes, Die Weltentstehung des Platonischen Timaios nach den antiken Interpreten, Leiden, 1976, esp. pp. 43–120, who suggests that Galen was strongly influenced by the ideas of Plutarch and Atticus. See also A. J. Festugière, Le Compendium Timaei de Galien, Revue des Etudes Grecques 65, 1952, esp. pp. 99–105 (repr. in: A. J. Festugière, Etudes de philosophie grecque, Paris, 1971, pp. 489–495), and Dillon, pp. 157–158; 242–244; 252–253; 286–287.

Thirdly, Galen was prepared to concede that there might be powerful arguments in favour of the eternity of the world: the observations of astronomers over the centuries had revealed no alteration in the size of the sun or any other change in the nature of the heavens.[1] Likewise, even in his youthful De exper. med. 19,3: pp. 122–123 Walzer, he was prepared to note the force of a counter-argument against creation, the so-called 'idleness' argument, see Sorabji, pp. 249–252 (the whole of Section III, pp. 193–286, offers an important guide to the debates on the creation and eternity of the world among thinkers of Antiquity and the Early Middle Ages).

Finally, Galen's position of agnosticism is a strictly logical one, and relates to a specific question, whether the world was created or not. In practice, he was a strong upholder of the theory of divine creation, see Larrain, in: Galens Kommentar zu Platons Timaios, pp. 184–186, and R. J. Hankinson, Galen and the best of all possible worlds, Classical Quarterly, n. s. 39, 1989, pp. 206–227. But although most believers in a literal interpretation of Plato's Timaeus and in the activities of a divine creator, Plato's Demiourgos, would have agreed that both the world and matter were created, there were others among Galen's contemporaries who denied that matter itself began and that the world's creation implied of itself such a beginning, cf. Sorabji, pp. 193–195; 268–283; 312–318. Subsequent authors in the Christian, Islamic, and Jewish traditions all took issue with Galen on this point (see above, pp. 39–40). Most notably, Maimonides in his Aphorisms 25,40 criticised Galen's views on

[1] Cf. al-Ghazāli, *Tahāfut al-falāsifā*, p. 82 Bouyges (transl. p. 55 Kamali); Kraus and Walzer, in: Gal. Compend. Tim. Plat., p. 11 (from the alchemical Corpus Gabirianum).

cosmogony (and on the soul) at length for contradicting the Scriptures. But, even here, he was prepared to make a significant concession to Galen; his doubts, the result of his considerable logical ability, could not be resolved by logic alone, but only by the addition of faith, see M. Meyerhof and J. Schacht, Maimonides against Galen on philosophy and cosmogony, Bulletin of the Faculty of Arts of the Egyptian University 5, 1939, pp. 53–76. Cf. also, for a general survey of Arabic criticisms of Galen on this point, Bürgel, pp. 276–290.

P. 56,13: Elsewhere, lines 13 (utrum^{II}). 18; pp. 76,26; 78,23; 80,2, "utrum" is balanced by "aut" or "uel"; here and p. 116,24. 27, it stands alone. Since Ibn Falaquera has "or not", the words may have stood in his Arabic source, but they could easily have dropped out in the transmission process.

P. 56,13 et utrum – 14 extra: The debate between the various philosophical sects on the existence of worlds beyond our own is singled out by Galen at De animi cuiusl. pecc. dign. et cur. 7,8–11: CMG V 4,1,1, pp. 67,8–68,4, as a prime example of a worthless discussion that lacks any compelling argument or demonstrative diagram (as in geometry). It was a topic discussed by Plato in his Timaeus (55 c/d) and reported by all the doxographical writers, see Diels, Doxographi Graeci, pp. 291,10–292,19; 327,7–329,5. The Peripatetics and Platonists considered the cosmos a unity, with nothing outside it, cf. Arist., De caelo I 9: 279 a 9–12; [Gal.], Hist. philos. 32 (7): Diels, Doxographi Graeci, p. 617,4–7 = XIX 249,6–10 K.; the Stoics posited the existence of void beyond the cosmos, cf. M. Pohlenz, Die Stoa. Geschichte einer geistigen Bewegung, 3rd ed., Göttingen, 1964, vol. I, p. 65; vol. II, pp. 37–38; the Epicureans accepted both the existence of void beyond the cosmos and a multiplicity of other worlds beyond our own, see Epic., Epist. ad Herod. 45, and Usener, Epicurea, fr. 301; 304; 306: pp. 213,6–214,4; 214,13–33; 215,4–9.

P. 56,17 de – 19 incorporeum: Once again, Galen draws attention to a common division between the schools. The Middle Platonists of his day believed firmly that God was incorporeal, see e.g. Plut., De def. orac. 29: 426 B; Alcinous, Didasc. 10: p. 25,33–26,14 Whittaker; Justin, Dial. cum Tryph. 1; the Epicureans and most Stoics were equally certain that their gods were corporeal. For a variety of opinions, see Diels, Doxographi Graeci, pp. 292,20–293,1; 301,21–307,3; 464,11–12; 567,7–572,19, and S. R. C. Lilla, Clement of Alexandria, Oxford, 1971, pp. 44–50.

P. 56,20 scilicet – deitatis: Although Galen often talks of the Creator god, he does not use the phrase "divine power" or "powers" to refer to the Creator, although others did (cf. Alex. Aphrod., Quaest. II 3: pp. 47,28–50,25 Bruns). These words are thus likely to be the result of expansion within the process of translation.[1] Nonetheless, Galen's train of thought is clear; he cannot say where God is to be found, but things take place in the world which can come about only through a Creator, who is God (an identification accepted by Galen throughout his writings). The monotheist trend in Galen, who

1 For other examples from the school of Ḥunayn, see G. Strohmaier, Ḥunayn ibn Isḥāq et le serment hippocratique, in: Arabica 21, 1974, pp. 322–323 (repr. in: Strohmaier, Von Demokrit bis Dante, pp. 220–221).

stressed the role of the Divine Creator[1], helped to smooth the transition of Galenism to the Christian and Muslim worlds.

P. 58,1 sicut – 5 earum: The sophist Protagoras of Abdera, c. 490–420 B.C., famously declared that he was unable to know whether the gods existed or not, or what they were like: περὶ μὲν θεῶν οὐκ ἔχω εἰδέναι, οὐθ' ὡς εἰσὶν οὐθ' ὡς οὐκ εἰσὶν οὐθ' ὁποῖοί τινες ἰδέαν (Protag., fr. B 4: II, p. 265,7–8 D.-K.). The evidence of Ibn Falaquera confirms that Galen's original reference to Protagoras survived into Arabic, but the mistaken change to the far more famous Pythagoras of Samos is a simple one and could have been made any time in the subsequent process of transmission in Arabic as well as in Latin.[2] Given the uncertainty over how Pythagoras came to replace Protagoras, I have retained "Pictagoras", a common mediaeval Latin form of Pythagoras, in the text. The feminine forms, "earum", "ipse", "earum", look back to "uirtutes" (line 44) and are another example of the tendency of Arabic translators to avoid suspicions of polytheism.

This particular comment by Protagoras was well known in the second century, being quoted by Diogenes Laertius (De clar. philos. vitis IX 51), Philostratus (Vitae sophist. I 10: II 13,9–12 Kayser), Diogenes of Oenoanda (fr. 16 Smith), and Sextus Empiricus (Adv. math. IX 55). Both Diogenes and Sextus wrongly interpreted the scepticism of Protagoras to indicate a belief in atheism, and Galen may be seeking here to distinguish his own variety of agnosticism from another that was liable to be so misunderstood. He thus makes an important distinction between knowledge of the existence of God and knowledge of God's essence. Galen recognises the activities and existence of God, but denies, at least for the present, that we can know what His essence is. How far this disjunctive argument was original to Galen is not clear, but it differs from those of Philo, who acknowledged the ultimate incomprehensibility of God, even through mystical experience, and of Alcinous / Albinus, who allowed that one might know what God was not, see Sorabji, pp. 158–159.

P. 58,5: "regimen" corresponds to an original Arabic *tadbīr*, which translates both Greek δίαιτα, "regimen" or "lifestyle", and διοίκησις, the general organisation of the body by the Creator, cf. the use of "regere" for διοικεῖν at p. 116,25. But although "regimen" in mediaeval Latin frequently means "rule", its far more usual meaning in medical texts is that of "regimen" or "diet", and a translator who was well acquainted with medical writings was certainly offering a hostage to fortune if he translated a word for "organisation" with one that carried an alternative and more specifically medical meaning.

P. 58,6–7 in diuinationibus et in sompniis: In his acceptance of "divination and dreams" Galen is typical of his contemporaries in the Ancient world.

1 See G. Strohmaier, Galen als Vertreter der Gebildetenreligion seiner Zeit, in: Neue Beiträge zur Geschichte der Alten Welt, ed. E. Ch. Welskopf, Berlin, 1965, pp. 376–377 (repr. in: Strohmaier, Von Demokrit bis Dante, pp. 95–96).

2 Indeed, one manuscript and the editio princeps of Ibn Falaquera's Hebrew both give the wrong reading "Pythagoras".

His whole career had been determined by the "clear dreams" in which Asclepius had appeared to his father Nicon and changed the course of Galen's career from philosophy to medicine (see De praecogn. 2,12: CMG V 8,1, pp. 76, 29–78,3, with parallels); he had been led to revise his plans for studying the eye as a result of a dream (see De usu part. X 12: II 93,5–10 Helmr. = III 812, 14–813,2 K.); and on more than one occasion his treatment of patients was influenced by what he had seen in a dream or by what others had had confirmed for them in a vision (see e.g. De cur. rat. per venae sect. 23: XI 314, 18–315,4 K.; Meth. med. XIV 8: X 971,5–972,5 K.). Although he was prepared to interpret some dreams as indications of a physiological state[1], he was also convinced that others manifested the direct intervention of a god or gods. Indeed, given Galen's attachment to Asclepius[2] and the importance of the great shrine of Asclepius at Pergamum, where sufferers would sleep overnight and receive visions, it is hard to imagine him doing otherwise. At In Hipp. Iusiurandum comm., fr. 1 c: Rosenthal, p. 60, he reports that many people have been cured through dreams and visions sent by Serapis or Asclepius, at Epidaurus, Cos, or Pergamum, his home city, and that 'people in general bear witness to the fact that God has given them the craft of medicine through inspiration in dreams and visions', cf. also Artemid., Onir. IV 22: p. 255,9–13 Pack, for an identical comment, and, somewhat more sceptically, Diog. Oenoand., fr. 15 Smith, who remarked that some believed that φάσματα ἐναργῆ reveal the existence of a Creator. See in general, Kudlien, pp. 117–130; H. Müller, Ein Heilungsbericht aus dem Asklepieion von Pergamon, Chiron 17, 1987, pp. 193–233; O. Weinreich, Antike Heilungswunder. Untersuchungen zum Wunderglauben der Griechen und Römer, Gießen, 1909 (Religionsgeschichtliche Versuche und Vorarbeiten VIII 1), pp. 77–81. Artemidorus (Onir. IV 22: pp. 255,9–258,2 Pack) goes out of his way to emphasise that the gods in healing visions, at Pergamum, Alexandria, and elsewhere, offer cures that are "entirely in line with proper medicine and in no way alien to medical reasoning".[3] Any that cannot be explained in medical terms are the result of incompetence, quackery, and ignorance on the part of the dream-interpreters, not the gods. This is an attitude that would have earned Galen's vigorous approval.

More problematic is "diuinationibus". Ibn Falaquera's "divination, augury" is an expansion of the Arabic, which probably corresponds to an original μαντική. In general, Galen rejects the validity of mantic divination and augury within medicine, whether it involves observing entrails or the flight of birds, horoscopes, or the interpretation of chance events, see, in particular,

1 In Hipp. Epid. I comm. III 1: CMG V 10,1, p. 108,1–24.

2 Whether by calling himself a θεραπευτής of Asclepius Galen was indicating that he had performed a (minor) role in Asclepius cult at Pergamum when a boy (which would have been entirely appropriate for someone of his social class) or merely that he was a worshipper is still disputed; cf. Kudlien, pp. 120–121.

3 There is the possibility that Galen was acquainted with at least some of the works of Artemidorus, if the writer on dreams from Daldis is the same man as the Ἀρτεμίδωρος ὁ Φωκᾶς, who wrote on divination, see Gal., In Hipp. De victu acut. comm. I 15: CMG V 9,1, p. 129,31–33, but the identification is far from certain.

De praecogn. 3,7: CMG V 8,1, p. 84,5–10, with the comments on pp. 169–172. One might imagine, too, that Galen was not entirely in favour of the custom, certainly prominent in his own lifetime, of seeking medical assistance through consulting oracles like that of Apollo at Claros in Asia Minor or the pseudo-prophet, Alexander of Abonuteichos, see L. Robert, Trois oracles de la théosophie et un prophète d'Apollon, Comptes rendus de l'Académie des Inscriptions 1968, pp. 568–599 (repr. in: Robert, Opera minora selecta, pp. 584–615); idem, A travers l'Asie Mineure, Athens, 1980, pp. 393–430; D. Clay, Lucian of Samosata: four philosophical lives (Nigrinus, Demonax, Peregrinus, Alexander Pseudomantis), in: ANRW II 36,5, Berlin and New York, 1992, pp. 3406–3450; S. Mitchell, Anatolia. Land, men, and gods in Asia Minor, Oxford, 1993, vol. II, p. 13. But evidence is constantly accumulating from new discoveries of papyri and inscriptions that Galen's restraint was far from being universal, and, indeed, might well have been a minority view, see, e.g. C. A. Faraone and D. Obbink, Magika Hiera, Princeton, 1991; P. Athanassiadi, Dreams, theurgy and freelance divination: the testimony of Iamblichus, Journal of Roman Studies 83, 1993, pp. 121–127, cf. also R. Gordon, M. Beard, J. Reynolds and Ch. Rouché, Roman inscriptions 1986–90, ibid., pp. 148–150; P. Athanassiadi, Philosophers and oracles, pp. 45–62. Philostratus (Vita Apoll. III 44: I 118,5–22 Kayser) mentions the belief that medicine derives from mantic divination, an idea which the slightly later Iamblichus shared (De myst. 3,3). But Galen's rejection of mantic divination does not necessarily involve a denial of all belief in the possibility of divination or refuse all credence to prophecy. Rather it is based largely on his view that often such divination was used inappropriately or was founded on somewhat shaky premisses, especially when applied to medicine. Had his discussion on dreams, astrology, divination, and the interpretation of signs within the eight books of his exposition of the medicine of Asclepiades survived (see Gal., De fac. nat. I 12: Scr. min. III 121,23–122,3 Helmr. = II 29,7–11 K.; De libris propr. 8: Scr. min. II 115,2–3 Müller = XIX 38,6–7 K.), we would have had a clearer idea of his opinions, but his denunciation of Asclepiades and his followers, who would have included the Methodists[1], for 'despising' such things and for claiming that the gods were indifferent to men, implies at least a certain degree of acceptance.

P. 58,7 sed – 9 suam: Ibn Falaquera's Hebrew version and the Latin differ widely, and it is not easy to decide which preserves Galen's original thought. According to Ibn Falaquera, Galen is here using the providence of God towards his creatures in general as evidence for his existence. The Latin version, as presented in the manuscripts, although requiring emendation, gives a slightly different sense: proof of God's existence can be found through his activities on our behalf when we are in deep trouble. Of the emendations to the Latin proposed in the apparatus, that of J. Kollesch and D. Nickel is perhaps the neatest, and I have followed it in my translation. But, whatever the original Greek, the general thrust of Galen's argument can still be made out.

[1] Note the prescription of the Methodist Soranus for the ideal midwife, Gyn. I 4,4: CMG IV, p. 5,28–30: 'she should be free from superstition, so as not to be distracted from her necessary duties by any dream, portent, customary rite or vulgar religious belief'.

Divine intervention in the world in saving those in need, e.g. sufferers from disease or those in danger of shipwreck, proves that gods exist.

P. 58,10 curauerit – 11 habui: At the end of his life, Galen declared that he had been a worshipper of Asclepius ever since the god had cured him of an abscess (De libris propr. 2: Scr. min. II 99,9–11 Müller = XIX 19,1–3 K.). Scholars have generally identified this with the incident reported in De cur. rat. per venae sect. 23: XI 314,18–315,7 K., when in his youth, and suffering from a chronic pain in the area where the liver met the diaphragm, he had been instructed by two 'clear dreams' (a standard phrase in Asclepius cult) to carry out the extremely dangerous procedure of an arteriotomy in the space between the right index finger and thumb. This may also have been the occasion, around 148 A.D., on which Galen suffered the first of several successive attacks of illness brought on, so he thought, by eating the wrong foods and so severe that he needed to be bled. After his father's death, he suffered a recurrence of the same acute condition, which then recurred annually until he was 28, and which involved at least the threat of an abscess at the point where liver and diaphragm touch. Galen treated it by bleeding, until he finally cured himself by a change of diet (De bonis malisque sucis 1,16–19: CMG V 4,2, pp. 392,25–393,20.[1] It is possible that these passages all refer to the same incident and to the intervention of Asclepius in a dream to give Galen advice on venesection the first time he fell ill, advice which he then followed in subsequent years. But it is also clear from Galen's own account that, dramatic though it may have been, the god's intervention was only partially successful, and eventually Asclepius' recommended method had to be replaced by dietetics.

P. 58,11 et – 14: The Hebrew of Ibn Falaquera provides the key to resolving most of the problems in the second part of the Latin sentence; a compendium "ui^{2}" for "uidetur" was misunderstood as "uir(um)", with a subsequent alteration of "in liberatione" to provide a verb.

That gods could send signs or appear in person to guard or to warn would have been accepted by most of Galen's contemporaries, cf. Diog. Oenoand., fr. 15 Smith. The belief in protecting deities, whether of cities or of individuals, was widespread, and many testimonials survive to the appearance of a god or gods to mortals in time of need, see especially Lane Fox, pp. 102–167. Virtually any god could be hailed as 'Saviour' (see A. D. Nock, Essays on religion and the Ancient World, Oxford, 1972, pp. 720–735) and those rescued from danger, especially drowning, often commemorated their escape by affixing to a temple wall a painted or inscribed tablet, see especially Horace, Carm. I 5,13–16, with the further examples assembled by R. G. M. Nisbet and M. Hubbard, A commentary on Horace: Odes, Book 1, Oxford, 1970, p. 78.

1 D. Gourevitch and M. D. Grmek, Medice, cura te ipsum. Les maladies de Galien, Etudes de Lettres. Revue de la Faculté des Lettres de l'Université de Lausanne, Janvier / Mars 1986, pp. 45–64, confuse the issue by citing, p. 53, a long section from the commentary on Hippocrates' De humoribus (II 2: XVI 222,10–16 K.). This is a renaissance forgery, and the text cited is here made up from the passages already quoted from De libris propr. and De cur. rat. per venae sect.

Cicero (De nat. deorum III 89) tells a nice story of how Diagoras, the notorious atheist, was shown, as proof of the gods' concern for mortals, votive tablets hanging on the temple walls. His response was neat: "That is only because there are none painted for those who are not saved or who die in shipwreck."

If one supposes the same subject in the two "quod" clauses, the subject of "uidetur", too, will be the god. There may then be a particular reference here to Asclepius and to Pergamum, where the god Asclepius was worshipped as 'Saviour', and where at least one of the votive inscriptions at the shrine (no. 63 Habicht) recorded how Asclepius had been instrumental in saving someone from drowning.[1] The rescue by the god of Aemilius Sabinus and Aemilius Herennius from the 'outer sea' (i.e. the Atlantic) and its barbarians occurred within Galen's lifetime, to judge from the lettering on the stone, and such an unusual incident may not have gone unnoticed by Galen.

Still more likely, given their acquaintance, at least at a distance (see Gal., In Plat. Tim. comm. IV: CMG Suppl. I, p. 33), is Galen's familiarity with the nautical adventures of the orator and hypochondriac Aelius Aristides. In many of his speeches, Aristides referred to dangerous incidents during a variety of voyages. In the earliest of his orations to survive, he celebrated his salvation from a storm at sea by the god Sarapis (Or. 45,32). A few years later, when sailing between the two Asia Minor ports of Clazomenae and Phocaea, he was only saved from shipwreck by making a vow to Zeus (Or. 43,2–3), and by the direct intervention of Asclepius (Or. 48,12–14). On yet another occasion, off Delos, he was again caught in a storm, from which he had to be rescued by Asclepius (Or. 48,68). No wonder then that, towards the end of his life, in one of his formal addresses to Asclepius, he emphasised how Asclepius had often appeared to sailors in trouble and stretched out his hand to help (Or. 42,10). The words of Aristides also found expression on stone, for a florid inscription from the Asclepieion (no. 145 Habicht) bears one of his hymns to the god, in which, in recherché language, he describes (lines 5–8) his encounters with storm and near-shipwreck; see also R. Herzog, Ein Asklepios-Hymnus des Aristeides von Smyrna, SB d. Preuß. Akademie d. Wiss., phil.-hist. Kl. 1934, Berlin, 1934, pp. 753–769, whose arguments for Aristides' authorship still remain convincing despite the criticisms of C. A. Behr, Aristeides and the Sacred Tales, Amsterdam, 1968, p. 52 n. 44.

However, Ibn Falaquera appears to distinguish the two subjects; the former relates specifically to the cure by Asclepius, the latter, "what (can be seen)", to the sign, not to Asclepius. G. Strohmaier in his review of Zonta's book (Orientalistische Literaturzeitung 92, 1997, cols. 368–369) takes this distinction still further. He quotes al-Bīrūnī, who explains in his Chronology how many scholars, including Galen, interpreted the appearance of St. Elmo's fire around the masthead of ships as a sign of divine intervention. Except for the fact that in antiquity this phenomenon was associated with the Dioscuri, not

1 Habicht also notes the frequent naming of ships after Asclepius, presumably to secure his assistance in times of danger. Cf. also P. Oxy. 1381, a dedication to Imouthes, often identified with Asclepius, from a man saved from shipwreck; and Inscriptiones Graecae XII 5,712 (Syros), a dedication to Asclepius to protect from shipwreck.

Asclepius, Strohmaier argues, the rather sceptical Galen cannot be referring here to a miraculous apparition of Asclepius[1] but to an observation of St. Elmo's fire that he had made himself and to a belief in the saving consequences of that sign. The whole thrust of Galen's argument is that the existence of divinity is revealed by certain interventions and actions in this world, a formulation that encompasses Asclepius, although it is by no means confined to any one god.

P. 58,17 et – 20 firmius: Since there were no specific laws regulating religious belief in Galen's time, it is unlikely that when he declared his intention of 'following the law' he had a particular religious doctrine in mind. Nor need we see here an allusion to Socrates' decision in 399 B.C., argued at length in Plato's Crito (50 b–54 c) to accept the laws of Athens and his condemnation for impiety, even though he considered himself entirely guiltless. Rather, the parallel passage in De placitis Hippocratis et Platonis (IX 7,13–15: CMG V 4,1,2, p. 588,22–29) suggests that Galen is referring to Socrates' comments, reported by Xenophon in his Memorabilia (I 1,11–16), on the uselessness of many types of philosophical inquiry. Many questions about the natural world, e.g. on creation and decay, were, in the opinion of Socrates, incapable of resolution and were likely to lead only to frenzied and futile argument. If forced to choose, he was prepared to follow "customary usage", νόμος. The Arabic equivalent, *sunna,* covers both customary religious usage and legal prescript; Ibn Falaquera's "religion" keeps the right nuance, while the Latin translator's version is less satisfactory.

P. 58,22 Sed – 60,6: Much of this treatise is taken up with questions relating to the soul; as well as chapters 3 and 7, the final chapters also discuss the soul and its activities. Such a concentration of effort is particularly striking in an author who on many occasions claims to eschew such speculation as irrelevant, impractical, and non-medical. If one also considers that the years after 185 also saw his works De moribus, De affectuum et peccatorum dignotione, and probably also Quod animi mores corporis temperamenta sequantur[2], then Galen must have devoted a considerable amount of time in his old age to reflecting on this inscrutable theme, alongside other more strictly medical topics. Even though, throughout his life, he continually professes ignorance of the soul's essence and immortality, these are questions to which he often returns, sometimes even in whole treatises, see below, pp. 142–144, comm. to p. 60,3–6, and always inconclusively. All this implies a certain inquietude in Galen, although it would be going too far to see in him a prime

1 Cf. Kudlien, p. 127.

2 For the date of De moribus see Walzer, New light, p. 83 (repr. in: Walzer, Greek into Arabic, p. 144), with the comments of S. M. Stern, Some fragments of Galen's On dispositions (Περὶ ἠθῶν) in Arabic, Classical Quarterly, n. s. 6, 1956, p. 97 n. 1 (repr. in: S. M. Stern, Medieval Arabic and Hebrew thought, ed. F. W. Zimmermann, London, 1983, no. III). A positive reference to the behaviour of slaves under torture following the failure of the revolt of Perennis (185 A.D.) is hardly likely to have been made public until after the death of the blood-thirsty emperor Commodus in 192. The later De moribus is dated, the later the others that cite it.

example of an inhabitant of E. R. Dodds' 'age of anxiety'.[1] Given his reluctance to commit himself to any sectarian opinion and the difficulties involved in discussing many of these part-religious, part-philosophical topics, such uncertainty is hardly surprising, and it did not prevent him from investigating other questions in this area to which he was confident that firm solutions could be found.

P. 58,23 secundum – 60,1 populus: It is one of the strengths, as well as one of the weaknesses, of Galen's philosophical position that he preferred to take as his starting point in debate 'what everybody knows', or, as he liked to put it, 'what is clearly visible', τὰ ἐναργῆ or τὰ ἐναργῶς φαινόμενα. It came close to, although it did not entirely coincide with, his claim that the axioms of a science must be self-evident and self-guaranteeing (see Gal., Inst. log. 1, 4–5: p. 4,8–22 Kalbfleisch). It was an index of Galen's metaphysical realism, as Hankinson (Galen, On the therapeutic method, pp. 123; 131) puts it, that if, as seems likely, Galen intended the phrase to be understood in the strong sense that such a proposition would be agreed by all fair-minded participants in the debate, or even by everyone, there could be no disagreement about the foundations of any subsequent argument deriving therefrom. The preference for starting from 'what everyone knows' was one of Galen's weapons against Scepticism, see Ph. De Lacy, Galen's response to skepticism, Illinois Classical Studies 16, 1991, pp. 283–306; Hankinson, Galen on the foundations, pp. 15–29, and would have been readily welcomed by Peripatetics and Stoics, cf. Clem. Alex., Strom. VIII 7,3. Others would have been less certain of the value of such 'common notions', cf. Plutarch's tract On common notions, against the Stoics (De communibus notitiis contra Stoicos: 1058 E–1086 B), which points to the possibility that what everyone knows is not necessarily true. Besides, as Lloyd points out, many of the premisses that Galen chooses to regard as evident are frequently open to challenge, and many of his impeccably logical constructions rest on dubious foundations.[2] But, in Galen's defence, it can be argued that by accepting as a starting point something agreed with an opponent, he was allowing the possibility of dialogue between them in the pursuance of truth. This procedure comes close to that advocated by another distinguished scientist of the day, Ptolemy, see P. Manuli, Claudio Tolomeo: Il criterio e il principio, Rivista critica di Storia della Filosofia 36, 1981, pp. 64–88; A. A. Long, Ptolemy On the criterion: an epistemology for a practising scientist, in: The question of eclecticism, ed. J. M. Dillon and A. A. Long, Berkeley, 1988, pp. 176–207. Given that, in the absence of modern investigative tools, scientists in Antiquity inevitably relied on logic to explicate, develop, and, indeed, go beyond empirical evidence, any investigation that took as its starting

1 See E. R. Dodds, Pagan and Christian in an age of anxiety, Cambridge, 1965, pp. 45–50; G. W. Bowersock, Greek sophists in the Roman Empire, Oxford, 1969, p. 74. Galen's individual soul-searching is not affected by the demonstration of R. MacMullen (The Roman government's response to crisis, New Haven, 1976; Paganism in the Roman Empire, New Haven, 1981, pp. 49–73) that Dodds and Bowersock exaggerated the extent of the political and spiritual crisis.

2 G. E. R. Lloyd, Theories and practices of demonstration in Galen, in: Rationality in Greek thought, ed. M. Frede and G. Striker, Oxford, 1996, pp. 255–277.

point what was then universally known or agreed was more likely to lead to fruitful results than one that did not.

P. 60,1–3: Galen regularly links voluntary motion and sensation together, especially since they are, in his (and Aristotle's) opinion the two features that distinguish animals from all other living beings, and he treats their cause or origin as identical.[1] In his claim that "all men" called their source the soul, he is rejecting by implication the objections of Sceptical philosophers to any such formulation. Such 'boorish Pyrrhonism' (cf. Gal., De praecogn. 5,15: CMG V 8,1, p. 98,8), a reluctance to concede any of the basic premisses on which Galen believed his (and any) medical science should be constructed, he opposed vigorously both in theory and when he met it in real life. His broad formulation, however, is designed to include Stoics, Peripatetics, Platonists, Epicureans, and medical investigators, even if their individual interpretations of this common definition might differ considerably. Epicurus' understanding of the soul as a blend of four elements (Usener, Epicurea, fr. 315: p. 218,20–31), two of which are ultimately responsible for movement (pneuma) and sensation (the "unnamed element"), can hardly be reconciled with the unitary views of the Stoics or with the Platonist, and largely Galenic, opinion that related both voluntary motion and sensation to one part of the soul and to pneuma alone.[2]

P. 60,3–6: Galen's agnosticism about the substance of the soul was a conviction that he expressed throughout his life (see the testimonia), even if, in practice, he was inclined to favour a physicalist interpretation, most notably in Quod animi mores corporis temperamenta sequantur, as one that corresponded best both to what Plato had written and to the data of medical experience. Like most doxographers, Galen mentions first the question of the substance of the soul, and then the question of the soul's mortality, with the implication that if the first and simpler question cannot be resolved[3], it is unlikely that the latter, more difficult one can be so.[4] The presentation of arguments in this way, as a series of either / or divisions, is singled out by Mansfeld, Doxography, as a characteristic of Aetius and the so-called Vetusta placita, but there is no reason to think that Galen was here relying directly on a handbook to organise his thoughts.

The question of the mortality or immortality of the soul was standard in the doxographical tradition, if not in ancient philosophy in general, and it

1 The reading of C γ (uoluntarius), which wrongly identifies the cause with motion and sensation, depends on a scribal misunderstanding of "motus" as nominative; that of ε (uoluntarii) is a correction that corresponds to the sense.

2 For the difficulties in interpreting the view of Epicurus, see G. B. Kerferd, Epicurus' doctrine of the soul, Phronesis 16, 1971, pp. 80–96; Long and Sedley, vol. 2, pp. 68–69.

3 At one point in his writings, De trem., palp., convuls. et rig. 6: VII 616,4–617,2 K., written between 169 and 176, Galen's agnosticism weakens and he identifies the soul or nature with the body's innate heat. But his formulation here is that of an aside, and could merely indicate the opinion that he thought most plausible for his present purposes and one wherein one "might not go far wrong".

4 Cf. the scheme for ordering such questions put forward by Ioann. Philop., In Arist. De anima comm.: CAG XV, pp. 32,30–33,15.

provided an opportunity for debate even within individual philosophical schools.[1] That Plato had believed in an immortal soul was widely accepted, but what precisely he had meant by this was far from clear, even among Platonists (cf. Procl., In Plat. Tim. comm. V: III 234,8–18 Diehl). There was considerable dispute over whether Plato had advocated the introduction of an immaterial and incorporeal soul into the body (see Galens Kommentar zu Platons Timaios, fr. 6: p. 67,1–5 Larrain) and whether he had believed that each part of the tripartite soul was equally immortal. Indeed, it was hotly debated whether the word "mortal" was to be taken in a literal or a figurative sense (see Gal., De plac. Hipp. et Plat. IX 9,8–14: CMG V 4,1,2, p. 600,4–30). Modern scholars on the whole agree with Galen's somewhat despairing conclusion that Plato was not totally self-consistent in his ideas on the soul. See also pp. 104,15–106,2.

Galen, although confident of the tripartition of the soul, takes a line apparently independent of all other Platonists. Whereas most interpreters of the Timaeus had argued for the immortality of the irrational as well as the rational soul, Galen seems to have moved from an agnostic view of the immortality of *all* parts of the soul (De plac. Hipp. et Plat. IX 9,8: CMG V 4,1,2, p. 600,5–10) to that expressed in De moribus (2: p. 248 Mattock) and Quod animi mores corporis temperamenta sequantur (3: Scr. min. II 36,16–19 Müller = IV 773,3–6 K.), which asserts the mortality of the two lower, irrational, parts of the Platonic soul as argued in the Timaeus (cf. also Compend. Tim. Plat. XVII a. c: pp. 72–73; 74 Kraus-Walzer). This was an interpretation favoured especially by Atticus and by Galen's teacher Albinus (so Procl., In Plat. Tim. comm. V: III 234,8–18 Diehl); see De Lacy, in: CMG V 4,1,2, p. 707, the note to p. 600,7–10, for possible qualifications. For a variety of Platonic views, cf. Dillon, pp. 256; 260; 292; 315–317; 350; 377; P. A. Vander Waerdt, Peripatetic soul-division, Posidonius, and Middle Platonic moral psychology, Greek, Roman, and Byzantine Studies 26, 1985, pp. 373–394; A. S. Mason, Immortality in the Timaeus, Phronesis 39, 1994, pp. 90–97. But Galen seems to go further than most in his criticisms of arguments for the immortality of the rational soul, allowing in De moribus (2: p. 40 Kraus) for a belief in the total mortality of the soul, and in Quod animi mores corporis temperamenta sequantur (3: Scr. min. II 37,16–39,4 Müller = IV 774,7–776,10 K.) accepting some strong criticisms of the Platonic position. Not only does he make fun of Plato's belief in immortality, but he points out the logical implication of interpreting the Platonic soul in an Aristotelian way – all its parts must be mortal.[2] Whether this represents a change of position on the part of Galen, or the

[1] See Mansfeld, Doxography, especially pp. 3965–3092. Galen's attack on Asclepiades' views on the essence of the soul, De libris propr. 8: Scr. min. II 115,3–4 Müller = XIX 38,8 K., which would have given an insight into a non-Platonic theory, is now lost.

[2] The conclusions of this hypothesis are spelled out again strongly in three lines deleted by Müller, p. 38,2–4, and ascribed by him, p. XXXVII, to the zeal of a schoolmaster wishing to make his point clearly. But these lines were already present when the Arabic translation was made (see p. 43 Biesterfeldt), and I am inclined to view them as genuine. It should perhaps be pointed out that a claim that some parts of the soul are not immor-

logician in him pursuing the consequences of a hypothesis without necessarily assenting to it, there is, at the least, an alteration in the tone of Galen's answers over the years, and he is no longer the dutiful adherent of Plato that he appears in his earlier writings. See, for important discussions of this shift, L. García Ballester, Alma y enfermedad en la obra de Galeno. Traducción y comentario del escrito Quod animi mores corporis temperamenta sequantur, Valencia and Granada, 1972 (Cuadernos hispánicos de historia de la medicina y de la ciencia XII, ser. A), pp. 181–200; P. L. Donini, Tre studi sull'Aristotelismo nel II secolo d. C., Turin et al., 1974 (Historica – Politica – Philosophica. Il pensiero antico – Studi e testi 7) , pp. 134–139; Moraux, Der Aristotelismus, vol. II, pp. 773–791; Lloyd, Scholarship, pp. 13–19; Singer, pp. 41–55; Hankinson, Galen's anatomy of the soul, pp. 197–233.

P. 60,8–62,2: De placitis Hippocratis et Platonis, one of Galen's greatest works, was a restatement in Platonic terms of the consequences of his own anatomical discoveries. In this book, he took strong issue with the Peripatetics, Stoics and Chrysippus, especially for their belief in a unitary soul, relying on his own anatomical observations on the three major organs (and, in his opinion, the three independent systems) of the body to confirm the truth of the tripartition asserted by Plato in the Republic and the Timaeus. Since Plato had commended Hippocrates' method of dialectic and praised him for being a great teacher, Galen saw no difficulty in taking the next step and arguing that Plato's medical knowledge derived from that of Hippocrates. To prove this, he produced a variety of texts from the Hippocratic Corpus which showed, to his own satisfaction, if not to that of modern scholars, that the great Hippocrates also believed in tripartition. But Galen's belief in tripartition did not depend on what Hippocrates or Plato had said, although the support of these witnesses gave added authority to his own pronouncements, but on what he thought he had observed in practice and on his own arguments from first principles. Together they moved the argument from the merely plausible to the certain. See Lloyd, Galen on Hellenistics and Hippocrateans, in: Lloyd, Methods and problems, pp. 398–416, and in: Galen und das hellenistische Erbe, pp. 125–143.

Galen's conviction that many of the ideas that he attributed to the historical Hippocrates could also be found in Plato, and vice-versa, had a significant consequence, which is exemplified here. Galen slides from talking about the soul's mortality or corporeality to a statement of the location of the three sources of activity, and then to a discussion of various bodily processes. In his view, as expressed at De plac. Hipp. et Plat. VI 8,57–58: CMG V 4,1,2, p. 418, 29–35, this shift presented no problems. He was merely talking in medical language about what a philosopher, speaking to philosophers, would think of as powers or faculties of the soul. There was an underlying unity of doctrine, even if it was expressed in different ways. Not everyone would be convinced, see above, pp. 141–142, the note to pp. 58,23–60,1, and, as this treatise shows, Galen's frequent moves from a strictly medical topic to one less medi-

tal does not exclude the possibility that they may survive the separation of soul and body for a considerable time.

cal are disconcerting for those who do not share his view of the close relationship between medicine and philosophy. See P. N. Singer, Levels of explanation in Galen, Classical Quarterly, n. s. 47, 1997, pp. 525–542.

P. 60,8–10: Since the opening of De placitis Hippocratis et Platonis has been lost, it is impossible to tell how Galen there justified its composition, and whether this is a direct quotation from it. Certainly he was familiar with the Platonic phrase, εἰς τὸ λήθης γῆρας (Phaedr. 276 d), for he used it at least twice in his works, De puls. diff. III 3: VIII 657,10–11 K.; Meth. med. VII 1: X 456,10–11 K. Only in the latter passage does he use the same verb as Plato (θησαυρίζεσθαι), but in both instances he refers to the treatise in question as a ὑπόμνημα. The presence of "memoria" in the Latin suggests that the same word appeared in the original Greek here. G. Strohmaier supposes that the phrase "defensio et memoria" represents a hendiadys, *ḥifẓ wa-dhikr*, in the Arabic version, because *ḥifẓ* can mean both defence and memorial.

P. 60,10–12 epate: From the substance and mortality of the soul, Galen makes a standard transition to consider the individual parts of the soul, see Mansfeld, Doxography, p. 3084.

P. 60,11 et – incorporea: The corporeality or incorporeality of the soul was a question that was separately debated from its mortality or immortality. Most Platonists, e.g. Harpocration, Albinus, Alcinous, and Numenius, considered it, either in whole or in part, incorporeal or immaterial (see Dillon, pp. 261; 293; 375); the Epicureans believed that it was something material (Epic., Epist. ad Herod. 63); and the Stoics identified it with *pneuma*. The doxographical tradition placed Aristotle firmly among those who considered the soul to be incorporeal, as the enmattered form of the body, but several of the Peripatetics, arguably rightly, interpreted Aristotle in such a way as to eliminate any suggestion of a body / soul dualism. Galen's contemporary, Alexander of Aphrodisias, for example, believed that it was the result of a mixture of the bodily elements (e.g. Alex. Aphrod., De anima: p. 24,21–24 Bruns; but cf. Quaest. II 9: p. 54,24–26 Bruns); see P. L. Donini, L'anima e gli elementi nel De anima di Alessandro di Afrodisia, Atti della Accademia di Scienze di Torino, Classe di Scienze morali, storiche e filologiche 105, Turin, 1970, pp. 1–47. Galen, as already noted above (pp. 143–144, the note to p. 60,3–6), seems to favour corporeality, at least in his last writings, and his arguments there are similar to, although not identical with, those of Alexander, as the eleventh-century Aristotelian commentator Michael of Ephesus observed (In Arist. Parva nat. comm.: CAG XXII 1, p. 135,22–30); cf. also Moraux, Der Aristotelismus, vol. I, pp. 132–134; vol. II, p. 742 n. 223. Galen returns to this question more fully at pp. 116,20–120,14.

P. 60,11 principium – 12 epate: As he goes on to make clear (p. 108,4–8), Galen is not talking here of movement in any spatial sense, for plants also have this movement, but of movement in the widest sense, including both voluntary and involuntary movement; the heart is the source of pulsation, the brain of volition and sensation; see Gal., De plac. Hipp. et Plat. II 8, 24–25; VI 3,4–5: CMG V 4,1,2, pp. 160,36–162,6; 372,29–374,4.

P. 60,14–18: That the nerves, the conduits of voluntary motion, took their origin from the brain, not the heart, was demonstrated by Galen anatomically. In his syllogistic argument on the soul, this formed the minor premiss of what he called the "only scientifically formulated argument". The major premiss, "agreed by all physicians and philosophers", was that the governing part of the soul was located where the beginning of the nerves was (see Gal., De plac. Hipp. et Plat. I, III–V: CMG V 4,1,2, pp. 66,13–68,25), and Galen's conclusion, directed against Chrysippus and the Stoics, was that this was the brain, or, at least, not the heart alone.

That voluntary movement and sense perception come from the brain is a commonplace in Galen's writings. "perceptio que est omnium sensibilium" should correspond to αἴσθησις πάντων τῶν αἰσθητῶν; cf. Gal., De plac. Hipp. et Plat. VII 8,1: CMG V 4,1,2, p. 474,31, and the thrust of Galen's argument is thus that perception is brought about in a similar way to voluntary motion in that external sensibilia are perceived as a result of activity and movement coming from the brain; cf. Gal., De plac. Hipp. et Plat. VII 8,3–4: CMG V 4,1,2, p. 476,3–11.

P. 60,18–19 motus operationis pulsus: Galen talks of the source of "pulsative motion", De plac. Hipp. et Plat. VI 3,5; VII 3,2: CMG V 4,1,2, pp. 374,1–2; 440,2–3, and of "motion in the pulses", ibid. II 4,49: p. 128,4. These parallels suggest that we should keep both "motus" and "operationis" ("movement involved in pulse activity"), and that the readings of C and B represent attempts to simplify the ungainly series of genitives. C omits "motus"; B inserts "et" and deletes "quod^I" (line 19), making "pulsus" the subject of the following sentence.

P. 60,19 quod^I – 62,2: Galen's view of pulsation is significantly different from that of modern physiologists. In his view, just as the nerves communicate sensation from the brain, so the arteries communicate a pulsative movement from the heart to the rest of the body. But this movement is not, as in modern physiology, one within the arteries, but is contained in the actual coats of the artery, which are so constructed as to have the potentiality for expansion and contraction, just like the heart itself. Indeed, the heat and the consequent sooty waste produced within the heart actualise these potentialities within the arterial coats and the heart at one and the same time; one might think of a pulse impulse in the same way as of a nerve impulse. Both heart and artery thus expand and contract simultaneously in accordance with the pulsative power that reaches them together (see Gal., An in art. nat. sanguis contin. 7,3; 8,4: pp. 176,3–4; 178,27–180,1 Furley-Wilkie = IV 730,16–17; 733,17–734,1 K.; De usu puls. 4,2: p. 208,17–210,13 Furley-Wilkie = V 163, 17–164,13 K.; De fac. nat. III 14: Scr. min. III 249,14–16 Helmr. = II 204,11–13 K.). The innate heat, which helps to sustain all parts of the body, is largely retained in the left ventricle of the heart, where one of its functions is to prepare the thinner arterial blood from the thicker venous blood as well as the *pneuma*, which in turn acts both as nutriment and as coolant. It is the innate heat which is the source of physiological activity (and as such is not confined to the heart). Galen uses, with appropriate caution, the simile of the innate heat as a fire, sustained by blood and *pneuma* (De respir. usu 3,8–9: pp. 106, 13–108,10 Furley-Wilkie = IV 490,12–492,10 K.) and it is the action of the fire, blazing up and down, and producing smoky residues, that Galen sees as the prime cause of pulsation. For Galen's ideas on the pulse, see Harris, pp. 397–431.

But we are still some way from linking anger with innate heat, and from ascribing a belief in their physicality to Plato and Hippocrates. That courage and anger were located in the heart was the view of Plato, especially in the Republic and the Timaeus, and in his major discussion at De plac. Hipp. et Plat. VI 1: CMG V 4,1,2, pp. 360,4–366,30, Galen explained how Plato's spirited soul, as revealed in anger or grief, could be interpreted in terms of the movement of the pulse. This strongly physicalist interpretation of the diagnosis and cause of passions was confirmed for Galen by what he had seen in his clinical practice, for he claimed, especially in De praecognitione (CMG V 8,1) and in his final commentary on Epidemics VI: CMG V 10,2,2, pp. 485,17–487, 36; 494,8–495,2, that he was an expert in understanding the interrelation between psychic and physical imbalance, see, above all, García Ballester, pp. 117–152; Pigeaud, pp. 153–183; P. Manuli, La passione nel De placitis Hippocratis et Platonis, in: Le opere psicologiche, pp. 185–214.

But if Galen found no difficulty in moving directly from a discussion of the cause of the pulse to a comment about the physical causes of anger or in locating the seat of anger within the heart (cf. Gal., In Hipp. Epid. II comm. VI: CMG V 10,1, p. 361,7–43) – for, in his view, Plato had merely expounded in a philosophical manner the facts of medical knowledge –, it required some ingenious exegesis to relate this to Hippocrates and to innate heat. Leaving aside De corde (6: IX 84,9 L.), a late tract in the Hippocratic Corpus not utilised by Galen, the words τὸ ἔμφυτον θερμόν are found only at Aphorisms I 14. 15: IV 466,8. 15 L., in a famous passage that describes the decline in "innate heat" between growth and old age, cf. p. 64,11–13. This was enough for Galen to conclude that Hippocrates himself had believed in the importance of innate heat, and together with an observation in Epidemics II 5,16: V 130,18–20 L., that a man whose vein pulsated at the elbow was more likely to be angry than one whose vein did not, it established to Galen's satisfaction that the connection between anger and pulsation was well known to Hippocrates (cf. De plac. Hipp. et Plat. VI 8,42–47: CMG V 4,1,2, p. 416,16–36).[1] There was thus no doubt in his mind that both Hippocrates and Plato were talking about one and the same thing, albeit in slightly different language, and Galen could assert without further comment that a greater amount of innate heat had been given to the heart than the liver precisely in order to assist in the production of anger (In Hipp. Epid. VI comm. V 5: CMG V 10,2,2, p. 274,3–5). In turn, his belief that the heart and, in particular, the pulse, help to maintain the proper level of heat throughout the body (cf. De usu puls. 3,3; 8,1: pp. 206,2–3; 226, 6–7 Furley-Wilkie = V 161,2–3; 179,6–7 K.), provides a physical counterpart to the Platonic role of the second part of the soul as the soul's regulator.

P. 62,1 tamen – quantitas: The agreement of C and O confirms the reading "tamen", which in its standard abbreviated form (t̃m) was very easily misread as "cum". But if the subject of the sentence is heat, we should expect

[1] Given that, in Hippocratic Greek, the word φλέψ meant simply "vessel", Galen's equivocation of vein and artery is less surprising than it might seem at first sight.

"hic", not "hoc", and the genitive "parue quantitatis" is difficult to construe. The simplest solution is to follow β in making "parua quantitas" the subject, and to supply "de".

P. 62,3: "motus" is used in the sense of active change (cf. Gal., De fac. nat. I 2: Scr. min. III 105,15–16 Helmr. = II 7,2 K.), in particular in growth and nutrition. Galen, following a generally Aristotelian line, distinguishes these vital properties, which are common to all living things, and some even shared with inanimate objects (e.g. the lodestone has the capacity to attract certain objects), from the 'psychic' powers peculiar to the higher orders of creation.

P. 62,4 in tribus dictionibus: Not three separate treatises, but one treatise in three books, On the natural faculties (Scr. min. III 101–257 Helmr. = II 1–214 K.). The word is a neat rendering of the Arabic *maqāla*, which is cognate with *qāla*, "he said".

P. 62,5 uirtus[I] – 7: The manuscripts are inconsistent both between themselves and in their own readings as to the case of the relative (qua / que) that follows "uirtus". Since Galen views these faculties as instruments in the process of nutrition and growth rather than as performing the process themselves, the instrumental ablative case is preferable to the nominative, and I have regularised to "qua". The reflexive "sibi" (lines 5. 7) also points the same way, and indicates that the unnamed subject of the relative clause is the living thing, not the faculty.

P. 62,8–12: Galen expresses his agnosticism about what exactly forms the embryo in the womb in several places and he returns at greater length to the subject in chapter 11. His formulation here does not correspond exactly to what he says elsewhere in his writings. In particular, although he is convinced that everything living has the four natural faculties, this is the only place where he floats the possibility that the formative substance of the embryo is made up solely of the four faculties. However, at De sem. I 6,1–2: CMG V 3,1, p. 84,16–20, he declares that the semen that enters the uterus possesses all four properties, and has congenial material to work on in blood and pneuma. Hence, if one followed the (generally Aristotelian) line that semen gave form to the matter of menstrual blood, one could argue that it was not the semen as such, but the faculties contained therein that actually formed the embryo. But Aristotle did not choose to speak in terms of faculties, let alone the four later identified by Galen. At De fac. nat. I 6: Scr. min. III 111,24–112,4 Helmr. = II 15,10–15 K., Galen himself posits a "shaping faculty" different from the other four natural faculties, and "artistic" in the sense that it does everything for a purpose. But neither here nor anywhere else in his writings does he finally decide on what this "shaping faculty" is, and he returns again in ch. 11,1 (p. 90,18–20) to the identification of this "more subtle substance". Some of his agnostic arguments are further expounded in the final section of De foet. form. 6: IV 700,5–701,7 K. On the one hand, Galen cannot believe that something purely material or even the soul contained in semen can have produced such a marvellous work of art as Man, for that required wisdom and reason. On the other hand, the likeness of children to their parents suggests a material cause, as does the inability of the rational soul to control and organise the body completely after birth.

P. 62,10 istarum quatuor uirtutum: "uirtus", "faculty", is one of the most difficult concepts in Galenic physiology to define, not least because it encompasses a series of overlapping meanings. It is firstly the cause of some active change or motion; as a good Aristotelian Galen was well aware that something could happen only if there was also the potentiality, capacity, or faculty for it to do so. But at the same time it is also a shorthand term used by Galen to denote a cause whose true essence is unknown; see De fac. nat. I 4: Scr. min. III 107,14–20 Helmr. = II 9,13–10,1 K. So there is a blood-making faculty in the veins, and a pulsatile faculty in the heart, and a special faculty in every other part corresponding to the activity of that part (cf. pp. 86,17–88,5 / 86, 19–88,5). From one point of view, Galen is merely multiplying entities unnecessarily, for two different actions might well be brought about by the same, but unknown, cause, and his followers, particularly in the Renaissance, were roundly criticised for what seemed to their opponents a mere passion for tautology. But this is unfair to Galen, not least because of his implication that if the essence of the particular cause were to become known, it would no longer need to be called a faculty. It is also important to note that he takes a physicalist view of faculties: they are the result of a particular combination of elements or qualities at the remotest micro-level of the organism (see De fac. nat. I 3; III 7: Scr. min. III 106,4–107,7; 221,24–222,4 Helmr. = II 7,15–9,6; 167,4–11 K.). There is no way that Galen could 'see' such a faculty, and his hypothesis is the result of a logical meditation on the ideas of philosophers and physicians. As such, it is far from foolish. Since he favoured a definition of illness in terms of a damage to function, he could explain it in terms of not only gross anatomy, but also invisible changes taking place within the living body. The discoveries of modern bio-medicine, above all of DNA, have shown how many disease conditions can be traced back to the very micro-level of an organism. Not only obvious genetic disorders, like spina bifida or Down's syndrome, but many cancers and diseases that manifest themselves only at a later stage, e.g. Alzheimer's disease, are now shown to have an origin in the ultimate genetic make-up of the individual. Galen's faculties, it can be agreed, had no immediate value in therapeutics – but neither, as yet, does the knowledge that Down's syndrome is the result of a chromosome defect help in the treatment of a Down's syndrome child, once born –, yet as an explanation for changes taking place (or not taking place) within the body they were neither foolish nor unwarranted.

Galen believed that in his treatise De facultatibus naturalibus he had proved that every living thing has these four faculties or powers, "uirtutes", at a very minimum, although the number of such faculties is limited only by the number of effects whose cause is unknown. At times Galen's own names for them confuse as much as they enlighten, not least when turned into Latin. As p. 108,17 shows, the translator, somewhat unfortunately, translates δύναμις ἀλλοιωτική, the alterative faculty, as "uirtus digestiua". In De fac. nat. III 1: Scr. min. III 204,8–13 Helmr. = II 143,3–8 K., Galen treated the nutritive faculty as a specific type of alterative faculty, whereas earlier at I 7: Scr. min. III 112,11–15 Helmr. = II 16,6–10 K., he had regarded the two as separate "handmaids" of the faculty of growth. Here (lines 7–8) the "digestive faculty" is declared to produce growth, and there is no mention of the nutritive faculty or of the faculty of growth. But this may be only an apparent contradiction, the result of leaving out several stages in the argument in order to proceed quickly to the next point, for at De fac. nat. I 7–8: Scr. min. III 114,4–17 Helmr. = II 18,12–19,8 K., Galen had declared that growth was impossible without nutrition, and that the nutritive faculty was a special form of the alterative.

P. 62,12–15: The comparison between plants and the embryo (cf. p. 90, 19–20) is one of the major features of Galen's embryology, see Nickel, pp. 22–27; 79–80. He was by no means unusual in this, as his attempts to clarify his own terminology show. Platonists, Aristotelians, and Stoics, all made use of the same comparison, even if they disagreed on the terminology to be used. The first two, according to Galen (De plac. Hipp. et Plat. VI 3,7: CMG V 4,1,2, p. 374,13–19), declared that in plants there was something that controlled nutrition and growth, which they called "soul", qualifying it as "nutritive" or "vegetative" or "reproductive" (the Aristotelians) or "appetitive" (the Platonists); the Stoics, by contrast, reserved the term "soul" for animals, preferring to speak instead of "nature" in plants (cf. Chrys., fr. 710–712: SVF II, p. 204, 11–24). Galen typically regards the problem as purely one of semantics, in that he is prepared to go along with whatever name his opponents wish to use, and at times he shows no hesitation in linking all the formulations together (see De Lacy, in: CMG V 4,1,2, p. 662, the note to p. 374,18–19). He does, however, point out at De foet. form. 3: IV 665,7–13 K., that the term "nature", used by the Stoics even in specific discussions of psychology, is the "common expression", and he prefers it in most circumstances as being the 'normal word' (cf. De fac. nat. I 1: Scr. min. III 100,5–15 Helmr. = II 1,7–2,5 K.).

P. 62,14 reuac: Nowhere in the discussions cited in the previous note does Galen say that he is using the term "natura" because it corresponds to "reality" (rem ueram), the reading of C, or to "reason" (rationem), that of β. Besides, the sentence structure and the parallels elsewhere in Galen indicate that there should be here a reference to the Stoics. At p. 84,5 the word for "Stoics", translated into Arabic as *firqat al-riwāq*, "the sect of the pillared hall", was transliterated as "reubach". A similar transcription was here quickly emended away and replaced by words that appeared to give some sort of sense.

P. 62,16 in libro – 17: "medici populares" here means "doctors in general" (οἱ πολλοὶ τῶν ἰατρῶν), not mediaeval town physicians, who are occasionally so designated, or "physicians of the people". It is possible that the Arabic word *mutaṭabbib*, "healer", was here used by Ḥunayn, a word which later came to bear the connotation of a lesser physician than the Galenic *ṭabīb*, but there is nothing in De facultatibus naturalibus to indicate that that tract was aimed at any specific group of physicians, let alone lesser healers. An audience including doctors is implied in the brief reference at De ord. libror. suor. 2: Scr. min. II 84,13–17 Müller = XIX 54,18–55,3 K. to the value of De facultatibus naturalibus for one who has been trained in anatomy, but there is no indication of a dedicatee. The opening chapters suggest that Galen has a broad public in mind. One glossator in B added to "hoc libro" in the margin "s. presenti" to inform his readers that Galen was referring here to De propriis placitis, not to De facultatibus naturalibus. He was wrong, but at least he was aware of the difficulty of the phrase.

P. 62,19 demonstraui – 20: Galen's claims for Hippocrates as the first to declare that bodies resulted from a mixture of the four elements are fundamental to his whole system of medicine. But his brusque formulation hides a variety of unproven assumptions. Firstly, Galen was convinced that the historical Hippocrates wrote at least the first section, chapters 1–8, of De natura hominis, the very foundation-stone of Galen's Hippocratic medicine. Others disagreed, either attributing authorship to someone else (see Gal., In Hipp. De nat. hom. comm. I prooem.: CMG V 9,1, pp. 8,20–22; 9,15–19) and refusing to accept this treatise as genuine, or ascribing different doctrines to Hippocrates.[1] But, even granted Hippocratic authorship, Galen's claim is far from watertight. He may have thought that Philistion, who certainly believed in a theory of four elements (Anon. Lond. XX 25–30), and Petron, who favoured four primary opposites (Anon. Lond. XX 1–6), came after Hippocrates, and he may never have himself read the Hippocratic De carnibus, which has a different four-element theory (2: p. 2,10–18 Deichgräber = VIII 584,10–18 L.).[2] But he was well aware that Empedocles had argued that the human body was composed of elements. However, in Galen's opinion, the Empedoclean four elements, like bricks in a wall, were subject to no mutual interaction (see Gal., De elem. ex Hipp. sent. 9,11: CMG V 1,2, p. 130,8–10; Arist., De generat. et corrupt. II 7: 334 a 26–30; and above, p. 116,9–12). Hence, his claim for Hippocratic priority rests on the narrow definition of the body being created from a mixture of elements (cf. In Hipp. De nat. hom. comm. I 13: CMG V 9,1, p. 27,20–27).

But there is a further difficulty. Galen was convinced that he could derive his theory of the four elements from De natura hominis: In Hipp. De nat. hom. comm. I 18: CMG V 9,1, p. 32,1–9; cf. De elem. ex Hipp. sent. 5,32; 9,25: CMG V 1,2, pp. 100,19–24; 134,13–15. But the author states that the body is made up of blood, phlegm, bile, and black bile, which are later linked with the four primary qualities of hot, cold, wet, and dry. Nowhere does he declare that the body is made up of the four elements; indeed, after chapter 1 these four simple elements are never mentioned at all. A non-Galenic believer in Hippocrates could easily claim that he had deliberately rejected elements in his explanation of the workings of the body (as indeed some Hippocratics did, see Gal., In Hipp. De nat. hom. comm. I 14: CMG V 9,1, p. 28,23–27). But since Plato in the Timaeus (82 a) had also spoken of four elements as the ba-

1 Aristotle, Hist. anim. III 3: 512 b 12–513 a 7, had ascribed a description of the blood-vessels very similar to that in chapter 11 to Polybus (or Polybius); cf. H. Grensemann, Der Arzt Polybos als Verfasser hippokratischer Schriften, Akademie d. Wiss. u. d. Lit., Abh. d. geistes- u. sozialwiss. Kl. 1968,2, Wiesbaden, 1968; for a different account of Hippocratic ideas, see Anon. Lond. V 35–VI 43, with J. Jouanna, in: Hippocrate, Des vents, De l'art, ed. and transl., Paris, 1988 (Collection des Universités de France), pp. 39–49.

2 Galen nowhere cites this tract directly, except for citations in his Hippocratic glossary: Ling. s. dict. exolet. Hipp. explic.: XIX 72,11; 79,6 K. But he could well have taken over these entries from an earlier lexicographer, and not read the work himself.

sis of the physical world and of the human body, and since, according to Galen, Plato had learned from Hippocrates, Galen saw no difficulty in bringing together elements, humours, and qualities, and ascribing a belief in elements to the historical Hippocrates; see Lloyd, Galen on Hellenistics and Hippocrateans, in: Lloyd, Methods and problems, pp. 406–409, and in: Galen und das hellenistische Erbe, pp. 134–136.

P. 62,21: The repetitive "de hoc quod iudicauit" is guaranteed by its presence in C B, two manuscripts rarely found in agreement in bad readings against the rest (e.g. p. 100,6. 8). They probably derive from the repetitive style of the Arabic translation, and their omission in other manuscripts is the result of homoioteleuton.

P. 64,5–7: This definition of heat shows how much Galen was indebted to Aristotle for the vocabulary and the concepts of his physics, although he does not regard this doctrine as specifically Aristotelian, but as a widely recognised basic concept of natural philosophy. The four elements are so called, in Galen's phrase, "obviously because they have simple and unmixed qualities" (In Hipp. De nat. hom. comm. I 14: CMG V 9,1, pp. 28,8–29,17). Heat is at its hottest in fire, for example; wetness at its wettest in water. Cf. also Moraux, Der Aristotelismus, vol. II, pp. 736–739, and Alex. Aphrod., Quaest. II 17: pp. 61,29–62,14 Bruns, for a contemporary discussion of the definition of heat. This specific usage of "the hot" is then modified to allow for a more general definition, a substance in which hotness predominates over other qualities.

P. 64,7–10: The third meaning given to "heat" is that of innate heat, and is once again justified by Galen by an appeal to custom and usage. But the role of innate heat is far more important than might at first sight appear from this comment. Not only is it present in the body from its very creation, but its maintenance is, for Galen, essential if life is to continue (see e.g. De locis affectis V 1: VIII 298,7–10 K.). It plays a prime part in the creation of life and in the formation of the foetus (see De marcore 4: VII 678,5–7 K.) and at De trem., palp., convuls. et rig. 6: VII 616,11–617,4 K., Galen comes very close to identifying it with soul or nature as a substance eternally mobile and self-moving.[1] This contradicts his normal agnostic stance on the soul (p. 60,3–6), and its unusual bluntness may simply be the result of it being an aside within a broader discussion, an interesting idea whose consequences Galen does not have time to pursue.

P. 64,10–16: The Latin translation presents two difficulties. "bethenem", the reading of ε (= Parthenius), cannot be right, for the text in question was written against Lycus of Macedon, and looks like a scribal rationalisation of a word hard to understand. The manuscripts of the β-group appear to agree on the transcription of the opening letters (which would have suggested the expansion in ε), but the reading of C (boelius) is closer to the original "Lycus", especially if transcribed from a badly written Arabic original (LYQWS 〉 BLYWS).

1 This disproves the contention of Siegel, p. 165, that "Galen was never inclined to regard heat as a vitalistic force".

Whether Galen was referring to one or to two tracts is harder to determine. The Latin translator undoubtedly had two Arabic words in front of him, which he carefully distinguished in his version as "in uno librorum" and "in dictione". But nowhere else in this tract is Galen so vague in referring simply to "one of my books", especially when he immediately follows with a precise reference to another tract. Although Galen often refers to his view of the problem, he reserves his longest discussion for the commentary on Aphorisms I 14: XVII B 404,8–415,6 K., and it is probable that a specific reference to this passage has fallen out, either in the Arabic or, as J. Kollesch suggests, in the Latin.

Lycus of Macedon was Galen's older contemporary, a Hippocratic, and a pupil of Quintus, albeit for less than a year, with a keen interest in anatomy and in Hippocratic exegesis. In Galen's eyes Lycus can do very little right. His anatomical works are full of error, and he goes on far too long, talking about pathology instead of the results of dissection (see Gal., De musc. dissect.: XVIII B 927,3–7 K.). His belief that urine was the residue of the nutriment supplied to the kidneys could be easily disproved by the facts of observation, and was based on a misunderstanding of Erasistratean physiology (see Gal., De fac. nat. I 17: Scr. min. III 152,13–153,6 Helmr. = II 70,7–71,6 K.; De atra bile 6,13: CMG V 4,1,1, p. 84,20–22). His Hippocratic exegeses, which were unknown to Galen until the middle 170's, are treated with similar roughness. They are filled with misunderstandings of every kind; they are based on poor texts; and show a fundamental ignorance of Hippocratic doctrine (see Gal., In Hipp. Epid. VI comm. V 14: CMG V 10,2,2, p. 288,16–26; Adv. Lycum 7,21–22: CMG V 10,3, p. 29,12–21; In Hipp. Aphor. comm. III prooem.: XVII B 562, 1–10 K.; In Hipp. Epid. III comm. I 4; III 72: CMG V 10,2,1, pp. 13,4–17,21; 154,13–15).

But, at times, even Galen seems to have respected him. Certainly his anatomy book is mentioned once with apparent approval as a reasonable representation of the teaching of Quintus (see In Hipp. De nat. hom. comm. II 6: CMG V 9,1, p. 70,13–17). Galen also made in two books an epitome of all his anatomical treatises and implies that he had found them "useful" (see De libris propr. 3: Scr. min. II 104,9–14 Müller = XIX 25,5–10 K.). For a vigorous defence of Lycus, see W. D. Smith, pp. 65–69; 116; 130–131; 155–156, building on the arguments of F. E. Kind, art. "Lykos" (no. 52), in: RE XIII, 1927, cols. 2408–2417.

P. 64,13 cum – 15 naturalis: At Adv. Lycum 6,1. 4–19: CMG V 10,3, pp. 18,18–22; 19,12–23,22, Galen quotes at length from Lycus, who took the line that the text referred to the effectiveness of the hotness, not to any specific substance, "innate heat". If Galen's quotation is accurate, Lycus did not comment directly on the word ἔμφυτον, except to say that it applied to heat that was found throughout the body, and, presumably, in its natural state. There is no suggestion that he was thinking of a specific substance within the body, as Galen does. His interpretation is not without its merits, for, except for the late reference in De corde 6: IX 84,9 L., the words τὸ ἔμφυτον θερμόν are found only in this Aphorism (I 14: IV 466,8 L.) and could easily bear the meaning attributed to them by Lycus. At the very least, even if Galen's point is conceded, the notion of "innate heat" does not bulk large in the Hippocratic Corpus. See also above, p. 147, the note to pp. 60,19–62,2.

P. 64,14 non – 16: Galen's account of innate heat, both here and in his attack on Lycus, is somewhat obscure; innate heat is linked with its own substance, which is sperm and (menstrual) blood; and generation results from the interaction of these two substances, which are the carriers of this heat. Innate heat is not some third, independent, substance, infused from outside into the newly generated body.

P. 64,23 et – 66,7: In De elementis ex Hippocratis sententia Galen says nothing directly on the question of the differences between the innate heat of children and adults, and Galen's reference is a mistake. He says more at De temp. II 2: pp. 47,3–56,9 Helmr. = I 582,18–598,5 K., in which he typically presents himself as resolving a very difficult debate. One side, arguing that blood was the hottest humour and that, at the moment of conception, the foetus was almost all blood, posited a gradual falling off of innate heat over the course of life. The other side, with almost equally plausible arguments that were not easy to refute, countered that young adults had within them both more blood (witness their numerous outpourings of blood in menstruation and in nose bleeds) and more yellow bile, the hottest of the humours. Galen admits that, despite having examined thousands of children, young persons, and adults, he cannot decide whether one is 'hotter' than any other, although there may be a perceptible difference in the quality of the heat, that in adults being drier and more biting. His solution, which hardly qualifies as a demonstration, is to say that they are hot for different reasons, and that the young child is hottest because it is closest to the moment of generation, i.e. has more innate heat, while the adult has more acquired heat.

P. 66,2 ὥσπερ – 8: Whether Galen has any empirical basis for this suggestion, that the less the amount of natural heat, the more dangerous the fever, is unclear. At In Hipp. Aphor. comm. I 14: XVII B 413,17–414,11 K., he claims that the elderly do not suffer from acute fevers as often as young children, but that when they do so, the outcome is more likely to be fatal: for the cold body of an old person to attain febrile heat requires a considerable change and an equally considerable cause. It is, of course, impossible to assign a modern diagnosis to these fevers, for the word itself merely signifies a hot disease in general, and does not carry any of the specific modern connotations of the term. But Galen, and others like him, may well have noticed the preponderance of diarrhoeal disorders among young children, and, since many ancient fevers might be classified as modern infectious diseases, longevity may also demonstrate an acquired or an inherited immunity.

P. 66,8 εἶναι – 11 θερμόν: How Galen decides on the differences between the quality of the heat is not easy to determine. He had no thermometer, and could judge the heat of a fever only by touch. His division is vague, and, it might be argued, ultimately circular, yet it is one that Galen believed capable of empirical demonstration. Innate heat is what feels right to the touch, acquired heat does not. But, at the same time, what he felt when he touched the body was also influenced by his conception of the role of the two sorts of heat: innate heat is universally good, and hence lacks any negative qualities ("not biting", "not painful"), acquired heat is more destructive. The acquired heat, especially in fever, behaves like a fierce fire, producing smoke and fumes as if from wood; natural heat tends to create vapour, as if from moisture. Since the body of the young child is wetter, less solid, and less earthy than that of the adult, the result of the action of its innate heat will resemble steam more than dark smoke. And, just as a fire gives off different smoke and fumes according to what is burning, and individual materials react differently to heat, so the body's different exhalations in heat reveal the underlying elemental make-up. One can thus use empirical evidence gained from observing and touching the patient to proceed φυσικώτερον to an understanding of the body's elements (see Gal., In Hipp. Aphor. comm. I 14: XVII B 407,10–413,6 K.).

P. 66,10 ἄδηκτον – 13 πυρετούς: The Latin translation (or its source) omits the second part of the contrast between the two types of heat, and begins again with a subordinate clause (quia). The Greek manuscripts of this extract, however, offer the odd formulation of a definite article c. acc. c. inf. following κατά, a main clause being absent. Helmreich wrote κατάδηλον instead of the transmitted κατά γε, but that word is rare in Galen, who, in this tract at least, eschews such loose formulations in favour of "I have shown" or "I have proved". Since there is no convincing explanation for the corruption I have decided to delete the words κατά γε τὸ.

P. 66,14 ὧν – 18: Galen regularly attributes all fevers to a change in the natural heat of the body (see In Hipp. Aphor. comm. I 14. 16: XVII B 414,2–3; 426,5–6 K.), expressed both quantitatively (there is more heat) and qualitatively (there is a different sort of heat); cf. ibid. I 14: XVII B 408,11–15 K.; De diff. febr. I 1: VII 275,5–276,7 K. His division of fevers into three main types is not easy to follow. Ephemeral fevers are defined as those that last only for one day (see Meth. med. X 2: X 666,14–16 K.; In Hipp. Aphor. comm. IV 55: XVII B 734,1–4 K.) and are particularly associated with buboes. Galen is inclined to identify their cause simply with the production of heat, e.g. through over-exercise or getting angry (De diff. febr. I 7: VII 295,14–296,5 K.). The other two types mentioned here are both longer lasting, and differentiated according to their origin within the body. "Hectic" fevers, so called either because they are long-lasting or because they attack the body's general make-up (ἕξις), originate in changes in the solid substances of the body; putrid fevers in the putrefaction of its humours (see ibid. I 9: VII 304,3–10 K.). Although these two have different causes and seats, their courses and consequences are often more akin to each other than to those of the ephemeral fevers, and hence they are often considered together by Galen (cf. In Hipp. Aphor. comm. I 14: XVII B 408,13–15 K.).

P. 66,20–21: The manuscripts are divided as to whether it is the types (modi) or the temperaments (complexiones) that are composite. The presence of the same (wrong) reading in C B (D) (compositi) might suggest that it was already in the archetype, but the textual corruption from -te to -ti is very easy, and the same error could have occurred independently in three manuscripts.

Although the Latin translator is not entirely consistent in the words he uses for 'mixture', he generally follows the division adopted by translators after 1200 who used "complexio" to refer to a mixture of qualities or humours, "commixtio" to refer to one of elements, see D. Jacquart, De crasis à complexio: note sur le vocabulaire du tempérament en latin médiéval, in: Centre Jean Palerne, Mémoires 5: Textes médicaux latins antiques, ed. G. Sabbah, Saint-Etienne, 1984, pp. 71–76.

P. 66,23–25: In De temperamentis, Galen had argued that his belief in four composite temperaments was shared with the "most important doctors and philosophers", and had excoriated those who had accepted only two and who had denied the possibility of a temperament dominated by the warm and wet or by the cold and dry (De temp. I 2: p. 2,4–21 Helmr. = I 510,16–511,15 K.). As so often in this treatise, Galen here repeats his earlier conclusions dogmatically and includes little of his earlier argumentation.

P. 68,4 τὴν – 7: At De temp. I 3: p. 9,20–10,3 Helmr. = I 523,4–17 K., Galen made it clear that his prime target was Athenaeus of Attaleia and his followers, who appealed to Aristotle, Theophrastus and sundry Stoics to support their claim for the superiority of the moist and warm temperament over all others. Establishing the truth of these assertions is not easy, for Galen is the sole source for these views of Theophrastus, Athenaeus, and the Stoics.

P. 68,14–19: If the report of their arguments given by Galen at De temp. I 3: p. 9,20–10,3 Helmr. = I 523,4–17 K. is accurate, his opponents certainly made the comparison between the live body and corpses, but except by implication in referring to "life" (ζωή), they did not mention plants. Later on in the same treatise (I 5: p. 18,5–9 Helmr. = I 536,15–537,3 K.) Galen ascribes the discovery that animals are warmer and wetter than plants to "the ancients", but it is unclear whether this formed part of the argument of Athenaeus.

P. 68,20–24: His opponents' derivation of the warm and wet temperament of the seasons from that of the body is roundly attacked by Galen as a foolish use of metaphor (De temp. I 5: p. 17,13–21 Helmr. = I 535,12–536,3 K.). Besides, in his opinion spring is not predominantly warm and wet and therefore the best season, as they insist, but it has a perfectly equable balance of the four qualities (see ibid. I 4: p. 10,4–12,7 Helmr. = I 523,18–527,6 K.; cf. In Hipp. Epid. I comm. I prooem.: CMG V 10,1, p. 7,7–13). Their mistake lies in assigning a pair of qualities to each season, and in assuming that because, in comparison with winter, spring is warmer, and, in comparison with summer, wetter, this must indicate a predominance of these two qualities in spring. As Galen rightly says, on the same argument one could claim that spring was cold and dry, for it is colder than summer, and drier than winter. His second objection is that if one compares what Hippocrates said in the Epidemics (II 1,1: V 72,3–7 L.; III 2. 4. 7: I 224,7. 18–19; 225,18–20; 228,5–7 Kw. = III 66,14; 68,9–70,1; 72,7–74,1; 84,7–8 L., then one must conclude that a warm, wet spring would be most unhealthy – and since Galen's opponents believe in the healthiness of spring, they are to be convicted of inconsistency (De temp. I 4: pp. 13,5–16,23 Helmr. = I 528,14–534,10 K.).

P. 70,1 Ypocras – 2 Epidimiarum: Galen's use of Epidemics II is not without its problems, for he was well aware that other scholars, and possibly other Hippocratics, doubted whether Hippocrates was the author of this tract. Galen accepted the force of many of their arguments, but explained away any discrepancies between this text and the, in his view, certainly authentic Epidemics III by supposing that Epidemics II was written when Hippocrates was a young man (see De sept. partu 3: p. 347,118–124 Walzer). Modern philologists, even those who believe strongly in the Hippocratic authorship of Epidemics I and III, would disagree with this hypothesis, and set Epidemics II at least a decade later, cf. K. Deichgräber, Die Epidemien und das Corpus Hippocraticum. Voruntersuchungen zu einer Geschichte der koischen Ärzteschule, Abh. d. Preuß. Akademie d. Wiss. 1933, phil.-hist. Kl. 3, Berlin, 1933 (durch Nachwort und Nachträge vermehrter photomechanischer Nachdruck, Berlin and New York, 1971), pp. 74–75; J. Jouanna, Hippocrate, Paris, 1992, p. 537.

P. 70,2. 5 Epidimiarum . . . Elguefete: The Latin translator offers two separate versions of the Arabic title, one translated, the other merely transcribed. The normal explanation for a transcription is that the translator was unaware of the meaning of the word in front of him, and played safe by reverting to a less informative transcription. But it is then odd for the translator, having got it right a few lines previously, to revert to a transcription, and one might posit two separate versions of the titles in the Arabic, *Kitāb Abīdīmiyā* and *Kitāb al-wāfida.*

P. 70,7 in secunda dictione: Contrary to what the Latin translation might suggest, this quotation does not come from Book II of the Epidemics, but from Book III. The error, if such it is, can be explained palaeographically. A Latin abbreviation III^{a} may have been misread as II^{a}, and then expanded. The other, more likely, possibility is that the corruption occurred when Arabic *al-t͟hālit͟ha* (the third) was misread as *al-t͟hāniya* (the second) (G. Strohmaier). Given this possibility, emendation of the Latin is not necessary.

P. 70,13 complexio – 15 [anni]: The Latin translation presents several difficulties. C and B each undependently omitted "complexio – anni" through homoioteleuton. ε replaced "anni", which had wrongly entered into the text from line 13, with "etatis", which should be regarded as an unfortunate conjecture. Under the influence of the ε-tradition B^{2} filled the gap with "constructio . . . etatis". The problematic "anni" has been eliminated from the text.

P. 70,14 eodem – 18 ita: Galen here suggests that the divergence is apparent only; both sides are talking about two different things. The Latin translator tries to keep the nuance by first turning the dissension into something firmer: "it is possible to observe a difference", and then by qualifying it: "which is not so".

P. 70,19 membrorum radicalium: The translation of τὰ στερεὰ σώματα, the solid parts of the body[1], as "membra radicalia", "fundamental", "radical" or "root-like" parts is unexpected. Elsewhere, so G. Strohmaier informs me, e.g. in the Arabic versions of De elementis ex Hippocratis sententia and De symptomatum differentiis, the word στερεός is translated as *aṣlī wa-ṣulb* (fun-

1 I.e. bones, ligaments, membranes, arteries, veins, nerves, tunics, and flesh, Gal., De temp. II 2: p. 46,6–10 Helmr. = I 581,14–17 K.; cf. [Gal.], Def. med. 33: XIX 356,16–18 K.

damental and firm) or simply as *aṣlī* (fundamental), deriving from *aṣl*, "root" or "foundation". The Latin translator thus translated accurately his Arabic exemplar, although the resulting term was not familiar in medical sources.

P. 72,1 membri: The use of this word here and line 24; p. 74,8. 12. 14 as a translation for νεῦρα (νεῦρον) suggests that in the Arabic *ʿaṣab* (nerve) was read as *ʿuḍw* (bodily part) (G. Strohmaier).

P. 72,14 ἐρρέθη – 16: Given that Galen's comment (repeated e.g. De plac. Hipp. et Plat. VIII 1,1: CMG V 4,1,2, p. 480,10–11) was of little relevance in translation, and presented problems in expressing nuances of the two terms, the omission of this aside may be ascribed to the Arabic translator.

P. 72,17 et – 20: The Latin version here does not correspond to the Greek and is based on a misunderstanding (or, less likely, the corruption) of the underlying text. Where in the process of transmission this error was made is not clear.

P. 74,1 et – 4: It is a nice indication of the excerptor's priorities that he omits the empirical evidence to back up the statement that flesh is more sensitive to pain than nerves.

P. 74,5 Νομίζεται – 9 αὐτῶν: Galen does not make it clear who these "many doctors" are who take the severe consequences of inflammation of the nerves as evidence for nerves being more sensitive than flesh.

P. 74,7 propter – 76,19 nerui: Contrary to what the Latin translator, and the annotators in B and E supposed, "elchatir" (lines 8. 17; p. 76,18), as G. Strohmaier informs me, is not a disease, but a transcription of *al-khaṭar* (danger) or *al-khaṭir* (dangerous). This error colours the Latin version of the next sentence, and may also be responsible for the omission of καὶ φλεγμαῖνον (line 20) in the following sentence. "elchatir" is to be distinguished from "elchadir" (p. 76,2. 5) which is a transcription of *al-khadar* (numbness) or *al-khadir* (numb), an obvious source of confusion in the manuscripts. Although one can see how some of the Latin translation corresponds to the Greek, its overall message is very different, even when it is intelligible.

P. 74,9 ἐπιφέρουσι: The reading of P seems to have been ἐπιφέρει (so also W). But the singular form cannot be correct, since it requires τὰ νεῦρα as subject. But this is impossible, since they are the recipients of what is brought. The Latin version gives no help here, for it is some distance removed from the Greek. The traces of the correction of P², which Kalbfleisch, Zu Galenos, p. 691, read as .πιφέροι, can be taken, so J. Kollesch and D. Nickel suggest, as the remains of an original ἐπιφέρουσι. This would restore sense to the sentence, making the subject φλεγμοναί (inflammation).

P. 74,15 καὶ – 23: The conjunction of particles, καὶ μέντοι καὶ, emphasises the additional point that is about to be made to support the view that a cut and a damaged nerve present different levels of pain. Although Galen elsewhere talks of sensation in the nerves, he does not remark on the difference between the types of pain in flesh and nerve or between the consequences of inflammation, or on others' views on the topic.

P. 74,23 οὕτω – 27 φλεβὶ: At De anat. administr. III 9: pp. 187,14–189,8 Garofalo = II 395,1–396,7 K. Galen tells how an incompetent practitioner had sliced through three nerves while venesecting, an unfortunate incident that was only detected some time later when the patient could not move his hand. Others had done the same when opening a vein in the arm or the leg.

P. 76,10 et – 13: The Latin translator produces a text that is hard to reconcile with the Greek. His confusion was caused by a misunderstanding of the Arabic word *tašannağa* (so G. Strohmaier suggests), which means both to shrivel up and to go into spasm. That damage to the nerves resulted in spasm, and was often accompanied by inflammation, was familiar to Galen (see Meth. med. IV 6; VI 3: X 290,9–12; 406,14–18 K.).

P. 76,18–20: Neither reading offered by the manuscripts for this section is entirely satisfactory. If one follows the reading of C γ (magis sensibilis carne quam sit in se), Galen is here repeating the opinion of "many doctors" (p. 74,5–6 / 74,5), that the nerves are more sensitive than flesh; but the comparative clause "quam sit in se" then conflicts with "carne". ε, with the small emendation of D. Nickel, offers a more coherent and syntactically better reading (magis sensibilis cum carne quam ⟨si⟩ sit in se): the nerve is "more sensitive with flesh than if it were by itself". J. Kollesch suggests a parallel with De locis affectis II 2: VIII 74,7–8 K., where Archigenes is criticised for failing to realise that nowhere in the body does flesh exist by itself (αὐτὴ καθ' ἑαυτήν). But although this is what Galen undoubtedly believed, this truism corresponds fully neither to the criticism that follows nor to the common view announced earlier. A second point concerns the relationship of "et secundum . . . in se" to what comes before or after. C γ insert "et" before "ita", as if a new sentence began there. The comment of Fisedis is thus made into a general denunciation of any theory involving the sensitivity of nerves. The reading of ε, which leaves out "et", and links the criticism of Fisedis with "et secundum . . . in se", fits better syntactically, for the subordinate clause is further linked to the main clause by "ita".

P. 76,20 Fisedis – sensibilem: Who is the mysterious Fisedis? In this treatise Galen mentions several well-known physicians and philosophers, e.g. Hippocrates, Herophilus, Erasistratus, and Chrysippus, as well as the Stoics in general. He does not refer to what might be termed minor figures, and there is thus a presupposition that behind the garbled name hides a familiar doctor or philosopher. Posidonius could be a candidate, because the transition of Posidonius to Fisedis in Arabic would be possible. But did Posidonius hold this view of nerves? Galen, who in De placitis Hippocratis et Platonis makes much of Posidonius' differences with Chrysippus on psychology, says nothing about it there, and there is nothing elsewhere in the fragments of Posidonius that indicates that he held such a belief.

One author who certainly did was Asclepiades of Bithynia. According to [Rufus of Ephesus], De dissect. part. corp. hum. 72: p. 184,15–185,1 Daremberg-Ruelle, Asclepiades denied that there were sensory nerves, and Galen in his Methodus medendi (XII 7: X 852,9–853,2 K.) scornfully rejected what he considered Asclepiades' atomist explanation of pain and sensation (cf. Vallance, p. 37). At De locis affectis II 8: VIII 90,8–9 K. Galen reports Archigenes' criticism of Asclepiades for saying that nerves were without pain in arthritis because a nerve was entirely free of sensation. In terms of doctrine, then, the passage could well apply to Asclepiades. His name would then have been corrupted in Arabic from ʾSQLYBYDYS to FYSYDYS (G. Strohmaier).

P. 76,25–78,3: Galen returns again to the question of the soul, moving from a discussion of damage to the nerves and its consequence, a loss of sensation, to a discussion of the ultimate source of sensation, the soul. He begins by taking up the two points he had made in chapter 2 (p. 60,10–11) that he did not know whether the soul was corporeal or incorporeal, mortal or immortal. Nevertheless, he goes on to argue, even if the unlikeliest combination of these opposites turns out to be true, and the soul is both incorporeal and immortal, it still remains logically possible for such a soul to reside in the mortal body. If so, it remains a plausible option that the body is endowed with sensation, which it receives from the soul.

P. 78,5–6: Galen explains later (p. 116,5–19 / 116,5–23) just what he means by "mixture", but, for the moment, he emphasises that generation of the body depends on a mixture, identical[1] with the mixture of the elements.

P. 78,6–10: This is Galen's strongest assertion of the corporeality of the soul, and depends closely on his claims in his late treatise, Quod animi mores corp. temp. sequ. 3: Scr. min. II 37,16–38,4 Müller = IV 774,7–775,3 K., where he follows Aristotle's identification of the soul with the form of the body. This view, as many commentators have pointed out, is similar in many ways to that developed by Alexander of Aphrodisias a few years later, see Moraux, Der Aristotelismus, vol. II, pp. 740–742, with refs. But one should also note the provisionality inherent in this declaration: "if the soul . . ., then . . .", which leaves the way open for a reiteration of Galen's agnosticism.

P. 78,10–11: At De elem. ex Hipp. sent. 6,38: CMG V 1,2, p. 114,18–20, Galen, interpreting Aristotle's definition of matter, asserts that eternal matter, indestructible and uncreated, is totally without quality, and that any quality is both created and perishable. At Quod animi mores corp. temp. sequ. 3: Scr. min. II 36,23–37,1 Helmr. = IV 773,10–11 K. he declares that matter is conceptually without qualities, although it contains within itself a mixture of the four primary qualities. This doctrine is clearly restated here in the first part of this sentence, and hence the subject of "opinantur" should be Aristotle and his followers, or mankind in general.

P. 78,16: The essential word here for Galen is "sensibilem", for it is feeling or sensation that distinguishes the living body from the dead.

P. 78,16–19: Galen misrepresents himself slightly, for in the passage he cites from memory, De san. tuenda I 2,10–11: CMG V 4,2, p. 5,8–15, he concentrates on the drying out of the body, and says nothing about its increasing coldness; later, at I 5,50: p. 13,19–20, he mentions the gradual drying out and cooling of the body as responsible for the deterioration in the quality of life of the elderly. However, in De temp. I 3: p. 9,13–10,3 Helmr. = I 522,15–523, 17 K., he notes that Aristotle, Theophrastus, the Stoics, and the followers of Athenaeus of Attaleia all associated death with cold and dryness, even if their explanations and understanding of the phenomena left something to be desired. Later on in the same treatise, II 2: p. 46,10–47,2 Helmr. = I 581,17–

1 C's "eodem modo" puts the stress wrongly on the process of generation.

582,18 K., Galen describes death as the extinction of the body's innate heat, as, over time, the body itself becomes colder and drier.

P. 78,22–24 uult^{II}: Although Galen frequently declares that questions on the mortality and corporeality of the soul are irrelevant to practical medicine, he keeps returning to them, especially in this treatise. His agnosticism has here a double purpose: it enables Galen to withdraw gracefully from any discussion, once his position is threatened, and it contrasts him with those who believe strongly in one position or another, but who are content with assertions or with only that part of the evidence that is in their favour.

P. 78,23 ita – 80,1 spiritus: The repetition of "prout uult" suggests that Galen has no specific target in mind: 'it doesn't matter whether one wishes to say . . .'. But "iudicauit" is more precise, and refers to the Stoics, and Chrysippus in particular, who frequently declared that the soul was corporeal and identical with πνεῦμα, see Hierocles, Elem. eth. 1,5–33; Cleanthes, fr. 518: SVF I, pp. 116,32–117,14; Chrys., fr. 790; 841; 879: SVF II, pp. 219,24–28; 228, 18–40; 235,20–236,22. Galen's complaint here is that the Stoics did not make adequate use of the new anatomical discoveries of the Alexandrian physicians.

P. 78,23 substantia: Both C and O have the compendium "scia (scīa)", followed in C by "sua"; B ε have the simpler "anima", both readings are possible, for Galen talks sometimes of the soul itself, sometimes of its substance being incorporeal or corporeal, cf. p. 60,3–6. 10–11. Given the presence of this compendium in both branches of the tradition, and the ease with which a scribe, faced with a difficult compendium or simply through inadvertence, could have repeated "anima" from the previous line, I have followed C O.

P. 80,1 et – 6: Many of the details of the life and opinions of Erasistratus remain controversial, not least because his writings have almost entirely disappeared, and later authors, and Galen in particular, display an ambivalent attitude towards his very varied investigations. One thing stands out above all: on every aspect of the body he was constantly putting forward challenging ideas which derived from logical argument and from technically sophisticated practical investigations.

Although Galen was not impressed by his mechanistic physiology (or by the ideas on therapy attributed to him by his followers), he praised him highly for his work in anatomy, especially on the heart and the brain. Galen's formulation here is somewhat ambiguous, inasmuch as he endorsed none of the possibilities mentioned for the localisation of the soul's pneuma. Certainly Galen himself had strong reservations about the theory of pneuma as put forward by Erasistratus, as we shall see. But rather than himself proclaiming adherence to one particular theory, Galen may be emphasising here the methodical application of the results of anatomical investigation as a way of extending the insights of philosophy. He is contrasting what the Stoics and Chrysippus did not do with the ways in which the anatomical results of others might have been utilised.

Galen's paraphrase of Erasistratus (lines 2 spiritus – 3 concauitatibus) raises two major questions of interpretation. In the fragments of Erasistratus directly quoted by Galen, there is no mention of the soul, but only of spirit.

Given Erasistratus' preference for mechanistic explanations of the workings of the body, and despite the importance he gave to *pneuma*, Galen may here be modifying Erasistratean discoveries to fit his own preconceptions, see, for other examples, W. D. Smith, Erasistratus' dietetic medicine, Bulletin of the History of Medicine 56, 1982, pp. 399–409; Garofalo, in: Erasistrati Fragmenta, pp. 32–43. Erasistratus himself seems to have described the body as being administered by *pneuma* (or *pneumata*), as instruments of nature (fr. 86: p. 90 Garofalo) collaborating in the natural functions of the body. However, writers who drew on ancient doxographies asserted that Erasistratus had located the ruling part of the body in the meninges of the brain (fr. 40; 41: pp. 73–74 Garofalo), and Soranus the Methodist would appear to have discussed both the role of *pneuma* and the consequences of Erasistratus' discoveries in his book On the soul: see J. H. Waszink, in: Quinti Septimi Florentis Tertulliani De anima, ed. with introduction and commentary, Amsterdam, 1947, pp. 22*–34*; Mansfeld, Doxography, pp. 3099–3107. If Galen is wrong to introduce the soul into Erasistratus' argument, he at least erred in good company.

The rest of this section is far from easy to interpret. Given that Galen is dealing specifically with the *pneuma* of the soul, he would not appear to be talking here of *pneuma* as breath drawn in from outside the body, but as something that provides life and sensation for the animal organism. Elsewhere Galen contrasts the view of Erasistratus (which he himself endorses) that the source of sensation is found in the ventricles of the brain with that of Aristotle and some of his followers, who placed the controlling power in the heart, from which it communicated life and sensation through the major ducts of the body. Galen could be referring to this well-known debate here, particularly if "in concauitatibus" was translated as 'in the ventricles'. But as we have seen at p. 70,19, the "membra radicalia" (line 3) are the solid parts of the body, and the contrast will thus be between the view of Erasistratus that *pneuma* was present only in the cavities of the body, i.e. the ventricles of the brain and the interior of the nerves and arteries, with one that placed it also within the solid parts themselves. On this interpretation, "concauitates" is to be taken in a general sense, not, as might be first thought, as a reference specifically to the ventricles of the brain.

Although the repetition of "uel" (line 3) suggests that Galen is distinguishing between those who believed that the *pneuma* was contained only in the channels of the body, those who allowed it, when necessary, also to permeate to the solid parts of the body, and those who believed that it was always present in every part of the body, even in those that were solid, there are problems with this interpretation. This triple distinction is not found elsewhere in Galen; and only two names are given. It is easier, as J. Kollesch suggests, to take the second "uel" in an intensifying sense giving the preceding statement greater precision, to give an opposition between Erasistratus and "Elumerephilis".

Who lies behind "Elumerephilis" (line 4)? The letters could easily be interpreted as referring to Herophilus. Even without Galen's information that Herophilus had Praxagoras as his teacher (T. 10–11: pp. 54–55 v. Staden) one could have deduced that Herophilus attributed a considerable degree of importance in his physiology to *pneuma* (cf. v. Staden, pp. 252–267), and this passage from Galen would only confirm it. But G. Strohmaier points out that the initial "El-" (Arabic *āl* or *ahl*) of "Elumerephilis" signifies membership of a family or group in Arabic and that the actual name of Herophilus corresponds to ʾMRFYLS, an easy miscopying of ʾYRFYLS. Therefore, one should think of the Herophileans rather than their founder. His pupil Chrysermus talked of both a vital and psychic faculty being involved in the production of the pulse (T. 156: p. 331 v. Staden), and the distinction between natural and psychic *pneuma* was common in the early Hellenistic period.

P. 80,6–7: The variant spellings of the name "Chrasis" suggest that the Latin translator had originally written "ch^{7}sis", using a compendium for "r" with preceding or following vowel, which was expanded differently by the scribes within the two traditions. The "eb-" in C O represents a misreading of "ch-" such as could have been made by any scribe. At p. 82,15 all manuscripts have "chrosis" (crosis E). Behind these forms lies the name of Chrysippus, whose Arabic form *Khrūsibus* can be easily altered through a change of pointing to *Khrūsīs* (G. Strohmaier).

That Chrysippus is the author in question, and that Galen is specifically attacking his two-book work On the soul, is clear from the parallel passages in De plac. Hipp. et Plat., especially III 1,7–19: CMG V 4,1,2, pp. 168,26–172, 4. Galen's language might imply that he had written a treatise specifically in order to refute Chrysippus on this point, but he records none among his writings on Stoicism. It cannot entirely be excluded, however, that his (lost) De substantia animae secundum Asclepiadem (see Gal., De libris propr. 8: Scr. min. II 115,3–4 Müller = XIX 38,8 K.) was directed at least partly against Chrysippus as well as against Asclepiades. It is, however, more likely that in this section Galen was drawing on what he had written in De placitis Hippocratis et Platonis, whose third book, CMG V 4,1,2, pp. 168–232, was composed in response to the claim of an "eminent sophist" that Galen had not adequately refuted all the arguments of Chrysippus that the rational part of the soul resided in the heart. Galen's attack there concentrated on his opponent's anatomical errors and, as he also proclaims here, on his preference for irrelevant quotation over the sound evidence of anatomy, e.g. I 6,12–13; 10,2; III 2, 1; 4,7: CMG V 4,1,2, pp. 80,18–24; 96,16–18; 174,25–28; 192,32–37. It is not just Chrysippus's sins of commission that excite Galen's wrath, but also his sins of omission.

P. 80,7–10: Galen is referring to what he has said at the beginning of this chapter (pp. 76,25–78,3). He in general takes the line that the body, as made up out of elements and humours, is sensitive only potentially, and that it is through the provision of 'psychic spirit' that these potentialities inherent in the construction of the body are actualized.

P. 80,10–13: Galen followed Erasistratus in his view of the brain, and repeated many of his experiments in order to trace the course of the nerves back through the pia and dura mater into the ventricles of the brain. Although locating the formation of the psychic spirit in the ventricles, he denied that the psychic spirit was anything more than the instrument of the soul.[1] His reasons were typically Galenic, the consequences of meditating on an anatomical experiment (see Gal., De plac. Hipp. et Plat. VII 3,19–22: CMG V 4,1,2, pp. 442,36–444,11): pressure on, or incision of, the ventricles results in the loss of sensation and motion, which return once the pressure has been removed or the incision closed. If the *pneuma* that escaped through the incision or was squeezed out was the soul itself, it is hard to see why the animal should have continued to live in the absence of a soul. Although Galen immediately reiterates his agnosticism about the actual substance of the soul, his preference for a physical location of the soul within the body of the brain reveals his sympathies.

P. 80,14–82,7: The connection between these two chapters is not immediately obvious, as it relates less to the specific questions under discussion than to the proper methodology to be employed in their investigation. Not only are both the location of the soul and the size of the sun appropriate questions for a philosopher-doctor convinced that the Creator's purposeful design extends to all aspects of the universe, microcosm as well as macrocosm (see Gal., De usu part. III 10: I 174,19–177,13 Helmr. = III 238,5–241,15 K.). Both are matters distinguished by a plethora of arguments based on insufficient or wrong premisses and analyses. Yet, Galen insists, a careful attention to the evidence of observation and the logic of demonstration can lead the lover of truth to certitude.

The same sequence of ideas occurs at De plac. Hipp. et Plat. VIII 1,20–21: CMG V 4,1,2, p. 484,22–33, and, since other arguments from that treatise appear also in these sections of On my own opinions, it is tempting to see Galen in old age composing his philosophical autobiography with the aid of at least some of his writings and picking out from his bookrolls a few choice paragraphs for insertion in his new work. But although Galen does follow at times the order of arguments, and often the wording, of other treatises, the overall impression is not one of a 'scissors-and-paste' doxography. Rather, this switch from soul to sun and back to soul suggests that the similarity of Galen's exposition here to that in other passages derives from the recurrence of similar 'triggers': the illogicality of Chrysippus demonstrates the failings of philosophers and doctors in general, exemplified by the debate over the size of the sun. Even if the concepts and language often remain the same, that is no proof that they have been taken over directly from another written text. Rather, over a career extending over at least fifty years, Galen more and more tended to repeat himself and to revert to the same formulations when dealing with the same or a similar topic.

P. 80,15 secundum – 16: There is a serious contradiction within the transmitted text. Galen's general point is that many of the arguments put forward in debate are 'unscientific', because they lack logical rigour and because their propounders have neither investigated things for themselves nor tested

1 The reading of ε, "principium" instead of "primum" (p. 80,12), cannot be right since Galen is talking about the psychic spirit, not the actual ventricles themselves; the phrase "first instrument of the soul" appears four times in De placitis Hippocratis et Platonis: VII 3,21. 23. 27. 30: CMG V 4,1,2, pp. 444,7. 15. 32; 446,13.

the arguments offered to them by others. The validity of this typically Galenic sally does not depend on the truth or falsity of the propositions in question, for his comment relates strictly to a principle of methodical procedure, not to its results, but it would be surprising if Galen were to choose as an example of unsafe argument a proposition with which he agreed. But as the Latin stands, Galen is attacking two entirely different and, indeed, opposed groups: those "who do not believe" (presumably that the sun is bigger than the earth) and those who "prove" that hypothesis. Besides, while one can see why Galen should attack the first group, the word "probare" and its Greek equivalents have a generally positive connotation, unless qualified to the contrary. The fact that "credunt" lacks an object, except by implication, is also disconcerting.

The easiest way to resolve the problem is by emending "et" to "eis". This has the advantage of restoring an object to "credunt", and places Galen firmly in the camp of those who argued that the sun was larger than the earth.

P. 80,16 quod – terra: There can be little doubt, although he nowhere states this explicitly, that Galen believed that the sun was larger than the earth. This had been the view of most astronomers since at least the fourth century B.C., although they might disagree over the relative sizes, and it is unlikely that Galen, who had a considerable knowledge of astronomy himself, would have dissented.[1] Only the Epicureans continued to argue in favour of the appearances[2], and Galen had little but contempt for their cosmology. See in general, J. L. E. Dreyer, A history of astronomy from Thales to Kepler, 2nd ed., New York, 1953, pp. 171–190; O. Neugebauer, A history of ancient mathematical astronomy, Berlin, Heidelberg, New York, 1975, pp. 109; 325–327; 417–426; 634–643; J. Barnes, The size of the sun in Antiquity, Acta Classica Universitatis Scientiarum Debreceniensis 25, 1989, pp. 29–41, concentrating on the philosophical and logical questions involved.

P. 80,16–19: The sequence of thought is clear: the true philosopher does not approve or reject a proposition without first spending some time in investigating its proof, but the Latin is at times problematic. "affirmet" (line 17) lacks a clear subject, and "eam" (line 17) is ambiguous. The philosopher himself can hardly be the subject, since it is his response that is in question, and if "affirmet" bears the same meaning as the subsequent "affirmantem" (line 18), the discovery cannot of itself declare anything, or 'confirm the truth' (if "eam" refers to "ueritas"). Besides, the philosopher would be foolish if he rejected something, if he thought that it affirmed or confirmed the truth. The easiest way to understand this passage is to suppose that the subject of "affirmet" is vague, "someone", as in the next sentence, and that its absence here is due to the process of translation.

What then does the philosopher do? Merely to have him listen to a proof

1 See Strohmaier, Hellenistische Wissenschaft, esp. pp. 160–162 (repr. in: Strohmaier, Von Demokrit bis Dante, esp. pp. 102–104), where a rare reference to Ptolemy the astronomer is made. At In Hipp. Epid. I comm. I prooem.: CMG V 10,1, p. 11,1–4, Galen accepts that certain things about the sizes and distances of the sun, moon and earth can be properly demonstrated by geometrical reasoning.

2 See Epic., Epist. ad Pyth. 91, and Demetrius Laco, as presented by C. Romeo, Demetrio Lacone sulla grandezza del sole (PHerc. 1013), Cronache Ercolanesi 9, 1979, pp. 11–15.

for a long while is weak, since one expects a verb that implies some direct involvement with the question of proof, perhaps corresponding to σπουδάζειν. Although "agit" instead of the transmitted "audit[II]" (line 18), as suggested by J. Kollesch and D. Nickel, gives better sense, I have chosen to obelise and to assume that the repetition of "audit" from the subordinate clause replaced another verb. It is also unclear whether "post longum tempus" (line 19) should be taken as a single prepositional phrase "after a long time", or, as the sense would suggest and Galen almost certainly wrote, as two adverbs, "then a long while".

P. 82,1 in ipsam: The agreement of C B guarantees the correctness of these two words; the fact that O ε both have "immanem", but in different places, suggests that the word appeared in β as a variant.

P. 82,2 et[I] – multum: Galen frequently claims not to want to spend time in refuting the wrong ideas of others; his practice was very different, as his opponents and posterity pointed out.

P. 82,3–5: At first sight, the phrase "hunc meum librum" would appear to be referring to the present treatise. But since Galen here rarely offers a proof for his beliefs, but merely lists them in order to avoid misinterpretation, it can hardly be said that this book was written to train others in proof. It is much more likely that he is referring, as he often did, to the fifteen books of his treatise De demonstratione. The loss of this important treatise is greatly to be deplored, for it contained what Galen saw as some of his major contributions to logic, especially his views on its role and value in scientific investigation. Many of the references to this treatise were brought together by I. v. Müller, Über Galens Werk vom wissenschaftlichen Beweis, Abh. d. k. bayer. Akademie d. Wiss., I. Cl. 20,2, Munich, 1895, pp. 403–478. Other fragments have been added by S. Pines, Rāzī critique de Galien, Actes du VIIe Congrès International d'Histoire des Sciences, Jérusalem (4–12 août 1953), Paris, s. a. (Collection des travaux de l'Académie Internationale d'Histoire des Sciences 8), pp. 480–487 (repr. in: S. Pines, Studies in Arabic versions of Greek texts and in mediaeval science, Leiden, 1986 [The collected works of S. Pines, vol. II], pp. 256–263); M. Mohaghegh, The Shukūk of Rāzī against Galen and the problem of the eternity of the world, in: Proceedings of the XXVII International Congress of Orientalists, Ann Arbor, Michigan, 13th – 19th August, 1967, ed. D. Sinor with the assistance of T. Jacques, R. Larson, M.-E. Meek, Wiesbaden, 1971, pp. 240–242; G. Strohmaier, Demokrit über die Sonnenstäubchen. Ein neues Fragment in arabischer Überlieferung, Philologus 112, 1968, pp. 4–6 (repr. in: Strohmaier, Von Demokrit bis Dante, pp. 6–8); Kraus and Walzer, p. 14; al-Rāzī, Shukūk, pp. 3–24; 29; 35; 43; 57; 67 Mohaghegh (G. Strohmaier); but much still remains uncollected in Arabic sources. Although not all have agreed with v. Müller's distribution of the various fragments to particular books, there can be no doubt that Galen ranged widely over medicine and science.[1]

[1] See J. Barnes, Galen on logic and therapy, in: Galen's Method of healing, pp. 50–102; idem, Galen and the utility of logic, pp. 35–38. Further important studies of Galen's logic include Hankinson, Galen on the foundations, pp. 15–29; and Atherton, pp. 175–214.

P. 82,5–7: What are the "propositiones" and what is Galen claiming to have banned? "Naming" (denominatione D) and "denoting" (denotatione E) propositions, although a feature of the mediaeval schoolroom, seem out of place here, and although "inuentione" might be considered suspect as a wrong anticipation of "inuentionibus" ("trying to find", line 6), it has both stronger manuscript support, and a greater relevance to Galen's current argument. The context suggests that Galen is unwilling to allow others to indulge in syllogistic argument about "istae propositiones", because all that it is strictly necessary to know is that there are three principles in man, each with its own distinctive method of activity. But what are these "propositiones"? It is possible that these are the propositions of Galen's opponents, i.e. that "istae" looks back to "eorum contradicentium" (lines 1–2), and that he is dissuading his readers from either seeking arguments in support of these contrary positions or wasting time in using syllogistic logic against them (a typically Galenic repetition of what he has just said in line 2). The present tense of the verb appears to rule out a reference to what was said in De demonstratione. Alternatively, the propositions are Galen's own, arguments that might be put forward or discussed at length in the appropriate context, but which are irrelevant to the practising physician. "istae" then looks back to the sort of questions already mentioned at pp. 78,22–80,6, and serves, again in typically Galenic fashion, to round off the short excursus on logical argument. See, for this type of argumentative structure, E. García Novo, Composition et style du traité de Galien De inaequali intemperie: avantages et désavantages pour la transmission du texte, in: Storia e ecdotica, pp. 145–147; 152–153.

P. 82,5 sillogismorum: Galen was particularly interested in syllogistic logic, and wrote two tracts specifically on its problems, see De libris propr. 11 (12); 15 (16): Scr. min. II 120,7; 123,15–16 Müller = XIX 44,9; 47,14–15 K. Later logicians credited him with the discovery of the fourth figure of the syllogism, see in particular N. Rescher, New light from Arabic sources on Galen and the fourth figure of the syllogism, Journal of the History of Philosophy 3, 1965, pp. 27–41; Moraux, Der Aristotelismus, vol. II, pp. 687–728; J. Barnes, Uma terceira especie de silogismo, Analise 2, 1985, pp. 35-61; idem, Galen and the utility of logic, pp. 33–51; Atherton, pp. 450–456.

P. 82,6 bonitatum anime: At first sight Galen's switch to discussing the ἀρεταί, "bonitates", of the soul is disconcerting. But in contrast to Aristotle, for whom no virtue could be a power (see Eth. Nic. II 5: 1105 b 19–1106 a 12), Galen follows the Platonic line of a strong interlinking of physical and moral well-being. His tripartite soul is not only necessary as an explanation for human ethics, but is also justified on anatomical grounds. He himself sees no difficulty about talking about the three parts of the soul, the rational, spirited, and desiderative, and the three physical systems dependent on the brain, heart, and liver, as if they were almost interchangeable (cf. In Plat. Tim. comm. III 2: CMG Suppl. I, p. 12,15–21). His proposed refutation of Chrysippus's De differentia virtutum in a treatise that was to bear the same title certainly would have included anatomical argument (see De plac. Hipp. et Plat.

VII 3,1–3: CMG V 4,1,2, pp. 438,24–440,8).[1] In this section Galen slips from a description of the physical body to talking about "virtues", the three parts and locations of the soul, and finally to what is valuable for physicians to know. Opponents might argue that Galen was deliberately taking advantage of some ambiguities of language to disguise the weaknesses in his own argument, yet for a Platonist, these ambiguities only served to confirm the close interrelationship between the physical and the moral activities of the soul.

P. 82,7–8: Galen's reference to the cure of the diseases of the soul suggests that he has moved in his argumentation from morality to medical practice. The diagnosis and explanation of mental illness (and of physical symptoms arising from mental turmoil) was one of Galen's specialities, see García Ballester, pp. 117–152; Pigeaud, pp. 153–183. But the diseases of the soul are also defined by Galen as passions, anger, wrath, fear, grief, envy, violent lust, excessive affection or hatred (De animi cuiusl. pecc. dign. et cur. 3,1: CMG V 4,1,1, pp. 6,25–7,5), all of which arise from an irrational impulse of the soul. They may have physical consequences that the doctor should note, but, equally, Galen leaves their treatment to an educator, a moral guide, not necessarily to the physician, and admits that they too might be classified by others as 'errors of the soul', which, to him, were the result of false opinion.

P. 82,10–15: "per operationem" (lines 10–11) represents an original ἔργῳ (in fact).

in libro suo: Somewhere in the process of transmission a reference to Plato's Republic has dropped out. This treatise which Galen regarded as a first attempt to investigate the soul contained only some of the arguments that Plato might have marshalled. The rest he left to his longer and more detailed exposition in the Timaeus (see De plac. Hipp. et Plat. II 7,19: CMG V 4, 1,2, p. 156,10–12).[2]

quod – corde: Galen's observation is correct. Plato in the Republic talks of the three parts of the soul, beginning at 442 b, but he does not go on to specify where in the body they were located. Indeed some commentators have argued that, in the Republic at least, Plato was thinking only metaphorically, and that to suggest a physical division is here "grossly misleading", see R. C. Cross and A. D. Woozley, Plato's Republic. A philosophical commentary, London, 1964, p. 128. On this interpretation, either the anatomical details in the Timaeus are equally speculative, part of the "likely story", or Plato's thought develops between the Republic and the Timaeus. Galen, on the other hand, sees no such change in outlook, and considers that the physiology of the Timaeus has its basis in the reality of this world. He assumes a very close relationship between the two treatises (Plato himself had represented them as conversations held on two successive days, see Tim. 17 a; 19 a; 27 a), and argues that Plato's silences and omissions are either deliberate or dictated by the different foci of the two dialogues. The Timaeus thus does not represent a

1 According to an avowedly later addition at De plac. Hipp. et Plat. VIII 1,47–48: CMG V 4,1,2, p. 490,1–9, this treatise was eventually written, but no such title is listed by Galen in his bibliographies.

2 Cf. Singer, pp. 41–55.

development but an amplification of Plato's earlier statements in a fashion appropriate to a work dealing with natural philosophy. Cf. further, pp. 104, 20–106,2.

P. 82,15–18: Galen returns to the complaint about Chrysippus and the Stoics that he had delivered in the previous chapter, but in a slightly different way. He acknowledges that they did indeed suggest a physical location for the ruling part of the soul, but he does not take direct issue immediately with their view of a unitary soul located in the heart. Instead, he attacks them indirectly, for failing to provide what would most help those interested in "philosophia scientie et philosophia pratice". The second type of philosophy is easy to define: whatever most helps in the practicalities of daily life, e.g. in medicine or in navigating (cf. Gal., De plac. Hipp. et Plat. IX 9,9–10: CMG V 4,1,2, p. 600,14–19). This was a common theme among some Middle Platonists, who, like Galen, contrasted their philosophy with that of the Stoic sage far removed from the practical cares of the world; see P. L. Donini, Le scuole, l'anima, l'impero; la filosofia antica da Antioco a Plotino, Turin, 1982, pp. 43–45. But the first is harder to pin down. The most frequent opposition in Galen is between a practical and a theoretical philosophy, and, since "scientia" elsewhere, e.g. pp. 14,53/55; 15,42/49, corresponds to θεωρία, this is what is most likely here rather than any interest in epistemology.

P. 82,18: The presence in C and O of the unintelligible "mutant" confirms that it stood in α, and that "narrare" is an emendation, taken over by B² from the ε-tradition. It is possible that the Latin translator wrote originally "nominare", cf. line 11, but "omiserunt" occurs on its own without a verb at line 17, and other solutions are possible.

P. 82,19 quod – 84,3: As the newly discovered Commentary on Hippocrates, Airs, waters and places, shows, Galen had a remarkable knowledge of meteorology, astronomy and geography, which he had gained from both reading and experience.[1] In his other medical writings he merely hinted at his learning in passing comments. So, for instance, his views on the origins of thunder and lightning appear in an exegesis of a Hippocratic sentence about the quality of water in various atmospheric conditions, and he insists there on the right, indeed almost the necessity, for the doctor to understand similar 'natural science' (see Gal., In Hipp. Epid. VI comm. IV 20: CMG V 10,2,2, pp. 229,22–231,3). If, as K. Deichgräber briefly indicated in the testimonia to p. 229,23, his explanation for thunder and thunderbolts is basically that of the Stoics (cf. Zeno, fr. 117: SVF I, pp. 33,33–34,2; Chrys., fr. 699; 701–704: SVF II, pp. 202,26–31. 39–203,26), it may then seem odd that he should criticise them for not providing all that the practical philosopher might require. But in his commentary on Epidemics VI Galen stresses the need for proper "demonstration", and in his brief reference to the reliability of theories about the sun

[1] See Strohmaier, Hellenistische Wissenschaft, pp. 157–164 (repr. in: Strohmaier, Von Demokrit bis Dante, pp. 99–106). The full commentary remains as yet unpublished, but the mediaeval Hebrew translation of some parts of it was edited by A. Wasserstein, Jerusalem, 1982. Cf. also G. J. Toomer, Galen on the astronomers and astrologers, Archive for History of Exact Sciences 32, 1985, pp. 193–206.

and moon in his preface to the commentary on Epidemics I (In Hipp. Epid. I comm., prooem.: CMG V 10,1, p. 11,1–5) he emphasises the crucial importance of demonstration and the geometric method. These were what he accused Chrysippus of lacking in his psychology, and Galen may be simply here extending the same criticism to Stoic natural philosophy in general. It may be no coincidence that Posidonius, whom Galen calls the "most scientific" of all the Stoics because of his geometrical logic (De plac. Hipp. et Plat. VIII 1,14: CMG V 4,1,2, pp. 482,33–484,1), put forward a similar explanation to Galen's for thunder and lightning (Posid., fr. 135 Edelstein-Kidd) and also discussed earthquakes, hail and snow, rainbows, and haloes (Posid., fr. 12; 230; 136; 134; 133 Edelstein-Kidd).[1] In all this, he (and Galen) responded to the agenda set by Aristotle in his Meteorologica (III 2: 371 b 19–373 a 32).

P. 84,4 et – 5: For "reubach" see above, p. 150, the note to p. 62,14. Galen wrote a total of six treatises (in seventeen books) against aspects of Stoic logic (see De libris propr. 15 [16]: Scr. min. II 123,12–17 Müller = XIX 47,11–16 K.), but in only two is an opponent, Chrysippus, named in the title. But, given that he has just been mentioned (p. 82,15), he may not be the anonymous Stoic here referred to. Galen's formulation, however, does not necessarily indicate a work devoted entirely to an examination of Stoic logic, for he could well have used the follies of a Stoic logician as the starting point for one of his own tracts on logic or demonstration.

P. 84,7–8: We pass from a reiteration of what the doctor needs to know about the philosophical debate over the controlling agent of the body to a medical problem that many doctors have neglected. Whereas practitioners could be excused from taking part in the former debate on the grounds that much of it was irrelevant, now Galen moves to an area of discussion that is central to medicine, how drugs work. If he is thinking of any specific group, then he is attacking the Empiricists, for whom an interest in causation was strictly limited or non-existent, and who were not concerned to discover why or how a drug worked, but only to establish that it did so in a particular case and might work again in a similar one (cf. Deichgräber, Empirikerschule, pp. 301-305).

P. 84,8–11: The crucial word here is "active", for Galen follows the Aristotelian line that, although there are many qualities, only the hot, cold, wet and dry are fundamental, responsible for change and for influencing an essentially quality-less matter (see Moraux, Der Aristotelismus, vol. II, p. 708; Harig, Bestimmung der Intensität, pp. 38–51).

P. 84,11 cum – actiue: Galen includes as drugs that work through their total substance all purgatives, and many epispastic or drawing drugs, some deadly poisons, and not a few counter-poisons or antidotes (see De simpl. med.

[1] See, in general, on the meteorology of Posidonius, M. Laffranque, Poseidonios d'Apamée. Essai de mise en point, Paris, 1964, pp. 214–239. Given that Posidonius was famous for his theories about tides (see Posid., fr. 214–220 Edelstein-Kidd), it is tempting to see the reading of C at p. 84,1 "terre maris" as the remains of an original "terre motus et maris".

temp. et fac. V 1: XI 705,14–17 K.[1]). They work through having a mixture of their primary qualities that has some direct affinity with the substance of the particular body or bodily part affected. Like all nutritious foodstuffs (see ibid. IV 9: XI 650,9–15 K.), whose mixture is such that they can be easily taken up and assimilated, they can be taken in directly and work swiftly. Counter-poisons occupy a sort of middle position, for they are related both to the body which receives them and to the poison that they drive out. Otherwise, according to Galen, they would either fail to act or damage the body to which they are given (see ibid. V 18: XI 761,6–764,9 K.).[2]

This explanation shows Galen at his best and worst. One can applaud his insistence on relating the assimilation of drugs to that of nutriment, while wondering whether his category of drugs that work by the totality of their substance was not a catch-all for anything or everything that could not be included in his other categories. The fact that it was the actual combination or mixture of substances within the individual drug that worked rendered fruitless any calculation of the cumulative effect of its individual ingredients, and opened the way to those who offered specific drugs for specific diseases without much concern for explanation, or to those who preferred to think in terms of antipathy, sympathy, and ineffable specificities. But Galen himself insists that he is not thinking in terms of secrets or mysteries, or of cosmic and magical sympathies. He is clear in his own mind which drugs are included in such categories, and derides those, like the Empiricists, who believe that any discussion of drugs in terms of causation is mere folly (see De comp. med. per gen. II 1: XIII 463,9–14 K.). But it would be unwise to believe that all ancient doctors shared his scruples, or confined this type of explanation to only a small number of medicaments (see Röhr, esp. pp. 96–133).

P. 84,12 Περὶ – 13 δυνάμεως: This form in which Galen cites his book On the properties of simples (XI 379–XII 377 K.) adds further weight to the suggestion that the book's original title did not include the words κράσεως καὶ found in the late manuscripts and in the printed editions of this tract (cf. Helmreich, Galeni fragmenta, p. 433, the note to lines 58/59).

P. 84,21 alterant: All manuscripts present this plural form as predicate to "genus medicinarum", a constructio ad sensum instead of the grammatically correct "alterat", unless this is an error influenced by the preceding plurals "alterant". Cf. the same construction ("genus animalium . . . habent") at p. 96, 17–18, where ε changed "habent" into "habet".

P. 84,22 ὄντα: I have deleted this word as a redundant duplication. Galen was enough of a stylist to avoid the horrible jingle that results if the word is retained.

P. 84,23 τὰ δηλητήρια – 86,7: The same distinction between "destructive" and "deadly" poisons (one might in English more clearly talk of 'deadly' and 'dangerous') is made by Galen at In Hipp. Epid. VI comm. VI 6: CMG V 10,2,2, p. 345,5–11, and at De simpl. med. temp. et fac. V 19: XI 767,7–768,2

1 The list at V 17: XI 760,12–17 K. mentions all purgatives, some antidotes, and, by implication, epispastics, and some poisons are added in chapter 19: XI 767,3–12 K.

2 See further, Harig, Bestimmung der Intensität, pp. 108–110.

K. He also is confident of providing an explanation for the θανάσιμα in terms of the action of the primary qualities. Elsewhere, at De simpl. med. temp. et fac. IX 1: XII 175,5–6 K., he seems to take τὰ δηλητήρια as a subdivision of the θανάσιμα, differing only in the extent of their toxic action.

P. 84,23–86,1 τὰ δηλητήρια καλούμενα / medicine que nominantur in Greca lingua guibentirie: At first sight there is little in common between the Greek δηλητήρια and the Latin "qui(n)bentime" (β) or "quebentime" (C), obviously the transmission of an Arabic transcription. Besides, δηλητήρια is not so rare or technical a word as to demand transcription at a first stage in the translation process. But the Latin translator is unlikely to have invented "in Greca lingua" for himself, and one may be sure that this phrase was present in his Arabic archetype.[1] In that case, Ḥunayn will have transcribed δηλητήρια to emphasise that he was using the Greek technical term. In the process of transmission, the Arabic DYLYṬYRY' became WYBNṬYRY', and the bilabial W was transcribed into Latin as "gu" (G. Strohmaier). Finally, this was misread as "qu", and the final strokes as "-me", to give a word far removed from the Greek.

P. 86,6 in parua quantitate: In the Latin version "parua" is misunderstood as applying to the quantity of drugs, not as in the Greek βραχεῖαν to the benefit to be gained, an error easier to make in the transition from Arabic to Latin than in that from Greek to Syriac or Arabic.

P. 86,7 οὕτω – 9: The use of opium, the juice of Papaver somniferum L., was widespread in Antiquity as an analgesic, and particularly for eye and ear trouble. Yet its toxicity was also well known, and Dioscorides (De mat. med. IV 64: I 218,6–221,21 Wellmann) and Pliny (Nat. hist. XX 200) report a debate about its safe administration that goes back at least to the time of Erasistratus in the early third century B.C. At Meth. med. III 2: X 171,4–6 K., Galen cautions against its indiscriminate use in eye diseases, but he recommends it in combination, e.g., ibid. XII 8: X 862,8–867,17 K. His contemporary, Apuleius, in his Apology (32), his public defence against an accusation that he was a poisoner, uses opium as one of his three examples of a dangerous drug that, given in moderation, will prove beneficial.[2]

P. 86,9 χρώμεθα: Kalbfleisch preferred the reading προσχρώμεθα instead of παρ.χρώμεθα P. Since Galen does not use this verb in his pharmacological writings, the simple χρώμεθα is more likely, and the prefix παρα- could be a wrong reading instead of πολλάκις.

P. 86,9–13 / 86,10–14: The Greek fragments and the Latin translation offer two opposed possibilities for the drugs whose workings Galen now describes. If one follows the Greek, Galen passes from the deadly via the merely dangerous to the beneficial drugs, which work on the principles described at the beginning of the chapter, either through one or a combination of two of the four primary qualities or, like purgatives, through the property of their

1 N. Serikoff tells me that he has found many examples of the phrase in Arabic translation literature.

2 In general, see J. Scarborough, The opium poppy in Hellenistic and Roman medicine, in: Drugs and narcotics in history, ed. R. Porter and M. Teich, Cambridge, 1994, pp. 4–23.

total substance. By contrast, the Latin translator apparently reverts to describing drugs that are non-beneficial. But there are two problems with his rendering: Galen is apparently excluding the dangerous drugs with a possible beneficial effect, and leaving only the truly destructive. But the action of the latter he has already explained as the result of the property of their total substance, and his comment that they bring about change through one or two qualities is self-contradictory. One way round this difficulty is to assume that by non-beneficial drugs Galen meant both the deadly and the dangerous when used to excess or alone, but Galen is usually clearer than this is his argumentation. It is also harder to see why the negative should have dropped out from the Greek than why someone should have added the negative in either the Arabic or the Latin.[1] A copyist, noting that Galen had just talked about the benefits to be gained from the use of opium, and seeing an adversative "sed", added the negative to distinguish the beneficial from the non-beneficial drugs that, in his view, Galen now discussed. Thus, although the Latin may provide evidence for a textual reading considerably older than that of any surviving Greek manuscript, in this particular instance it is a wrong reading. Nonetheless, there is no sound reason for deleting the negative from the Latin translation, which is, once again, faithful to its original in error.

P. 86,13 καὶ μέντοι καὶ – 23: Galen here spells out what he only alludes to elsewhere: how Nature produces certain of her effects or activities (for the possible equivalence of the two words ἔργον and ἐνέργεια, see De fac. nat. I 2: Scr. min. III 105,23–106,3 Helmr. = II 7,10–14 K.). Galen's humoral physiology is dominated by the four active qualities; every part of the body functions in its special way because of the way in which the four primary qualities are compounded in it (see ibid. II 8: Scr. min. III 187,3–8 Helmr. = II 118, 8–12 K.). Hence every natural effect is produced by the primary qualities, either singly or in combination. But Galen here appears to go beyond anything that he says in De facultatibus naturalibus or, as far as I can tell, elsewhere in the Galenic Corpus. He declares that coction in the stomach, blood-production in the liver, and nutrition and growth in every part of the body are activities based on the whole substance. In other words, the central functions of the living being are not determined by one or two of the primary Aristotelian qualities alone, but by their mixture, which cannot be described precisely in qualitative terms but which, if changed, results in an obvious loss of activity. Detractors of Galen might claim that this theory is tautologous nonsense, an explanation that explains nothing, but at least he should be given the credit for attempting a hypothesis. In this context it provides a link with the theory of drug action that he has just sketched. Just as the most deadly drugs are those that act through the peculiarity of their total substance, so the most significant parts of the body function in exactly the same way. Furthermore, only a drug whose combination is extremely powerful is capable of acting quickly on so vital a combination of bodily qualities. It is extremely dangerous, not only because of its own mixture, but also because it can attack the most important parts and functions of the body.

[1] Especially if, as in line 3, Galen had used μηδέποτε to avoid hiatus.

P. 86,16. 18 diuiduntur . . . adimplentur: G. Strohmaier suggests that γίνεσθαι was rendered by the Arabic translator with a hendiadys, *tuǧrā . . . tutammu* ("are brought about . . . are brought to completion"). A slight palaeographical change in the former gave *tuǧazza'u* ("are distributed"), which was then carried over into the Latin.

P. 86,21 et nutritio: The Latin translation does not give an equivalent to the Greek αὐξήσεις τε, either through inadvertence or because it was already absent in the Arabic archetype.

P. 86,23 διοικεῖν: Helmreich, Galeni fragmenta, p. 433, printed the correct reading διοικεῖν, with the infinitive depending on ἐδείκνυον, p. 84,22; but the manuscript reading at this point in fact is διοικεῖ. The Latin version, however, has "currit", which cannot be right, since it is "uirtus" within the part that flows, not the part itself. Whether we should read "regitur" or some other word, or whether the error goes back to the Arabic must be left open.

P. 88,6 Ἐπικουρίας – 12 δυνάμεων: Like a modern endocrinologist, Galen views the ideal body as maintained in homoeostasis, but instead of hormones and secretions, he sees as its regulators the three great organs of the body, heart, brain, and liver, each operating through its own independent system of powers or faculties. Just as the brain is the source of the psychic power, and the heart that of the vital, so the liver is the source of the natural power or faculty, i.e. that which supplies all the natural faculties for each and every part (see Gal., Synopsis libr. suor. de puls. 21: IX 492,8–11 K.). Given that later Arabic and mediaeval systematisers of Galen talked of three spirits, psychic, vital, and natural, corresponding to the three faculties, and that Galen himself in one of the last books of the Methodus medendi (XII 5: X 839, 10–840,1 K.) had floated the possibility of the liver as the source of a natural spirit, it is interesting that Galen does not use the word "spirit" in this section, but talks only of powers or faculties.[1]

P. 88,6 ad – 7 remaneant: C γ omit "ad hoc" after "indigent", ε includes it. The similar usage following "indigent" at p. 106,10 suggests that the latter is right, although in the later passage "ad" is followed by a noun, not a clause. At p. 90,6 "ad hoc quod" with subjunctive translates the similar εἰς τὸ c. inf. (p. 90,7).

P. 88,8 ἥπατος – 18: For Galen the liver is the source of the veins, through which it sends essential nutriment, the thicker food, contained in the blood (cf. De usu part. IV 15: I 234,3–8 Helmr. = III 318,14–18 K.). The liver not only prepares the food, but is in charge of its distribution (see Gal., De plac. Hipp. et Plat. VI 4,1–12: CMG V 4,1,2, pp. 384,1–386,9). It is also the source of all the vegetative functions that humans share with plants, the natural faculties. It is, in Platonic terms, the seat of the appetitive part of the soul; in Aristotelian, of the nutritive, vegetative, or reproductive (see ibid. VI 3,7: CMG V 4,1,2, p. 374,13–15; see also p. 102,17–19). The function of the liver and venous system resembles that of the root system of a plant, a simile that

[1] See O. Temkin, On Galen's pneumatology, Gesnerus 7, 1950, pp. 180–189 (repr. in: O. Temkin, The double face of Janus and other essays in the history of medicine, Baltimore and London, 1977, pp. 154–161).

goes back to the Hippocratic Corpus, if not earlier. The Hippocratic text De alim. 31: CMG I 1, p. 82,13, had called the liver the ῥίζωσις of the veins, but Galen here makes the comparison even more precise by specifying that he means the point at which the roots join the main stem of the plant.[1]

P. 88,18 οὐ μὴν – 90,6: Galen makes a neat distinction between the faculties of movement / sensation, and, in the next sentence, pulsation, which are produced and transmitted as and when needed, and the natural faculties, which remain innate in the substance of each part of the organism, and are sent out from the liver only as a supplement to what is already there. But elsewhere, e.g. In Hipp. Epid. III comm. I 40: CMG V 10,2,1, p. 58,18–21; In Hipp. Epid. VI comm. I 3: CMG V 10,2,2, p. 18,3–13; De plac. Hipp. et Plat. VIII 1,27–29: CMG V 4,1,2, p. 486,17–29, especially when speaking loosely, Galen uses the same words indiscriminately to describe the method of transmission of the three faculties from their sources including that of the natural faculties.

P. 88,19 quia – 24 hominis: The Latin translation must represent an Arabic translation which endeavoured to give the sense of the Greek text rather than an exact verbal correspondence.

P. 88,23 quorum – 26: The presence of the doublet "et – eorum" in both branches of the tradition, and the shared scribal error, "nutritur" (lines 24. 25), in C O, proves that it stood in the archetype of the Latin manuscripts: the absence of the words "hominis – natura^{II}" (lines 24–25) from B may be explained as an accidental omission through homoioteleuton. But "nutritur" makes no sense here, and hence ε emended to the palaeographically similar "mutatur". But how and where the mistake occurred cannot be determined.

P. 90,5 uerumptamen – 9 modicum: The Latin translator (and his source?) adds "epatis et", making it clear that Galen regarded both the 'natural' faculty in the liver and the 'vital' faculty represented in pulsation as essential for the maintenance and well-being of the organism. But the addition is not necessary, for Galen has just described the role of the liver, the brain, and the heart, and he comments in an aside that the faculty of pulsation is also of importance in maintaining all parts of the body, and not just the vascular system.

P. 90,12–17: Having explained the three ἀρχαί by which the body is organised (cf. p. 58,5–6 for the phrase "regimen animalium"), he raises the possibility that some one might wrongly think that he is talking about the two principles involved in generation (cf. p. 64,17 et demonstraui – 20 istius, for the same technique), asserts again his meaning more clearly, and then makes a neat transition to the topic that his putative audience might have wrongly

1 For a general survey of Galen's ideas on the liver and venous system, see N. Mani, Die historischen Grundlagen der Leberforschung, I. Teil: Die Vorstellungen über Anatomie, Physiologie und Pathologie der Leber in der Antike, 2nd ed., Basle and Stuttgart, 1965 (Basler Veröffentlichungen zur Geschichte der Medizin und der Biologie 9), pp. 65–70; Harris, pp. 323–332, neither of whom refers to this passage. Note also that the references adduced by Mani, p. 68, and by Harris, pp. 326 n. 3; 352 n. 5, to show the liver as the source of the natural faculties, derive from the commentary on the Hippocratic De alimento, which is a Renaissance pastiche.

assumed that he was already discussing. Galen's concern with correct meaning is not just a rhetorical device. The word ἀρχαί may apply equally to the organisation of the body in its normal state by the three main organs and to its creation within the womb by means of seed and blood; the precise significance of ἀρχαί depends largely on Galen's context.

P. 90,18–27: This chapter on embryology is among the most interesting of this book, because Galen here, unusually, confessed that, concerning one detail, he changed his mind during his lifetime. For Galenic ideas on embryology and generation see E. Lesky, Die Zeugungs- und Vererbungslehren der Antike und ihr Nachwirken, Akademie d. Wiss. u. d. Lit., Abh. d. geistes- u. sozialwiss. Kl. 1950,19, Wiesbaden, 1951; H. B. Adelmann, Marcello Malpighi and the evolution of embryology, 5 vols., Ithaca, 1966, pp. 744–748; Nickel, Untersuchungen zur Embryologie Galens.

P. 90,18–20: Galen's initial claim that there is a faculty responsible for the formation of the embryo at once puts him in opposition to the Epicureans and those who refused to believe in an argument from design (see De foet. form. 6: IV 688,4–7 K.). His second claim, linking the generation of animals to that of plants, goes back at least to Hippocratic times, if not to Empedocles (see Hipp., De nat. pueri 22–27: VII 514,6–528,25 L.; Empedocl., A 70: I, p. 296,16–20 D.-K.). At De sem. I 9,13: CMG V 3,1, p. 94,24–27, Galen accuses Aristotle, somewhat unfairly, of neglecting his own precept that one should consider the genesis of both plants and animals together.[1] This is not a charge which can be levelled at Galen, for his writings on embryology are filled with examples and with references, both real and metaphorical, to their similar growth and development (see Nickel, pp. 22–27, for excellent comments on Galen's methodology).

P. 90,21: "motus" here does not represent the active principle of motion that, as we have seen, Galen locates in the brain, but the movement, or rather the succession of movements, responsible for development within the foetus. Aristotle had argued (De generat. anim. I 2. 20: 716 a 4–7; 729 a 9–14) that the female provided the matter, the male semen the form and the principle of motion that created the embryo. Others went further: Galen ascribes to some Peripatetics the opinion that once the male semen has imparted the principle of motion to the menstrual blood, it is immediately ejected again (see De sem. I 3,6: CMG V 3,1, p. 68,18–20).[2] Galen himself holds the view that, as well as the matter in menstrual blood, both male and female seeds are necessary for generation, and both seeds contain this moving principle, albeit in different proportion, as does menstrual blood, although here the "active principle" is extremely weak, and the female seed becomes effective only when it is allied to the same power in the menstrual blood (see ibid. II 2,20–24: CMG V 3,1,

1 For a defence of Aristotle, see De Lacy, in: CMG V 3,1, p. 219, the note to pp. 94,27–96,2.

2 Aristotle himself argued (De generat. anim. II 3: 737 a 7–16) that the male seed dissolves and evaporates; this opinion was rejected by Galen (De sem. I 4,1–11: CMG V 3,1, pp. 70,27–72,19).

pp. 164,25–166,15).[1] But both Galen and Aristotle agree that matter is turned into an embryo as a result of some motion, just as milk is curdled by the addition of fig-juice or rennet, and Galen pours scorn on those who assume that this process could be achieved just by a single touch or glancing blow from semen. In his view, the generation of the embryo requires the continuous presence of the motive principle, which is responsible for a succession of movements (see ibid. I 5,10; 7,1: CMG V 3,1, pp. 80,24–26; 86,9–10).

P. 90,22–92,3: The apparent clarity of Galen's account of his (rare) change of mind hides a variety of difficulties. To begin with, although Galen does discuss the order of formation of the organs in the foetus in De usu partium (esp. XV 6: II 359,9–360,13 Helmr. = IV 241,1–242,13 K.), he does not report his change of mind there. He does, however, hint that since, in his view, the size of the liver, as observed in his dissections of animal foetuses, is far greater than that of the heart and brain, the liver is likely to have been formed first of the three major organs. This argument is repeated again at the end of his life in De foet. form. 3: IV 662,10–664,4 K., and further extended later in the same chapter (672,7–11 K.), where the order of formation is given as liver, heart, and brain. His anatomical observations are, in his opinion, confirmed by Hippocratic precedent, for he identifies as the still unformed liver the round red mass described by the Hippocratic author of De natura pueri (13: VII 490,15 L.). But later in De foetuum formatione (5: IV 682,14–18 K.) he appears to hold a slightly different view, one that sees the liver and heart, "the foundations of the house or the keel of the ship", as produced in a second step after the veins and arteries that bring the mother's blood to the foetus. The same development, first veins and arteries, then liver and heart, is implied at p. 94,6–10 ἧπαρ.

But the difficulties with Galen's memory do not end here, for in none of his extant works does he declare unequivocally that the heart was the first organ to be formed. At De plac. Hipp. et Plat. II 8,21–22: CMG V 4,1,2, p. 160,29–33, he says that others believe this, but without pronouncing on the truth of this assertion: he merely remarks that it is irrelevant to the argument for which it is generally used. His formulation is, at best, extremely cautious, and, taken in context, suggests that Galen did not himself believe in this theory. Certainly, later on in De plac. Hipp. et Plat. VI 6,32–56: CMG V 4,1,2, pp. 400,31–404,37, he concentrates on the formation of the liver as the prime source of the veins in a manner which would seem to indicate that he has already rejected the priority of the heart. At the very least, then, the evidence of De plac. Hipp. et Plat. II and VI indicates that before 166 A.D., the latest date for the composition of these books, Galen no longer believed strongly, if, indeed, he believed at all, in this theory. Or, to put it another way, Galen is likely to be right when he ascribes his belief in it to the days of his youth (i.e. before he was 30).

But did Galen ever believe in it? This passage is alone in stating this unequivocally, and, confusingly, when Galen elsewhere describes his change

[1] Cf. J. Kollesch, Galens Auseinandersetzung mit der Aristotelischen Samenlehre, in: Aristoteles – Werk und Wirkung, pp. 17–26.

of mind over the order in which the three major organs are created, at De foet. form. 3: IV 663,11–664,4 K., it is a change from a different opinion, that expressed at De sem. I 8,8–9,7: CMG V 3,1, pp. 92,4–94,6, cf. also De Lacy's note on p. 218 to p. 92,4–8, which imagines that all three organs are created and develop simultaneously. This view is certainly compatible with Galen's earlier comments in De placitis Hippocratis et Platonis, and may well have been held by Galen in the 160s, when Galen discussed embryology in the (lost) De demonstratione (see De usu part. XV 5: II 357,24–27 Helmr. = IV 238,17–239,2 K.). It was one that Galen came to doubt in the early 170s, between the composition of De semine and that of the last books of De usu partium (see De Lacy's dating in: CMG V 3,1, p. 47), and which he subsequently changed.

A commentator is here faced with a difficult choice between two alternatives, either of which has unfortunate consequences for Galen's reliability as an autobiographer. Galen may be right in his description of his change of opinion; he did believe, while young, that the heart was formed first, and, during the composition of the later books of De usu partium, he changed his mind and gave priority to the liver. But if so, he passes over in silence an opinion that he held for some time, discussed as a central part of one treatise, and, in the 190s or later, when he wrote De foetuum formatione, recalled as the opinion from which he was gradually compelled to dissent. Galen's fault is thus one of omission. The alternative is to believe that Galen is actually wrong in his recollection. Although he was well aware of the theory that gave priority to the heart, and referred to it in his writings, this was never one to which he adhered with any degree of firmness, and not the one that he had abandoned. Galen, in his old age, rewrote history.[1]

P. 90,23–24 ἀνδράσιν ἀξιολόγοις: By far the most famous of all who held this opinion was Aristotle, who believed that he had found confirmation for his view through observing the formation of the foetal chick in hen's eggs (see Hist. anim. VI 3: 561 a 11–13). It became the standard view among the Peripatetics and the Stoics, and was referred to by Pliny as almost universal (see the testimonia). Censorinus (De die natali 6,1: p. 9,2–3 Sallmann) traced the idea back to Empedocles, and the various responses to this problem formed part of the common stock of the doxographical writers. Indeed, in that tradition as represented by Aetius, the belief that the heart and with it the veins and arteries were formed first is ascribed simply to "the doctors" (Diels, Doxographi Graeci, p. 427,10–11).

P. 92,2 χωρὶς – 10: Galen's first argument is part logical, part morphological. For creation, the foetus requires blood, which comes through the bloodvessels of the womb. But the blood that reaches the heart via the veins has first to go through the liver: this can be seen anatomically and since in Galenic theory the liver is the starting-point of the veins, one can hardly ima-

[1] Cf. Nickel, pp. 80–82; A. Debru, L'ordre de formation des organes embryonnaires: la retractatio de Galien, Bulletin d'Histoire et d'Epistémologie des Sciences de la Vie 2, 1995, pp. 156–163. If Galen was writing from memory, confusion is perhaps more likely than deliberate omission of a major theory.

gine anything being produced from veins without a liver. Besides, the liver in the early foetus is the largest visible organ, and lies closest to the womb (see Gal., De foet. form. 3: IV 662,12–13; 672,8–9 K.; cf. Nickel, pp. 74–77). All these arguments indicate that the liver is formed at the same time as the heart, if not before it.

At De foet. form. 3: IV 664,4–8 K., Galen put forward two alternatives for the origin of the blood that forms the foetal heart: it comes either via the umbilical vein into the foetal liver and thence into the foetal venous system or from the mother's arterial system via the two arteries which eventually form the "great artery", or aorta (cf. De uteri dissect. 10,14: CMG V 2,1, p. 56, 9–14). Although he himself favours the first alternative, he is well aware that both veins and arteries co-exist in the foetus, and he does not entirely exclude the second, at least as providing an additional blood supply. The translation of ἀγγείων (vessels) as "uene", is over-precise, since Arabic *ʿirq* covers both veins and arteries. A translator also made a slight mistake in translating φλεβὸς as plural, not singular. Galen (wrongly) believed that there were two veins that passed from the mother to the umbilicus of the foetus, and then united together as soon as they had passed through the umbilicus to form a single umbilical vein going directly to the liver (cf. De usu part. XV 4: II 349, 11–16 Helmr. = IV 227,14–18 K.).

P. 92,11 licet – 12: The serious difficulties begin at "licet ueniat" and continue into the next sentence.[1] Although the manuscripts differ considerably among themselves, at least part of the sense is clear: the foetal arteries coming from the womb through the umbilicus[2] take a longer route to the heart than the foetal veins. The repetition at line 38 of the statement that the foetal arteries contain either pneuma by itself or a mixture of blood and pneuma suggests that C preserves the better readings. The translator's repetition of "spiritus" offered an obvious inducement to miscopying, and the varying position of "tantum", present in all manuscripts except O, suggests further scribal attempts to clean up a corrupt text.

But given that Galen so often inveighs against Erasistratus and his followers for thinking that the arteries contain only pneuma, could he have even allowed that possibility here? Could he have tried to include the Erasistrateans as supporters of his view of the course of the arteries, while not, for the moment, pointing out their errors? The answer must be no, for Galen insists strongly at De foet. form. 3: IV 664,7–9; 671,13–15 K., that the arteries carry both substances. He is well aware that the arterial blood in the foetus is much thinner and warmer than the venous (ibid.: IV 671,15–16 K.) and that the foetus receives its supply of pneuma from the mother through the arterial system, not via the foetal heart (see De usu part. VI 21: I 370,13–24 Helmr. = III

1 Although it is tempting to emend to "licet <et>" and to read "matre" for "matrice" at lines 11 and 13 (cf. the wrong reading "matrice" instead of "matre" in C at line 19, and the presence of "sua" at lines 11 and 13), to do so might be to improve on the translator.

2 At lines 20 and 26 the Latin word "diafragma" (barrier) corresponds to χόριον (chorion), but the parallels here indicate that Galen is not talking about the chorion but about the umbilicus, the ὀμφαλός.

509,3–13 K.). Besides, Galen is talking here about the transport of blood to the foetus as building material, and pneuma is irrelevant to the argument. At the same time, there can be no doubt that these passages stood in α, and probably also in the Arabic on which the Latin was based. A clue may be found in the fact that, both here and at line 19, the connecting relative is found only in ε, and looks like an attempt at emendation to give a smoother text. The offending sentences would then have stood on their own, perhaps as marginal glosses to explain the contents of the arteries, and would then have been taken over into the text.

P. 92,12–18: Galen's description of the course of the arteries in the foetus to join the aorta, which he had first set out in De usu part. XV 4: II 349, 16–351,25 Helmr. = IV 227,18–231,2 K., is remarkably accurate, and shows the results of some clever dissection (cf. Harris, pp. 291–293, and fig. 5; D. Nickel, Galens Untersuchungen zur embryonalen Blutbewegung, Communicationes de Historia Artis Medicinae 27 [93–96], 1981, pp. 25–35). But the manuscripts of the Latin translation present a text that differs in one important way from what Galen said there and at De foet. form. 3: IV 661,10–662,1 K. (cf. also De plac. Hipp. et Plat. VI 6,51–53: CMG V 4,1,2, p. 404,17–22; Simon, Gal. Anat. II, p. 163,9–13). According to the manuscripts, the foetal arteries that come together at the base of the spine then pass up the spine to join the aorta just below the shoulder blades before going to the heart; according to the quoted passages, they join the aorta much further down the spine, and there Galen carefully describes the "great artery", the aorta, not the arteries, as running the whole length of the spine, and it is the aorta too which enters the left side of the heart. The solution, as J. Kollesch and D. Nickel suggested to me, is to transpose the two clauses "et postea . . . pectoris" (lines 16–17) and "et postea . . . dorsum" (lines 15–16), which would then give a text entirely consonant with what Galen says in the parallel passages: the umbilical arteries join the aorta at the base of the spine, and the aorta, going along the spine straight to the chest region ("in directo pectoris", line 17, would correspond to εὐθὺ τοῦ στήθους, cf. for this construction with εὐθύ CMG V 3,1, pp. 114,12; 118,17) until just below the shoulder blades, would then turn inwards to reach the left ventricle, to which it distributes what remains of its contents.[1] The identical opening of each clause would make for an easy transpositional error, and the plural forms of the verb at lines 15–19 in ε would thus be an attempt by a scribe to regularise the grammar of the new sentence, in which arteries and aorta together reach the left ventricle.

P. 92,18–20: Galen is here talking about the substance within the foetal aorta and its source, which is the mother, not the womb itself, and thus the reading of β (matre) is to be preferred to that of C (matrice). When Galen re-

1 Although Galen knew that in the foetus the ductus arteriosus connected the aorta with the pulmonary artery, shrivelling up after birth, this passage implies that not all of the contents of the aorta took that path and that some reached the foetal heart, presumably the small amount necessary to ensure its living existence (cf. De usu part. VI 21: I 370, 18–23 Helmr. = III 509,8–11 K.).

peats himself later on (lines 20–21), he talks of the arteries receiving their contents "from the woman", a formulation that suggests that in his original Greek he had made a slight and elegant variation to avoid an exact verbal repetition while still maintaining the distinction between the womb as the starting-point of the arteries and the woman as the source of their contents.

P. 92,20–21: Galen's view, expressed at De foet. form. 5: IV 682,1–18 K., is that the chorion, the veins, and the arteries must be formed first. Only then can the next stage of generation, the formation of the liver and, subsequently, the heart, take place. Others, including Aristotle (De generat. anim. II 4: 740 a 1–23) disagreed.

P. 92,22 οὐ μὴν – 94,2: Galen repeats the anatomical argument he had used at lines 7–10. It is strengthened by the addition of σαφῶς: the passage of the vein first to the liver and then to the heart is something that is *clearly* visible to any one who cares to look.

P. 94,3 Ἔτι – 6: As Nickel, pp. 77–79, rightly says, Galen is primarily criticising the Stoics and Peripatetics (including Aristotle) who believed that the heart as the first part formed shaped all the other parts.

P. 94,4 et – 8: In the process of translation Galen's comment has become so garbled that it now says the reverse of the original Greek. The glossator in ε rightly identified "illud" with "cor", "prius . . . quam illud" corresponds to πρὸ αὐτῆς. This phrase at some point was misinterpreted so that instead of the formation of the vessels preceding that of the heart, it is the actual moment of generation that does so. The words εὔλογόν ἐστιν (line 9) have been omitted.

P. 94,12 ὅπερ – 17: The first of the views offered by Galen is that of Aristotle, the Peripatetics, and the Stoics (see the testimonia). It was, in his opinion, also that of Erasistratus and his followers (see De fac. nat. II 3: Scr. min. III 161,10–163,7 Helmr. = II 83,9–85,16 K.), although how far it was held by Erasistratus himself is a little more doubtful (cf. Garofalo's comment on Erasistratus, fr. 56: p. 79). It was not one with which Galen himself was in sympathy, and he wrote a specific tract dealing with the doctrine of Chrysippus on this point (see De foet. form. 6: IV 699,13–18 K.). Nonetheless, it is mentioned here as a possible explanation, not because Galen himself believes in it, but because as he says (ibid.: IV 700,2–702,4 K.), he can find no positive demonstrative proof in favour of any opinion at all. He is in a situation of *aporia*, unable to decide for certain just what it is that forms the embryo, and hence he is prepared for the moment to let this possibility remain, even though he himself believes that to think of seed or even the pneuma contained in it as the moulder of the embryo is unlikely to be right.

The second view is that the seed is a mere instrument, but an instrument of what? In De foet. form. 6, Galen rejects the idea that anything that is not endowed with wisdom could have moulded the foetus. By doing so, he opposes those who thought that the moulder is the soul contained in the seed, which the Aristotelians would call the vegetative soul, Platonists the appetitive soul, and the Stoics simply Nature, something which was, in his opinion, not only not wise but entirely without rationality. At the same time, the likeness of children to their parents suggests that seed must have something to do with the creation of the embryo. On the other hand, Galen cannot bring himself to believe that the rational soul, by which after birth one's whole life is run and organised, could be what moulds the embryo. One of his Platonist teachers had suggested to him that it was the World Soul that was responsible, an idea that Galen thought could well apply to man, but was close to impious if it referred to insects, worms, snakes and the like.[1] Besides, a material soul could not have the skill and ability to create complex organisms, and anyone who believed this risked falling into the trap of the Epicureans and those who rejected providence in favour of a mechanistic universe (cf. De foet. form. 6: IV 688,4–7 K.). But while Galen was firm in his negative arguments, all that he was prepared to say for certain on the positive side was that the cause that moulded living things was extremely great in power and wisdom.

P. 94,15 ἕτερον – 17 / 94,12 quod – 16: The neuter participle phrase τὸ διαπλάττον ("what moulds") is rendered in the Latin translation as an agent noun ("formator"), a change essential in Arabic, which lacks a neuter. This translation would not have seemed out of place to a translator familiar with Galen's Platonism and its demiurge or creator (cf. Larrain, in: Galens Kommentar zu Platons Timaios, p. 58; F. Solmsen, Nature as craftsman in Greek thought, Journal of the History of Ideas 24, 1963, pp. 473–496, repr. in: F. Solmsen, Kleine Schriften, vol. I, Hildesheim, 1968 [Collectanea IV], pp. 332–355). Indeed, Galen seems to go further in this direction when he characterises this unknown agent as ἕτερον . . . θειότερον, "something else more divine" than mere seed, but whether, as the Latin translation has it, he also called the "something more noble" "almighty God" is more doubtful. It is true that at De plac. Hipp. et Plat. IX 8,22; 9,3: CMG V 4,1,2, pp. 596,5–7; 598,7–10, Galen had seemed to talk in terms of gods who formed mankind, but he made it quite clear there that he regarded this as merely plausible, and as an idea of which even Plato himself was not entirely confident. Similarly, at De foet. form. 6: IV 687,12–688,2 K., while he was convinced of the moulder's wisdom and foresight, he refused to commit himself as to whether this was a god or a soul different from that of god. His appeal to philosophers to show him this moulder is clearly meant rhetorically. However much he might wish to believe, he cannot as yet accept any of the arguments so far put forward, and remains in a state of *aporia*. It is thus unlikely that in a treatise written not so many years after De foetuum formatione he should come out definitely in favour of a single creator, "almighty God". Besides, had so important a conclusion been in the Greek, it is hard to see why even the crassest or most cursory of excerptors should have left it out. G. Strohmaier suggests that it represents the Arabic translator's attempt to give a more theologically precise and acceptable interpretation of θειότερον.

P. 94,18–21: This is an unusually rough transition between topics. Ga-

1 This objection did not originate with Galen: it is used by Alexander of Aphrodisias against the Stoics (De mixt. 11: p. 226,28 Bruns; De anima libri mantissa: p. 113,12–16 Bruns) and may well have been a commonplace among the Peripatetics. I owe this point to R. W. Sharples.

len's rhetorical skills generally lead him easily from one theme to another, but here, having talked about generation and the foetus, he shifts abruptly to the four humours and to the treatises in which he has discussed them. The link in Galen's mind is probably to be gleaned from line 8. Having once declared his agnosticism about what it is that forms the foetus, he thinks about the building blocks of the body in sickness and in health, the four humours. But he stays only briefly on this point before going on to talk about drugs and their workings.

P. 94,18: C γ, manuscripts from both branches of the tradition, do not include the last of the four humours, which might imply that it had already been lost in Arabic. The addition of "et melancolia" in ε is thus another attempt at emendation; this is also suggested by the fact that at p. 98,7 and elsewhere in the translation the fourth humour is called "colera nigra", not "melancolia", which relates to the state, not the actual humour. If the error is thought to have occurred during the process of transmission in Latin, one might emend to "colera ⟨nigra, colera⟩ citrina".

P. 94,19 in – 21: In De elementis ex Hippocratis sententia Galen set out in detail for the first time his own explanations of the theory of the four humours, while in the late commentary on De natura hominis he explicated at length the Hippocratic treatise which more than any other proclaimed that theory. That other tracts in the Hippocratic Corpus known to and used by Galen promoted different views of the humours, in number, role, and identity, was less important to him than the fact that in his eyes (and in those of others, see Anon. Lond. VI 43 – VII 40) this was the central document of Hippocrates' teaching.

P. 94,22–96,2: Who these physicians ("quidam") were who thought that blood was the only substance like[1] and appropriate to nature is not made clear, nor does the author of De natura hominis attack those who believe this theory. Galen here merely categorises their opinion as "plausible", and contrasts it with the "more truthful" account of Hippocrates which depends on "probatio", "proof" (p. 96,2).[2]

Galen himself does not mention Thrasymachus of Sardis, fl. 380 B.C. (?), who is reported in the Anonymus Londinensis papyrus (XI 42 – XII 8) to have originated a theory that phlegm, bile, and pus were the results of malignant changes in the blood. His fluids are not the canonical quartet of the Hippocratics, and, given the variety of theories described in this papyrus and in the Hippocratic Corpus, let alone those that are now entirely lost to us, one can doubt Galen's picture of a world in which belief in his four cardinal humours was nearly universal.

P. 96,3 in alio libro: "post hoc" (line 9) would appear to rule out the treatise on purgatives, De purgantium medicamentorum facultatibus (XI 323–

1 The parallel with p. 96,18 shows that "similis" is here nominative, and that it is the nature of the body to which blood is similar. The phrase "similis nature et appropriatus ei" thus represents a hendiadys typical of Ḥunayn.

2 Galen also may be influenced by the account of the blood given by Plato in the Timaeus (82 c–83 a).

342 K.), as the book to which Galen refers for elucidation of his ideas on humours. Most likely is a reference to Galen's discussion of Hipp., De nat. hom. 5,3: CMG I 1,3, pp. 176,10–178,6 in his commentary on this passage (In Hipp. De nat. hom. comm. I 28: CMG V 9,1, p. 38,1–22) or at De elem. ex Hipp. sent. 13,1–10: CMG V 1,2, pp. 148,15–150,19.

P. 96,5–6: Galen argues that each purgative or emetic attracts one admixture in particular, although smaller amounts of one or two others can be removed at the same time. Given that there are four humours, why then does he apparently mention only three? Galen regards blood as the most appropriate of all the humours in man, and hence balance can be achieved by removing the other humours until that proper state is reached. This is what Galen appears to be claiming further on in this chapter, but it also implies an equivocation between blood as a humour and blood as the fluid in which all other humours travel round the body, cf. his definition at In Hipp. Epid. VI comm. II 40; IV 30: CMG V 10,2,2, pp. 109,12–15; 248,5–10. Galen, as we shall see (p. 100,11–12), is aware of this problem, but deems it irrelevant. It also comes close to the theory of the first group of "quidam" (p. 94,22) that he has just dismissed with the promise that his and Hippocrates' theory is even better. Besides, since only phlegm, bile, and black bile are attacked by pharmaka, there can be at most only two other admixtures removed by them.

P. 96,6–8: Galen here argues against those who thought that whatever drug was given attracted a certain amount of mixed humour from the body, which it then changed during the process of attraction either into its own nature or into itself (cf. De elem. ex Hipp. sent. 12,1: CMG V 1,2, p. 146,10–12; In Hipp. De nat. hom. comm. I 28: CMG V 9,1, p. 38,23–25; De atra bile 8,7: CMG V 4,1,1, p. 93,10–12; De purg. med. fac. 1. 2: XI 325,12–14; 329,10–13 K.). In other words, the type of fluid evacuated depended on what might be thought of as chemical or biochemical changes occurring as a result of an interaction between the drug and the fluid being extracted. This was an ingenious attempt to avoid the hypothesis that a specific drug could remove a specific fluid from within the body, especially if those fluids circulated together as and in blood. Galen quotes Julian the Methodist verbatim in support of this theory (Adv. Iul. 8,1–16: CMG V 10,3, pp. 62,16–67,22) which he frequently ascribes elsewhere (e.g. De purg. med. fac. 1–3: XI 324,3–335,18 K.) to Asclepiades and his followers[1], and to Erasistratus and the Erasistrateans, all of whom rejected or played down the role of humours in favour of a more mechanistic physiology.

P. 96,9–11: The tract De purgantium medicamentorum facultate (XI 323–342 K.) is cited only in treatises written in the 190s or later (see Adv. Iul. 8,1: CMG V 10,3, p. 63,1; In Hipp. De nat. hom. comm. I 28: CMG V 9,1, p. 38,26–27; Meth. med. XIII 6: X 893,16 K.; De ord. libror. suor. 2: Scr. min. II 85,19–22 Müller = XIX 55,17–56,2 K.). This suggests that it was written late in life, when he revived his particular interest in drugs. But Galen's interest here is not in establishing a chronology, and "post hoc" is simply a looser "later".

P. 96,12–15: Galen typically goes some way to meet his opponents, only

1 At p. 327,9. 18 K. read Ἀσκληπιάδειοι, -αδείους.

to use this apparent agreement as a further proof of the weakness of the alternative argument. He is prepared to accept that an actual drug can have an effect on the fluid attracted at the moment of attraction, i.e. that a drug that removes bile will make the fluid removed a little more bilious than it might otherwise have been, but, in his view, this effect is bound to be slight. But for his opponents, as we have seen, all or most of the effective change in the fluid removed occurred at or after the moment of attraction. Galen's concession of "slightly" would not have been acceptable to them. Nor would his explanation: that the change would be slight because it was largely bile that was already being removed. The Latin of the end of the sentence becomes difficult to follow, although the sense of the passage is clear. "in ipsa" refers back to the process of attraction already described. "inter omnes", on the other hand, is not easy to explain, and could well have come in as a repetition of the same words in line 16, where they make sense. It is possible, however, although somewhat unlikely, that Galen was intending here to emphasise that a small amount of another humour might also be evacuated at the same time, and, for that reason, I have not deleted the words. But what is missing is a reference to a cholagogue as specific to bile, and I suspect that "coleram" was lost either from the Latin, or, since all the Latin manuscripts agree in its omission and have "inter omnes"[1], at an earlier stage in the transmission.

P. 96,15–19: Although Galen asserts that blood *qua* humour is the most appropriate humour in sangineous animals, De elem. sec. Hipp. 10,1-3: CMG V 1,2, p. 138,15-140,2; De temp. II 3: p. 59,20-22 Helmr.= I 603,7-8 K., he mentions only once in a surviving treatise the fluid that takes the place of blood in bloodless creatures.[2] But Galen was familiar with Aristotle's definition of the various types of bloodless creatures as the testacea, crustacea, cephalopods, and insects in his Historia animalium I 6: 490 b 9, and with his long discussion of them at IV 1-7: 523 a 31-532 b 26 (see De usu part. III 2: I 130,4 Helmr.= III 177,13-14 K.), and he could well have commented on this specific point at greater length in a lost treatise.

P. 96,16: The agreement of C γ in reading "plus magis" confirms that these words stood in the translator's original manuscript. Unless these are authorial variants, the first comparative will simply strengthen the second, cf. p. 66,9–10 "magis minus".

P. 96,17–18 genus . . . habent: For this construction see above, p. 171, the note to p. 84,21.

P. 96,20 natura istarum medicinarum: The reading of ε ("natura") makes somewhat better sense than those of γ ("medicina") and C ("medicinas"), and corresponds better to what Galen probably wrote, πέφυκε c. inf. This formulation could have been rendered in Arabic by one that gave: "it belongs to the essential nature of the thing" (frequently attested in the Arabic version of De

1 The restoration by B² of the passage omitted in B (lines 15–16 "et – inter omnes" after "inter omnes") suggests strongly that "inter omnes" (line 15) was present in the exemplar of the corrector.

2 De nominibus medicis: p. 29,39 Meyerhof-Schacht, he calls it "blood-water" (Arabic *ǧubn*, but the Greek original is unclear).

elementis ex Hippocratis sententia), from which the Latin translator derived "natura" as subject (G. Strohmaier). The same idiom also appears in the phrase "natura medicine" (lines 6–7). The wrong readings of γ and C possibly derived from the following „medicinarum". Since the reading "medicina/as" goes back to α, the variant in ε must be a good conjecture based on the parallel in lines 6–7.

P. 96,21–98,2 stillea . . . iarcan . . . iarcan . . . listilia: The Latin translator transcribed the Arabic names of the diseases, *(al-)istisqā'*, "dropsy", and *yaraqān*, "jaundice", with consequent confusion. C preserves the best transcriptions, although even here one should note that at p. 98,2 C (or the translator himself) retains traces of the definite article *al-* which is dropped at p. 96,2. The confused text offered much room for speculation and invention, particularly in ε. At p. 96,21 the translator's "stillea" stood in β as "squilla", which was replaced by a gloss in B ε to give a familiar disease, "squinancia (-tia)", "quinsy". When the word reappeared ("listilia", p. 98,2), it was again misinterpreted as "lintissia" in γ and "leutissimam" in ε. The glossator of ε came up with the right answer, "yposarcam", "dropsy", but it is an open question how he reached his conclusion. Given his lack of success elsewhere, it is tempting to believe that he recognised traces of "leucophlegmasia" or "leucophlegmancia", standard transcriptions for one of Galen's types of dropsy.[1] If so, he was fortunate, for almost certainly, to judge from the parallel passages, especially at Adv. Iul. 8,14. 16: CMG V 10,3, pp. 66,19; 67,21, and De atra bile 6,10; 8,6. 7: CMG V 4,1,1, pp. 84,6; 93,1. 7, the phrase that Galen had used was οἱ ὑδεριῶντες, οἱ ὑδερικοί or a similar adjective. The glossator had better luck with "jaundice", correctly glossing it at p. 96,23, but he saw no need to intervene at p. 98,2 where his text had a plausible, if wrong, reading "artheticam", "arthritis".

P. 98,1–4: The sense of this sentence can be deduced from parallel passages (see Gal., Adv. Iul. 8,14: CMG V 10,3, p. 66,18–22; De atra bile 8,7: CMG V 4,1,1, p. 93,6–9; In Hipp. De nat. hom. comm. I 28: CMG V 9,1, p. 39, 5–8): one should observe what happens if one gives a hydragogue to a sufferer from jaundice, and a cholagogue to a sufferer from dropsy. The result would be disastrous, since none of the damaging humour would be removed, while, at the same time, a small amount of the humour related to the drug would be evacuated, to the detriment of the patient. This train of thought is only partially followed in the Latin, since the text at lines 3 medicina – 4 iuuamentum is seriously corrupt. 1. There is no qualification of "medicina" as a cholagogue (purgatiua colere) corresponding to the words "purgatiua aque" in line 2. 2. The expression "de humore simili sibi" lacks syntactical coherence. "de" probably expresses some partitive relationship (cf., at p. 96,23, the corresponding "de ipsa aqua") and depends on some form of "euacuare" that has dropped out in the process of transmission. In any case, the expression "simili sibi" must refer to the relationship of the humour to its corresponding drug

[1] See for examples of this equivalence in mediaeval texts, C. Du Cange, Glossarium mediae et infimae latinitatis, vol. V, Niort, 1885, p. 73 s. v. leucoflancia; and D. R. Howlett, A dictionary of mediaeval Latin from British sources, Oxford, 1987, vol. IV, p. 1193.

(cf. p. 102,5). 3. Since it is clear to Galen that only a small amount of the humour closely related to the contraindicated drug can be evacuated, the phrase "in magna quantitate" contradicts his reasoning, since one expects "in a small quantity". 4. After the phrase, "si contrario modo, per contrarium" (lines 1–2), it is inconceivable that comments on the application of contraindicated drugs should conclude with the notion that they are of some value (line 4). That this judgment is doubtful is proved by the parallel passages, which either reject the idea of any benefit or warn against the consequent additional damage. One expects at least a negative before "iuuamentum". That the text has not been transmitted intact is also evidenced by the omission of the copula "est" in C γ; in ε and B² the presence of the copula after "iuuamentum" depends on a later insertion. One must also wonder whether "non est" (ñ ē) has not dropped out after "euacuatione". The direct linkage of "illa euacuatione" with "iuuamentum est" (or "non est iuuamentum") is also suspect, and hence "in" has been inserted before "illa".

How far these corruptions have developed solely in the Latin tradition is not clear. At least where the problems are those of content rather than simply linguistic, it is possible that they go back at least to the Arabic tradition.

The glossators of D and E, faced with an obscure word (ysore ε), essayed a guess. In the margin of the manuscript E² put ".i. busbo"; D is very badly damaged at this point, and the letters inserted by D² above the line are almost illegible, but enough survives to indicate that the word was not "busbo", although what it was is impossible to say. "busbo", however, is an extremely rare word, not to be found in standard dictionaries of mediaeval Latin. It is a latinisation of a Flemish word "busboom", the box tree or the caper[1], and is thus a useful confirmation of the provenance of the glossator and of the manuscript in N. France and Flanders. But as a guess for the meaning of the word it is wide of the mark. Modern pharmacognosy has revealed the presence of steroidal alkaloids in the buxaceae family, including the common box tree, Buxus sempervirens, but these would not act as a cholagogue. The British Pharmaceutical Codex of 1907, the last major edition to concentrate on galenicals, notes that the leaves of the box tree could be confused with those of the bearberry, Arctostaphylus uva-ursi, which also grows widely in N. Europe, but bearberry leaves are a diuretic, used in diseases of the urine tract.[2] Neither box nor bearberry would have been of the slightest use in jaundice. Once again, the glossator has guessed wrongly.

P. 98,5–10 similitudine: Galen paraphrases rather than quotes Hippocrates directly here, and in a somewhat tendentious fashion. The author of De natura hominis strongly attacked those who believed that man was a unity, originally formed out of a single humour, and especially those who considered that man was composed of blood alone. In its place he set a theory of

1 This identification appears in a near contemporary Flemish manuscript, Utrecht, Universiteits-Bibliotheek 694, which identifies Capparis agrestis with "die vrocht van den busboom", see W. F. Daems, Boec van medicinen in Dietsche, Leiden, 1967, p. 279.

2 See G. E. Trease and W. C. Evans, Pharmacognosy, 11th ed., London, 1978, p. 115; British Pharmaceutical Codex, London, 1907, p. 1269.

the four humours, blood, phlegm, black and yellow bile, each of which predominated at certain times of the year, and each of which, in excess or deficiency, brought about its own range of diseases. But Galen's strategy here is to gain as much support as possible for his views, even from those who do not believe in the theory of the four humours. Hence, he grants the possibility that blood is the most appropriate substance in the body, and the most important of the humours, in order to show that others have observed the same phenomena as he, even if they have wrongly interpreted them. Besides, he is prepared to concede that the view of those who emphasise the role of blood is at least plausible, "uerisimile" (cf. De elem. ex Hipp. sent. 11,1–2: CMG V 1,2, p. 140,15–20; In Hipp. De nat. hom. comm. I 29: CMG V 9,1, p. 41,2–5) and goes on to say (lines 11–23) that it does not matter for the purposes of medical practice whether one believes that the four elemental humours were produced together or that blood was produced first, and subsequently the rest. Once again, the key to Galen's beliefs lies in his attitude towards proof and certitude. Hippocrates "has demonstrated" the existence of the four humours, but parts of the developed theory still remain at the level of plausibility.

P. 98,7: "causa" is preserved only by C, but it receives some support from O, which gives the feminine form of the relative ("que"), thereby suggesting that something has dropped out. The reading of B ε ("quod") thus represents a normalisation of the relative after the omission.

P. 98,8–17 corpore: Syntax and sense are hard to piece together in this section. The Greek excerptor excluded the crucial sentence ("et merito – similitudine"), although the Latin preserves enough of the sense to make the general argument clear, and in the process of transmission two Greek sentences have become one. "And rightly so, if . . ." forms a typically Galenic opening, emphasising and at the same time developing what has gone before, and "cum dictum sit" will refer back to what has been already said in the earlier part of the chapter, when Galen holds out an olive branch to believers in the primacy of blood (pp. 94,22–96,1). "si diuersificatur" is thus a slightly loose translation, where the "diuers-" element represents something that is 'special' rather than 'different'.

P. 98,17 εὔδηλόν ἐστι: These words do not appear in the Latin translation, but syntactically they are not required, and they may well have been dropped by a translator.

P. 98,21 ἐάν τε – 26 / 98,20 id est – 26: The clause ἐάν – φύσεως (lines 22–23) is missing from the Latin manuscripts, which also diverge considerably in their rendering of the final clause of the sentence. Their various readings throw considerable light on their interrelationship, as well as on the complex process of transmission. The fact that the Latin puts "secundum prius" (= κατὰ πρῶτον λόγον) before "et sunt in loco quatuor elementorum" (= στοιχειώδεις) strongly suggests that ἐάν – φύσεως had been lost either before or at the time of the first (Syriac) translation. This omission could not have been made in the Latin transmission or translation, for that text presupposes an Arabic text in which the word order had already been changed. Likewise, given the relatively similar linguistic structures of Syriac and Arabic, any omission involving a reordering of the text is unlikely to have taken place at the stage of translation from Syriac into Arabic. But whenever the error was made, the Latin translator was faced with an already corrupt text. ε offers readings that are very close to those in the original Greek, and I have mainly followed them in the text. But it then remains to explain the origin of the corruptions. If the archetype was both badly written and contained glosses, then the gloss on "omnium aliorum humorum" would have been taken into the text in C γ, while the apparently meaningless "suam", which corresponds to αὐτοῦ, was interpreted or glossed (correctly) in ε as "sanguinis".

P. 98,27–100,5: In De atra bile (esp. 6,4: CMG V 4,1,1, p. 83,1–3) Galen argued that changes in the spleen had profound effects on the body and would lead to an excess of melancholy. But this was not because this humour was produced in the spleen, but because the function of the spleen was to act as a sort of sump for the nasty residues of black bile from the liver (cf. De usu part. IV 4. 15: I 198,19–199,9; 232,16–233,5 Helmr. = III 271,7–272,3; 316, 15–317,11 K.). It purified the blood and the body of the potentially harmful black bile. This opinion Galen took back to "the doctors and philosophers of old" (see De fac. nat. II 9: Scr. min. III 197,5–18 Helmr. = II 132,8–133,1 K.; De atra bile 6,6: CMG V 4,1,1, p. 83,11–13). Modern investigations into black bile and melancholy have concentrated largely upon early Greek medicine and on Aristotle, e.g. W. Müri, Melancholie und schwarze Galle, Museum Helveticum 10, 1953, pp. 21–38; R. Klibansky, E. Panofsky, F. Saxl, Saturn and melancholy: Studies in the history of natural philosophy, religion and art, London, 1964; F. Kudlien, Der Beginn des medizinischen Denkens bei den Griechen von Homer bis Hippokrates, Zurich and Stuttgart, 1967, pp. 77–88; J. Pigeaud, La maladie de l'âme. Etude sur la relation de l'âme et du corps dans la tradition médico-philosophique antique, Paris, 1981, pp. 122–138; V. Langholf, Medical theories in Hippocrates. Early texts and the 'Epidemics', Berlin and New York, 1990 (Untersuchungen zur antiken Literatur und Geschichte 34), pp. 46–50; 267–269; Ph. J. van der Eijk, Aristoteles über die Melancholie, Mnemosyne 43, 1990, pp. 33–72. Galen's views are covered somewhat sketchily in H. Flashar, Melancholie und Melancholiker in den medizinischen Theorien der Antike, Berlin, 1966, pp. 105–117, and, with an over-enthusiastic desire to align Galen's diagnoses with modern medicine, by Siegel, pp. 258–321.

P. 100,5–7: Although all the Latin manuscripts put a stop after "probatione", Galen's train of thought runs on to "sillogismus", and I have punctuated accordingly. Both "debeat" and "dimittit" depend on "quod^{II}", the subjunctive representing an unfulfilled action. But the general connection of this whole sentence to what has gone before is not at all clear, and it is not easy to see why Galen should suddenly switch from recommending his book on melancholy to a complaint about logical inadequacy. Besides, the sentence itself lacks a main verb, unless "est" is to be understood (or has dropped out immediately after "est", line 5); and unless "hunc" stands for an indefinite "one", which is unusual, there is no name or person to which it can refer. Given that much of De atra bile was taken up with an attack on Erasistratus, Asclepiades, the Methodists and their followers, it is possible that at least one of these, probably Erasistratus, had been mentioned in a sentence that is now lost. Such a sentence would have run as follows: "But Erasistratus denied much that had been said by the ancients about black bile, and tried to show that it was wrong . . ." Finally, the construction of "debet" with accusative and infinitive is unusual, and may be the result of further textual corruption.

P. 100,6 reprobationem – 7: Since "sillogismus" is not connected with "probatio" throughout this treatise, the phrase "(reprobationem) sillogismi probationis" (C γ), "of a syllogism of proof" or "of a proof of a syllogism", is unlikely to be right, unless it represents a doublet within the translation process. One solution would be to delete the word as having crept into the text through duplication; another, which is followed here, is to emend to "probatione". Galen is thus criticising the logic of someone who attempts to overthrow a syllogism by an alternative (and, by implication, ineffective) proof, yet who does not bother to criticise the various premisses out of which the syllogism is constructed. Galen's argument is that one cannot attack a syllogistic argument without examining its individual premisses. For the importance of syllogistic logic in Galen, see above, p. 167, the note to p. 82,5.

Nonetheless, although Galen talks in De atra bile (7,6; 8,2: CMG V 4,1,1, pp. 86,10; 92,9–11) about the sophistic arguments of his opponents in their attempts to abolish black bile and boasts that those who followed the propounders of such novelties will in the end be compelled to acknowledge the refutation of these sophisms (ibid. 6,13: CMG V 4,1,1, p. 84,22–29) he does not refer to the necessity to examine the premisses of a syllogism. Indeed, his criticism of Erasistratus (ibid. 7,10: CMG V 4,1,1, p. 86,28–29) depends, ironically, on the fact that Erasistratus, contrary to his normal procedure, had been forced to develop an adequate syllogistic argument based on the phenomena. Galen is thus not paraphrasing here what he had said in De atra bile, as the context implies (lines 4–5), but developing a brief comment, only to return in a few lines to his original theme.

P. 100,7–9: Galen's attack may be directed against the Empirics (cf. Gal., Subfig. emp. 12: pp. 86,10–90,9 Deichgräber).

P. 100,10 quia – 11 duo: For the two meanings of blood, *qua* fluid in the veins and arteries, and *qua* humour, see above, p. 184, the note to p. 96,5–6.

P. 100,12 item – 15: At De atra bile 7,21: CMG V 4,1,1, p. 89,11–17, Galen states succinctly the view hinted at briefly elsewhere, e.g. ibid. 3,9: CMG V 4,1,1, p. 76,6–8, that melancholic humour (black bile) and bile are produced in the liver as a result of the digestion of foodstuffs. But equally, he is prepared to allow that yellow bile in particular can be turned into black by heating within the body, and that bodies that are hotter and drier are more prone to produce black bile (see ibid. 6,1–3: CMG V 4,1,1, p. 82,8–22). At In Hipp. Progn. comm. III 32: CMG V 9,2, p. 356,4–11, Galen also talks of thick blood being turned into melancholic humour simply through remaining in the veins, where it settles down like the lees in a wine-barrel or in an oil-jar.

P. 100,12 item – 13: The origin of black bile is one of the things that Galen believes that he can prove syllogistically. "item" thus refers back to line 10.

P. 100,15–18: The repetition of words and phrases has led to confusion in all the manuscripts. If my restoration is correct, Galen first explains that black bile is called black because it is a black humour, or fluid, and that this in turn refers to the sediment in blood which resembles that in wine or olive oil. But the transliterated Greek word for sediment ("ypostasma") has nothing to do with "conturbatio" or "turbatio". Indeed, the sediment forms precisely because the blood is not disturbed. But, as G. Strohmaier points out, since the Arabic word *'akar* can stand both for sediment and for something that is muddy or confused, the Latin translator thus adopted the wrong nuance in his version. More difficult is "ypostasma", for the word used by Galen in Greek is ὑπόστασις or ὑποστάθμη. Although the school of Ḥunayn often provided doublet translations consisting of a transcription plus translation, the manuscripts have the reverse order, and the translator's style usually does not admit a direct apposition. "dicitur" (line 16) is also misplaced. As J. Kollesch and D. Nickel suggest and I have followed in my text, both "dicitur" and "ypostasma" are to be removed, as a marginal gloss to "conturbatio" ("dicitur ypostasma") the two parts of which once stood at the end of two lines and were then integrated into the text at different places.

P. 100,18–19: In De fac. nat. II 9: Scr. min. III 199,17–201,22 Helmr. = II 135,15–138,15 K., Galen makes it clear that there are two types of black bile, and that the second, which is produced by the action of heat on the first, is more acrid.

P. 100,22–102,7: This is a very puzzling section, for, although the manuscripts are in general agreement, the sense of the passage and the way in which the arguments fit together are by no means clear. If we read "festinaui" with C, Galen's self-criticism is odd here, not least because there is no identifiable place elsewhere where he makes these comments, or claims that the veins that distribute food also carry black bile and sometime blood. The opening "ergo" also presents a difficulty, for there does not appear to be anything in either sentence to justify so emphatic a conjunction. Finally, the anacolouthon "uene . . . in illis" is unusual. The solution, with J. Kollesch and D. Nickel, is to posit a lacuna after "corpus" and to read "festinauit" with β. Galen's opponent, who may have been mentioned in the lost text, is thus denying that the splenic vein can attract black blood from the portal vein. Galen responds by accusing him of inconsistency: he accepts that each purgative attracts the relevant humour, but denies that the veins are able to do so although they are nourished by the humour appropriate to them.

P. 102,7–13: Galen returns to the plausible view he has mentioned earlier: that there is only a single fluid circulating within the body, blood. He points out that bloodless animals have a fluid that takes the place of blood and that provides them with nutriment. Blood is the main means by which the heat produced in the liver is transmitted to all parts of the body. But given Galen's belief that all living animals are to some extent dependent on heat for their very existence, he finds himself in difficulty when dealing with "bloodless animals". True, they are not perceptibly hot and there is no perceptibly hot animal without blood (see Gal., De foet. form. 3: IV 671,2–13 K.), but they must, *qua* animals, possess some form of heat. Hence Galen here posits a "natural heat" which takes the place of the heat produced in the liver of sanguineous animals.

P. 102,14–104,1: The discussion on heat in the living being leads on to a wider discussion about what it is that is responsible for life. Galen repeats his view that the heart is a source of heat, and that this heat is, in some way or other, distinct from that produced in the liver. The latter is involved in nutrition and the production of blood; the former in the production of θυμός (see Gal., In Hipp. Epid. VI comm. V 5: CMG V 10,2,2, p. 274,3–5).

P. 102,14 est loco illius: Although in line 12 "in loco" indicates a substitute ("in place of"), this cannot be the meaning of "loco" here, for the heart is the source and seat of natural heat, not its replacement. Instead, "loco esse" c. gen. represents an Arabic circumlocution for "as" or "like", so G. Strohmaier suggests.

P. 102,15–19: Whereas in chapter 3,5 Galen had argued that plants shared in the natural faculties or, in another formulation, the natural faculty that controls all living beings, he had not there talked about heat. Here Galen compares a type of heat in plants with a natural faculty, and goes on to say that one might follow Plato and Aristotle in saying that this is the same as the third, appetitive, part of Plato's soul and as Aristotle's nutritive soul. But although he here accepts the liver as the source of the natural heat and argues that it functions in animals rather like the root system of plants, he is not prepared to make the further move and identify soul with heat.

P. 102,18 et potes – 19: In chapter 3,6, Galen had equated the substance that controls plants with the soul of Plato and the Platonists. He now adds Aristotle to those who support his view. But to do this requires a certain amount of fudging of the issues. Aristotle had referred to various powers or properties of the unitary soul, especially those concerned with nutrition, reproduction, and growth (De anima II 3. 4: 414 a 32–33; 415 a 22–25). These three he ascribed to plants, as well as to animals, but he expressly rejected the idea that plants could have desire, since that presupposed sensation (cf. ibid. II 3: 414 a 32–b 2; Eth. Nic. I 13: 1102 b 29–31). Nonetheless, Galen claimed that Aristotle had merely made a category mistake: he had recognized the same phenomena as Plato, but had failed to see that his properties were parts of the soul, differing in type and location. His powers of nutrition, reproduction, and growth, or the "natural power", were thus identical with what Plato had termed the appetitive or desirous part of the soul (see Gal., De plac. Hipp. et Plat. V 4,3; VI 3,7: CMG V 4,1,2, pp. 312,29–34; 374,9–17). Galen thus is prepared to use the observations of Aristotle to support a theory to which he would not have assented. This amalgamation of Plato and Aristotle on this point may not have originated with Galen; cf. De Lacy, pp. 43–57; Singer, pp. 41–47; Moraux, Der Aristotelismus, vol. II, pp. 778–781. Nonetheless it fitted well with the 'eclectic' tendencies of second-century philosophy; cf. Dillon, pp. 174; 194.

P. 102,19–104,2: As he had declared at In Hipp. Epid. VI comm. V 5: CMG V 10,2,2, p. 274,3–8, Galen believed in two types of innate heat: one produced in the liver and involved with the production of blood, the other produced in the heart. The former, which Galen calls confusingly both σύμφυτος and ἔμφυτος (De foet. form. 3: IV 671,4. 12 K.), is described as a low heat present throughout the blood circulating in the veins. Galen says very little about this heat in his writings: at De marcore 3: VII 674,7–675,16 K., for example, he does not make clear where the heat under discussion comes from, and it is only the connection with nutrition and growth that would suggest that this heat is located in the liver. Similarly the source of the innate heat that is praised at De trem., palp., convuls. et rig. 6: VII 616,10–15 K. is not specified, although, given that this heat is described as ἀρχέγονον, the liver is somewhat more likely than the heart. More frequently, however, when he talks about the source of innate heat it is the heart to which he refers, e.g. De plac. Hipp. et Plat. VI 8,75: CMG V 4,1,2, p. 424,3–4. It is the innate heat located in the heart, the hearth of the animal, that, added to that already present in the blood, makes the blood and the animal feel properly warm (see De foet. form. 3: IV 671,3–13 K.). Plants, which lack the warmth of blood as well as the fire of the heart, are thus rightly termed colder than animals.

There are, however, two further problems in the text of this passage. Although Galen had earlier (p. 72,18 τὴν – 22) announced that hotter bodies were in general more sensitive than cold ones, "dat sensum" is unlikely to mean "provide sensation", i.e. render the organism more sensitive, at this point in the argument. It is the external perceiver who receives the sensation of warmth, and to whom the body feels warm to the touch; hence "calidum tactu" must go with "sensum". The presence in both C and γ of the second person singular "se(n)tis" further suggests that the intrusive "sentis corpus (calidum?)" was originally a gloss taken into the Latin, and then regularised to "sentit" in ε and by B[2]. Furthermore, since it is "calor" from the heart, not sensation or touch, that differs from the liver's heat, "qui" must be deleted.

P. 104,3–6 φυτά: The Aldine editors read the abbreviated and barely legible ending of διαφωνίαν in A as -ας and understood διαφωνίας as a partitive genitive, dependent on ἀξιόλογον, but the accusative is assured by other examples of the same abbreviation for the ending elsewhere in A. But whichever case is read, exactly what this disagreement is that is so important is not easy to discover. The Arabo-Latin tradition had the controversy taking place between the doctors and philosophers (an expansion of the vague τῶν λεγόντων as transmitted in A), but that is not the point at issue here. From the context, the apparent discrepancy arises over the meaning of hot and cold, when Galen declares that plants can be either hot or not hot. Galen goes on to explain (lines 6–14) that if one understands things correctly, there will be no divergence. But, rather than the statements of the vague τῶν λεγόντων J. Kollesch and D. Nickel suggest that it is Galen's own words that occasion this comment, and that, at a very early stage in the Greek tradition, ἡμῶν was corrupted to τῶν.

P. 104,7 ἀκριβέστερον – 14: The gaps left by the scribe of A indicate that he (or his exemplar) had relied upon a manuscript that was defective at this point. The Aldine editors took over the two supplements of A[2], but supplied the third by a conjecture (τῆς ἐσχάτης ἐπιστήμης) which left this part of the sentence without a verb. This was noted by an anonymous French reader of the late sixteenth or early seventeenth century, who inscribed in his copy of the Basle edition, now Cambridge, University Library, classmark Path. a. 72, λέγει vel λέγῃ after ἀκόλουθον, as well as by Goulston, who in the notes to his printed edition suggested that ἐπεξέρχεται or a similar word had fallen out after ἐπιστήμης. The solution may be found in the Latin version, "debet", which suggests that we should supply χρή. But this is not the only difficulty here, for neither A's ζητούμενον nor the Aldine ζητουμένῳ fits the balance of the sentence, where the parallel ὅταν clauses should take the form of verb with nominative participle. Hence D. Nickel's suggestion that we read ζητῶν.

The Aldine supplement at this point can be further improved with the aid of the Latin "ad firmam notitiam", which suggests that, at the very least, the adjective βέβαιος, a Galenic favourite, was involved, with or without an accompanying noun. The length of the lacuna in A suggests that more than the adjective stood there, and, unless it was a long verb, the choice should lie between γνώσεως and ἐπιστήμης. Both nouns are used by Galen with βέβαιος in similar contexts, the former more frequently than the latter.[1] The fact that at p. 114,21, "notitia" corresponds to an original γνῶσις and the phrase βεβαίαν ἔχειν γνῶσιν also occurs nearby (p. 114,17), leads me to prefer γνώσεως as a possible supplement.

Despite the textual difficulty, Galen's point is clear. If one is conducting a thorough investigation into a particular problem, one takes great care to secure a precise and secure formulation; a passing reference will simply carry the normal meaning, without any further implication.

P. 104,15–106,2 λέγοντος: Galen moves on from one example of a possible confusion caused by loose terminology and involving plants, whether they are hot and cold, to another, whether they are ensouled or not. Although the words are those of Galen, not of Plato himself, the view that living creatures, animals, are ensouled can be found throughout Plato's writings, from the Phaedrus, 245 c-e, to the Sophist, 219 e, and the very late Laws, X: 902 b. Plato, however, never uses the specific examples of stones, grass, wood, and plants as 'soul-less'. Nonetheless, such an inference could be easily made from such passages as Laws XI: 931 a, which describes statues as "soul-less", or Sophist 265 c, which refers to "things from the earth without souls" and which distinguishes these and plants from (ensouled) animals. Plato's wording here might suggest a certain ambiguity about whether plants have souls, for they are neither (ensouled) animals nor soul-less minerals, but his definitions elsewhere in his writings would appear to place them firmly among the 'soul-less'. At Euthydemus 287 d whatever has soul is also capable of thinking, and at Phaedrus 245 e, a section familiar to all Platonists and to many of their opponents, Plato defines the possession of a soul in terms of the capacity to move: everything that can move only by means of outside intervention is soul-less; everything that can move itself is ensouled. The apparent discrepancy

[1] For the former, see, e.g. De opt. doc. gen. 2,1: CMG V 1,1, p. 94,17 (εἰς βεβαίαν γνῶσιν ἥκειν); for the latter, De cris. I 16: p. 112,2–3 Alexanderson = IX 618,8 K. (εἰς ἐπιστήμην βεβαίαν ἥκειν).

between this theory and that of the Timaeus 77 a-c, which firmly attributes to plants, trees, and seeds the third part of the soul, was, presumably, among those discussed by Galen in his book De partibus et facultatibus animae; cf. De Lacy, in: CMG V 4,1,2, pp. 707–708, the notes to pp. 598,19–600,18; 600, 7–10; 608,8–9. This treatise is recorded by Galen among his works relating to Platonic philosophy (see De libris propr. 13 [14]: Scr. min. II 122,14–15 Müller = XIX 46,16–17 K.), and it is probably also to be identified with the tract in which Galen, as he said in De foet. form. 6: IV 700,1 K., "investigated discrepancies in Plato's views on the soul".

P. 104,18–19 καθόλου φάναι . . . πάντα: Goulston in his Dublin notes deleted καθόλου φάναι; the expression is not found in the Latin and might be thought over-emphatic here. But it is securely attested elsewhere, e.g. Gal., De difficult. respir. I 2; II 7: VII 757,15; 853,10–11 K.; De comp. med. sec. loc. VI 8: XII 963,15 K., all with plural forms of πᾶς, and should not be removed.

P. 104,20–106,2 λέγοντος: The Timaeus was for Galen, and for many other philosophers and physicians down to the sixteenth century, the most important of all Plato's writings. The author of the Anonymus Londinensis papyrus devoted extensive coverage to its medical ideas (XIV 11 – XVIII 8)[1]; it was translated into Latin by Chalcidius around 350 A.D.; and it became a major object of commentary in the later Middle Ages.[2] As well as including a summary of it among the eight books of his Summaries of Plato's dialogues, parts of which survive in Arabic and have been edited and translated by Kraus and Walzer, London, 1951, Galen composed a long commentary, in four books, on its medical sections. This survives only in fragments, edited partly by Schröder, CMG Suppl. I, 1934, and partly by Larrain, 1992. It held a central place in Galen's own medical theories and in his reconstruction of past doctrines, especially of Hippocrates, for a variety of reasons. First and foremost, it was Plato's longest and scientifically most interesting exposition of the natural world, φυσικὴ θεωρία, not least because, in its later chapters, its description of the creation of the human body and of its degeneration in disease is the most extensive treatment of the theme by an ancient philosopher. Secondly, although much of its teaching may have been Plato's own intellectual creation, it includes ideas similar to those found in the Hippocratic Corpus, especially in De natura hominis. Since Plato, a younger contemporary of the great Coan, knew some of his theories and praised him highly, it was an easy, if unwarranted, step to assume that the philosopher had learnt the medical views expressed in the Timaeus from Hippocrates, whom he had acknowledged as the best teacher of medicine. Hence, not only could Plato's medical ideas be interpreted by Galen in the light of surviving Hippocratic treatises, but they could also be used to throw light on (some would say, invent) the theories of Hippocrates that have not come down to us or to give a specifically Platonic slant to particularly obscure phrases from the Hippocratic Corpus.

1 This reference I owe to J. Longrigg.

2 See for a good summary of the influence of the Timaeus, T. Gregory, The Platonic inheritance, in: A history of twelfth-century philosophy, ed. P. Dronke, Cambridge, 1992, pp. 54–80.

Even though there is no cogent proof that Plato took his views on medicine as presented in the last sections of the Timaeus from Hippocrates or even from our Hippocratic Corpus (Philistion of Locri has a stronger, although far from exclusive, claim), Galen was only too eager to link one of his philosopher heroes with the great Hippocrates. Without the Timaeus, Galen's understanding of Hippocratic medicine would have been very different. See, for a bibliography of recent work on the importance of the Timaeus in Galen's writings, Lloyd, Galen on Hellenistics and Hippocrateans, in: Lloyd, Methods and problems, pp. 407–413, and in: Galen und das hellenistische Erbe, pp. 134–141; Ph. De Lacy, Galen's Platonism, American Journal of Philology 93, 1972, pp. 27–39; H. Diller, Empirie und Logos: Galens Stellung zu Hippokrates und Platon, in: Studia Platonica, Festschrift für Hermann Gundert zu seinem 65. Geburtstag am 30. 4. 1974, ed. K. Döring and W. Kullmann, Amsterdam, s.a., pp. 227–238; F. Ferrari, Galeno interprete del Timeo, Museum Helveticum 55, 1998, pp. 14–34, who rejects (p. 16 n. 6) Larrain's attribution of the recently discovered fragments to Galen's commentary.

All interpreters of Plato, including Galen, have struggled to reconcile the theories expressed in the Timaeus with those of Plato's other dialogues. Most recent scholarship has stressed the 'mythic' aspect of the Timaeus as a collection of very provisional hypotheses put forward for discussion, and has argued that the theories put forward in this dialogue were not necessarily all held or assented to by Plato; see e.g. Vlastos, Plato's universe. But Galen, and many other interpreters both before and since, saw no good reason to believe that Plato was not propounding theories to which he gave total credence, even if other problems then arose. To explain away discrepancies between the Timaeus and the other dialogues of Plato a variety of strategies have been employed. Many scholars have favoured a developmental approach, preferring to regard Plato's philosophy as changing over time, and setting the Timaeus either in the middle or towards the end of his long life.[1] Galen displays no interest in such chronological questions, but puts forward a view that resembles that of K. Gaiser, Platons ungeschriebene Lehre. Studien zur systematischen und geschichtlichen Begründung der Wissenschaften in der Platonischen Schule, 2nd ed., Stuttgart, 1968; J. N. Findlay, Plato: the written and unwritten doctrines, London, 1974; and H. J. Krämer, Plato and the foundations of metaphysics, Albany, 1990. These modern Platonists, following a hint in Aristotle (Phys. IV 2: 209 b 11–16) have suggested that Plato taught one thing in his written Dialogues and another, far more influenced by Pythagoreanism, in his private seances with his favourite students.[2] Although he does not go

1 G. E. L. Owen, The place of the Timaeus in Plato's dialogues, Classical Quarterly, n. s. 3, 1953, pp. 79–95 = G. E. L. Owen, Logic, science and dialectic. Collected papers in Greek philosophy, ed. M. Nussbaum, London, 1986, pp. 65–84, put forward strong arguments against what was then the standard view, that the Timaeus was among the last works of Plato. In Owen's opinion, the Timaeus was one of the middle dialogues, written after the Republic and Phaedo but before the Phaedrus. Contra, H. Cherniss, The relation of the Timaeus to Plato's later dialogues, American Journal of Philology 78, 1957, pp. 225–266 (repr. in: H. Cherniss, Selected papers, ed. L. Tarán, Leiden, 1977, pp. 298–339).

2 Most modern interpreters of Plato disagree with this approach, E. N. Tigerstedt, Inter-

quite so far, Galen asserts that the distinction between what Plato says in the Timaeus and elsewhere is a result of talking to different audiences in different ways. In the Timaeus he was addressing a very small number of hearers, capable of assimilating his complex theories[1]; in other treatises, he was speaking to a wider and less sophisticated audience. It was a distinction made clear also by the very type of language that Plato chose to use: concise and unadorned as opposed to his normal flowing richness (see Gal., Compend. Tim. Plat. 1 c: p. 34,14–16 Kraus-Walzer; cf. Galens Kommentar zu Platons Timaios, fr. 17: p. 123,1–10 Larrain; F. Walsdorff, Die antiken Urteile über Platons Stil, Bonn, 1927 [Klassisch-Philologische Studien 1]). Galen's argument, which was typical of Platonists of his day (cf. Apul., Apol. 12), brought with it several advantages. It was historically plausible, for the distinction between public and private discourse was familiar in the writings of Plato's pupil, Aristotle, and, in turn, of his pupil, Theophrastus (see p. 106,3–6 / 106,3–8); it preserved an overall consistency of doctrine throughout Plato's life; and, above all, it gave the Timaeus a privileged place among the Platonic Corpus as the bearer of Plato's most intimate teaching.

P. 104,24 ἀποχωρίσας / 104,23 dissentiebat: Both the Greek manuscript and, apparently, the oriental translator read ἀποχωρήσας, hence the Latin intransitive "dissentiebat"; but this leaves the accusative θεωρίαν (line 21) without a corresponding verb. The problem is resolved by the simple correction to ἀποχωρίσας.

P. 104,25 εἰς – 27 αὐτοῦ: Galen provides his own version of the words of Plato, Tim. 34 b: ψυχὴν . . . διὰ παντός τε ἔτεινεν. Alcinous, Didasc. 14: p. 33,6–7 Whittaker, similarly paraphrases Plato, using the compound παρεκτεῖναι. It is typical of Galen's somewhat inconsequential way of argument in this treatise that, although the opposition he is setting up between the Timaeus and the other treatises of Plato might lead us to expect the citation of Timaeus 77 a–b, the passage where Plato unequivocally declares that plants, trees, and seeds have at least the third part of the soul, he chooses instead to begin with a quotation that relates to the universality of the World Soul, and then proceeds as if he had cited the later section also.

P. 106,2 unumquodque – 3 quod: While the loss of "mundum" (p. 104, 26) in C γ may be attributed to a common carelessness, their agreement in the meaningless "unumquodque dicat arteriam secundum quod" cannot be explained except by positing an identical source. The omission of these words in ε is the result of emendation, for they stand in the same position in the Latin translation as do τἀνδρὸς . . . ὥσπερ in the Greek, which are otherwise absent from the Latin. If, with J. Kollesch and D. Nickel, we make the small pa-

preting Plato, Uppsala, 1977; G. Vlastos, Platonic studies, 2nd ed., Princeton, 1981, pp. 379–403.

1 Cf. for a similar description of the audience, Calc., In Plat. Tim. comm. I 1: p. 57,1–6 Waszink; Procl., In Plat. Tim. comm. I: I 22,21–23,16 Diehl. According to Procl., ibid. II: I 340,23–26 Diehl, the followers of Albinus and Gaius distinguished between the occasions when Plato offered possible truths and when he spoke "epistemonically", see T. Göransson, Albinus, Alcinous, Arius Didymus, Gothenburg, 1995.

laeographical change of "arteriam" to "contrarium", sense is restored to the translation.

P. 106,2 ὥσπερ – 6: The distinction between esoteric and exoteric writings is found often in the Aristotelian Corpus, e.g. Metaph. M 1:1076 a 28–29; Eth. Nic. I 13: 1102 a 26–27; Eth. Eud. I 8: 1217 b 22–23; Pol. III 6: 1278 b 31–32. But it would be going too far to hold that a distinction based upon form and audience carried for Aristotle the meaning of secret, as opposed to public, knowledge, however much later Aristotelians made that assumption.[1] Strabo, Geogr. XIII 1,54, the major ancient source for the story of the preservation and transmission of the library of Aristotle, implies that Theophrastus' esoteric writings were kept along with those of his master, and hence, like them, disappeared from view for two centuries or more, leaving only the exoteric works to circulate. Galen's contention that any divergence between the two groups of writings related to form and audience, not to overall doctrine, echoes that of Cicero, De fin. V 12, although he was prepared to concede differences of substance in certain areas as well. For recent discussions, see E. Howald, Die Schriftenverzeichnisse des Aristoteles und des Theophrast, Hermes 55, 1920, pp. 204–221; A. H. Chroust, The miraculous disappearance and recovery of the Corpus Aristotelicum, Classica et Mediaevalia 23, 1962, pp. 50–67; I. Düring, Aristotle in the ancient biographical tradition, Gothenburg, 1957 (Studia Graeca et Latina Gothoburgensia V), pp. 426–443; Moraux, Der Aristotelismus, vol. I, pp. 4–10; C. Lord, On the early history of the Aristotelian Corpus, American Journal of Philology 107, 1986, pp. 137–161; Gottschalk, pp. 1083–1097.[2]

P. 106,10 sensibus: Neither "cum fortibus" (β) nor "sorisibus" (C) makes any sense, and the former is an obvious attempt to give some meaning, albeit incorrect. Although "illius rei que percipitur" could by itself correspond to αἴσθησιν, the translator made the phrase more precise by adding "sensibus", whose *ductus litterarum* corresponds well to the reading of C.

P. 106,10 προσκρούει: This is a choice word, not otherwise found in this metaphorical sense in Galen, but entirely appropriate to the imagined situation of a lecturer performing in public. Philostratus, Vitae sophist. 8,2: II 84,27–29 Kayser, uses it of the disconcerting effect of a new-fangled and somewhat disconnected speech.

P. 106,12 πρὶν – 15 ἀφικέσθαι: Galen repeats in slightly different language what he had said before at p. 104,6–9 / 104,7–10 about the need for a proper, long, and careful argument leading to a coherent conclusion, and then continues with a relevant example of something that should not be enunciated lightly or casually. The Latin translation slightly misrepresents the Greek by stating baldly that "it ought not to be said that . . ." (lines 17–18), as if this was an opinion totally rejected by Galen.

P. 106,16 οὐδὲ – 24: The question what Plato had meant by the World Soul was (and is) hotly disputed. In the Timaeus (34 b–43 a) Plato had apparently argued for the World Soul as the immanent source of cosmic motion, re-

1 See most recently, Mansfeld, Prolegomena, pp. 24–26; 202–203.

2 I am grateful to R. W. Sharples for help with this note.

sponsible for the beginning and maintenance of unceasing and intelligent life within the universe. There is certainly an implication at Tim. 43 a that some portion of the World Soul is contained within the bodies of living creatures, but nowhere does Plato talk about the World Soul as being present in inanimate objects, except, again by implication, as a result of their very existence within a universe that is itself ensouled. Platonists in general linked the World Soul with that which preserved the life of the body, and hence refused to believe that it could be found in dead bodies or in inanimate objects (see Nemes., De nat. hom. 2: pp. 33,20–34,17 Morani).[1] The Stoics, however, developed the idea of the World Soul in ways that would have surprised Plato. The soul is not only to be found in all living things, including trees and plants (see, for example, Cic., De nat. deorum II 29–30; Chrys., fr. 826: SVF II, pp. 225, 39–226,13), but possibly in everything. According to Chrysippus, the upward or downward movement of fire and stones corresponds to assent and impulse in animals, activities in which, to a Platonist, the soul is certainly involved.[2] As R. W. Sharples points out to me, there may be here echoes of a contemporary debate, for Alexander of Aphrodisias regarded the internal source of motion of heavy and light elements as analogous to soul (being their Aristotelian form).[3] Such an opinion is unlikely to have pleased Galen, who had drawn the line at seeing the World Soul as great power involved in the creation of scorpions, spiders, vipers, worms and the like (De foet. form. 6: IV 700,17–701,6 K. with the discussion, above, pp. 181–182, the note to p. 94,12–17). Still less, then, could he accept the notion of stones and sand being animated by the World Soul, except in the very narrowest sense that they are all part of the ensouled universe. His hesitation about the World Soul is here patent. Not only does he go on to say that Plato's words, if understood in their normal meaning, would be rightly regarded as ludicrous, but he also refrains from basing his argument for the existence of a soul in plants (pp. 122,1–124, 18) on any universal penetration of the World Soul.

P. 106,20 εἰ – 24 / 106,21 et – 23: The Latin version omits ἁπλῶς – πολλῶν, and turns the single verb κατεγίνωσκον into an expanded doublet, "admirarentur . . . et dicerent quod esset insanus".

P. 106,24 ἐγὼ – 108,10: In this complex sentence, μὲν (p. 106,25) is taken up, after a parenthesis, οὐδὲ . . . φησιν, by μέντοι (p. 108,4) and by δὲ (p. 108,8).

Where Galen discussed just how Plato reached his opinion about the

1 Cf. Dillon, The Middle Platonists; Moraux, Der Aristotelismus, vol. II, pp. 577–579 (Atticus); J. Dillon, Alcinous. The handbook of Platonism, Oxford, 1993, pp. XVIII; XXIII; 126–127.

2 Nemes., De nat. hom. 35: p. 105,6–14 Morani, a polemical passage, perhaps deriving ultimately from Galen, and hence not entirely independent of what Galen says here.

3 Alex. Aphrod., De anima: p. 22,10–15 Bruns; De anima libri mantissa: p. 106,5–8 Bruns; and his interpretation of Aristotle as given in his Refutation of Galen's treatise on the theory of motion, p. 17 Rescher-Marmura. See R. W. Sharples, Alexander of Aphrodisias: Scholasticism and innovation, in: ANRW II 36,2, Berlin and New York, 1987, p. 1215. Gottschalk, pp. 1113–1114, would like to take this interpretation of Aristotle back at least to Andronicus.

World Soul is open to debate. He devoted at best only a few lines in the Compendium Timaei (4 a/b: pp. 42–44 Kraus-Walzer) to the role of the World Soul but without explaining Plato's method of argumentation. Schröder, in: CMG Suppl. I, p. VIII, assumed that Galen was referring not to his commentary on the Timaeus but to De placitis Hippocratis et Platonis or to the (now lost) De partibus et facultatibus animae. The latter must remain a possibility, but it is unlikely that Galen was alluding to De placitis Hippocratis et Platonis, since he nowhere there mentions the World Soul, directly or indirectly. Besides, Schröder's argument is now seriously weakened by Larrain's publication of new fragments (Galens Kommentar zu Platons Timaios) that relate specifically to this topic.

If these new fragments are genuine, it is clear that Galen did rather more than just report Plato's views. In fragment 11 (p. 95,5–14 Larrain), Galen appears to find likenesses between the substances within the human soul and those of the heavens, which can be interpreted in the strong sense to indicate that individual souls are formed from the same substances as the World Soul. In fragment 4 (p. 50,2–8 Larrain), Galen asserts that the logical part of the soul shares the two circuits of the World Soul, sameness and difference, in a way that marks it off from the two lower and mortal parts. More interestingly, in fragment 21 (p. 140,1–4 Larrain), Galen offers a criticism, or at least an explanation, of what Plato meant when he said that the World Soul was extended throughout the cosmos. Having quoted Plato, Galen adds 'but much better, I suppose, through the sun' (or 'sunlight'). Although the way in which Galen makes his suggestion is extremely hypothetical – the sentence begins with a conditional (εἴπερ), and δήπου is not emphatic –, traces of this interpretation can be found elsewhere in Galen, particularly in connection with sight (cf. fr. 22: p. 142,1–10 Larrain with the note; Gal., De plac. Hipp. et Plat. VII 7,24: CMG V 4,1,2, p. 474,20–22; Nemes., De nat. hom. 7: p. 59,2–19 Morani, perhaps through the intermediary of Porphyry). At the very least, even if Galen in the end neither assented to nor disagreed with Plato's views on the World Soul, he did rather more than his defensive formulation here suggests.

P. 106,27 in – iudicauit: The Latin manuscripts are divided on the translation of the typically Arabic expansion of συναποφηνάμενος (line 27); C γ have "hiis in quibus iudicaui", ε, in greater conformity with the Greek, has "hiis in quibus iudicauit". On account of the parallel passage, p. 108,26 ("prout ipse iudicauit"), the reading of ε has been accepted.

P. 106,29; 108,10 αὐτὸς ἐκεῖνος: For this phrase, common in Galen, see R. Janko, Αὐτὸς ἐκεῖνος: a neglected idiom, Classical Quarterly, n. s. 35, 1985, pp. 20–30, esp. pp. 29–30, where the Galenic examples are listed. It is frequently used, as also by Plato, to denote some remote figure of authority.

P. 108,2–3 ἄχρι τοῦ πιθανοῦ καὶ εἰκότος: Although Plato twice describes what he is doing in the Timaeus as providing an εἰκὼς μῦθος or τὸ εἰκός (29 c/d; 72 d) he does not use the adjective πιθανός. Nonetheless, Galen several times elsewhere characterises Plato's aims in this way (see De plac. Hipp. et Plat. IX 9,3. 6. 7: CMG V 4,1,2, p. 598,9. 20. 26; cf. also IX 9,12: CMG V 4,1,2, p. 600,22, where the adjective πιθανός alone is used). On the meaning of εἰκὼς μῦθος, see A. E. Taylor, A commentary on Plato's Timaeus, Oxford, 1928, p. 516, the note to 72 d 4–8; F. M. Cornford, Plato's Cosmology, London, 1937, pp. 28–31; Vlastos, p. 93.

P. 108,4 ὅτι – 10: Galen's formulations of Platonic doctrine here are not as consistent as one might like, and his customary precision of vocabulary is missing. Plato and the Platonists had associated the existence of a soul with the presence of some form of motion (cf. Cic., De nat. deorum II 32) and Galen apparently agrees with this proposition here and at the conclusion of this book (see pp. 122,1–124,22; cf. also In Plat. Tim. comm. III 2: CMG Suppl. I, p. 11,9–20).[1] Galen also allows that plants have some form of sensation, a proposition strongly denied by Aristotle, De iuvent. et senect. 1: 467 b 22–25; De anima II 3: 415 a 2–3; De part. anim. III 4: 666 a 34; De generat. anim. II 3: 736 a 30, and by the Stoics, for whom the possession of sensation was the distinctive feature of an animal (see Diog. Laert., De clar. philos. vitis VII 142–143), and who expressly denied that the vegetative faculty could be considered as soul (see Clem. Alex., Strom. VIII 10,4; Theodoret, Graec. aff. cur. V 25). Galen's acceptance of the Platonic position would also seem to run counter to his brusque presentation at De fac. nat. I 1: Scr. min. III 101,1–15 Helmr. = II 1,3–2,5 K., which firmly declares sensation and voluntary motion, the effects of the soul, to be peculiar to animals, and not to plants, and then repeats the same opinion in the end of the passage.

Galen's means of reconciliation is to appeal to context and language. In the opening section of De facultatibus naturalibus he notes that those who allow plants a share in soul are using the word "soul" in an unfamiliar way. Here he does not mention Plato's language as such, but argues that perhaps he did not take sufficient care to speak in a manner appropriate to the context. Had he done so, there would have been no discrepancy.

P. 108,11–18 ὀνομάζω: The Latin version ("nominabo", line 14) confirms that the Greek of A and of subsequent editions cannot be right, for in De facultatibus naturalibus Galen had demonstrated that all living beings, including plants, shared in the four natural faculties which determined the ability of any living organism to perceive and distinguish between what was suitable and unsuitable within the process of nutrition and growth (cf. also p. 62, 3–7). The possession alone of sensation and voluntary motion, which he there called effects of the soul, distinguished animals from plants. The first part of the sentence must thus end logically after κίνησιν (line 13), and the καὶ that follows introduces the second part of the sentence, not an additional distinguishing feature. Schröder, in: CMG Suppl. I, p. 41 in the note to p. 11,14–15, queried τε, presumably because he could find no subsequent connective particle, but more needs to be done. The simple change of ὀνομάζων to ὀνομάζω restores both sense and conformity with what Galen says elsewhere.

P. 108,15 ἄρτι: Galen is using the word somewhat loosely here, for his last reference to the four natural faculties is some way back, at pp. 86,23–88,

[1] There is no need to assume with K. Reinhardt, Poseidonios, Munich, 1921, p. 226 (cf. also pp. 105; 155; 355–357), that Galen took over this argument from Posidonius of Apamea. Mansfeld, Doxography, p. 3188, shows how widely known it was.

5. However, since he considered the perception of what was suitable or unsuitable (lines 6–7) as produced in some way by the natural faculties, he may be, equally misleadingly, referring to that.

P. 108,16. 18 scilicet . . . †tristiuam†: The Latin manuscripts again show descent from a heavily abbreviated exemplar. An abbreviated "scilicet" (".s.") could easily be misread as "sicut" (ε) or "sic" (C γ), and the variants for φυσικὰς (tristiuam β: cresciтuam C) clearly derive from the same exemplar. How the corrupt word in this exemplar had arisen is uncertain.

P. 108,18 μηδὲν – 25: Galen several times, both here and elsewhere (see the testimonia to p. 108,11–21), declares that the resolution of a particular topic is of little use either to medicine or to 'ethical' philosophy, or that one's choice of words is unimportant. At the same time, he is implying that what he has to say is often of direct relevance to one of the liveliest debates within Hellenistic philosophy, that of ethics, and thereby taking up a position within an ongoing controversy. According to Diogenes Laertius, (De clar. philos. vitis VII 39), the Stoics in particular divided philosophy into three types, 'physical', ethical, and logical (see K. Ieradiakonou, The Stoic division of philosophy, Phronesis 38, 1993, pp. 57–74). At least some of them kept the three distinct (cf. Diog. Laert., ibid. VII 40) but others certainly did not, especially Posidonius (see Posid., fr. 88; 90–91 Edelstein-Kidd) who began his courses of instruction with natural philosophy and progressed to ethics and logic. Galen adopts the same approach, going so far as (rightly) to talk about the "natural part" of ethical philosophy as represented in Plato. His own ideas on ethics and psychology, as we have already seen, have a basis in his ideas on physiology, for, especially in Quod animi mores corporis temperamenta sequantur, he adopts a strongly somatic interpretation of moral behaviour, and he is convinced that there is a role for the physician to play in investigating, and in controlling, moral behaviour. Psychology, properly considered, is a part of practical philosophy.[1]

P. 108,24 τινὰ μὲν – 110,3: Galen emphasises his own eclectic attitude towards Plato's natural philosophy: partly assent to what is certain; partly provisional acceptance as plausible; and partly suspension of judgment until at least plausibility is shown. It is worth noting that Galen does not reject any Platonic doctrine directly, although his third category can cover almost anything.

P. 108,26 et – 110,2: The Latin manuscripts agree in leaving out Galen's third category of response to Plato (καθάπερ – ῥοπήν, pp. 108,27– 110,1). The correct syntax of the sentence suggests that the omission occurred before the Latin translation was made, and perhaps even in a Greek manuscript.

1 For the debate on ethics, see J. Annas, Hellenistic philosophy of mind, Berkeley, Los Angeles, Oxford, 1992; M. C. Nussbaum, The therapy of desire. Theory and practice in Hellenistic ethics, Princeton, 1994 (Martin Classical Lectures, n. s. 2); and for Galen's own part in it, Hankinson, Galen's anatomy of the soul, pp. 197–233; idem, Actions and passions. Affection, emotion, and moral self-management in Galen's philosophical psychology, in: Passions and perceptions. Studies in Hellenistic philosophy of mind, Proceedings of the fifth symposium Hellenisticum, ed. J. Brunschwig and M. C. Nussbaum, Cambridge and New York, 1993, pp. 184–222.

P. 110,2 ἐπὶ – 3: Mansfeld, Doxography, shows how much the ancients' knowledge of earlier philosophy was organised around a series of 'disputed points', τὰ διαφωνούμενα, often expressed as a series of alternatives, hence τὸ ἕτερον, although we need not follow him entirely in his assumption that everything depended ultimately on a single source, the "Vetustissima placita".

P. 110,4 ⟨. . .⟩ ὥσπερ – 21: As the Greek of the manuscripts stands, the whole of the long passage depends on ὥσπερ, and serves as an example of a disputed topic on which Galen finds it impossible to decide in any way. Even for Galen, this is an extraordinarily complex sentence and forms by far the longest clause in the Galenic Corpus to depend on ὥσπερ. Besides, although in A there is an antecedent to which ὥσπερ refers, τῶν διαφωνουμένων (line 2), this manuscript places a full stop immediately before ὥσπερ, as if it began a new sentence, and all subsequent editors and translators have concurred. In the branch of the tradition represented by L and Nic., which starts here, the reader will seek in vain for a corresponding main clause that will bring the sentence to a grammatically correct conclusion. The emphatic οὕτω γοῦν (line 21) begins a new sentence that adds something further to the argument by providing an example of what has just been said, and does not correspond to ὥσπερ. One might argue that Galen has just lost himself in a labyrinth of his own rhetoric, and that the sentence has broken apart under the weight of superadded clauses, but the Arabo-Latin version suggests a neater solution. The Latin forms a syntactically correct series of sentences, and begins with words not in the Greek text which suggests that we should posit a lacuna in the Greek.

How much has been lost in the Greek, and where the lacuna should begin are not easy to determine. Given that the Latin opens with "De substantia autem uirtutum", it is tempting to suppose that περὶ τῆς οὐσίας τῶν δυνάμεων once formed part of a continuous text, and that the lacuna should be placed before ὥσπερ. A scribe might easily read this as a book title (cf. the title Γαληνοῦ περὶ τῆς οὐσίας τῶν φυσικῶν δυνάμεων in L and A), which would then lead to the circulation of the last chapters as a separate tract.

The Latin version also differs from the Greek heading in one significant way; it has no equivalent of φυσικῶν. In other words, Galen is talking about properties in general, not about the four natural faculties in particular. That the Latin is right on this point is clear from the structure of the immediate sentence and of the rest of the treatise. In his discussion of the soul, which forms the last sections, Galen here begins with the evidence drawn from human and plant activity which demonstrates the existence of various faculties. The specifically natural faculties do not appear until the very last chapter, where they constitute another argument for the existence of the soul. The supposition that some words were omitted would resolve many of the difficulties already indicated in the Greek, as well as restoring coherence to the general argument. The remaining sections of this book are concerned with the soul, not the natural faculties, and the reference to faculties is brought in for the purpose of comparison, not to serve as a guide to the remaining contents.

P. 110,4–6 ἐναργῶς: Galen uses a similar argument for the soul to that he had earlier used for the gods (p. 58,2–16). He appeals to 'what everybody knows', and to what is seen "clearly", i.e. these are premisses that only a foolish or a perverse opponent would wish to dispute; but, equally, they do not reveal or prove all that one might want, and a modern philosopher would undoubtedly wish to question both of Galen's starting points. But he is at least aware of methodological difficulties, and of how they might be overcome, as well as of the various points that might be reached on the way.

P. 110,7 τὰ – 10 πολυειδῶς / 110,8 operationes – 11: These activities are examples of voluntary motion and of perception, the two features Galen had declared earlier (see p. 108,11–13 κίνησιν) were peculiar to living creatures with souls. The similar list at De plac. Hipp. et Plat. VIII 1,2: CMG V 4,1, 2, p. 480,11–13, comprises extending and contracting the limbs, walking and running, and standing and sitting. Here Galen includes the more striking "wrestling". "surgendi" in the Arabo-Latin version represents either a misunderstanding by a translator or, less likely, a poor transcription of "currendi".

A, followed by all editors, inserts ἔσθ' ὅτε ("sometimes") after τρεχόντων, which, if right, would nicely point up the unexpected "wrestling". But elsewhere in Galen, e.g. In Hipp. Epid. VI comm. I 6: CMG V 10,2,2, p. 25,11–12. 29, the phrase has a further connective particle linking it to the following clause; otherwise the phrase would go with the preceding clause.[1] One solution to the problem would be to read ἔστι δ' ὅτε, a simple emendation, but the fact that the phrase is absent from the earliest witnesses, L Nic. and the Arabo-Latin version, suggests rather that we are dealing with an interpolation in A.

P. 110,12 ἐκ – 15 νοοῦμεν: The second argument in favour of the existence of a soul is the general principle beloved of Galen (and, he alleges, of all of us) that nothing happens without a cause. It is, he declares at Meth. med. I 7: X 49,18–50,3 K., a principle "universally admitted, requiring no demonstration" and "plain to the intellect" (cf. also ibid. I 4: X 36,18–19 K.; De plac. Hipp. et Plat. IV 4,36: CMG V 4,1,2, p. 258,13–14: "commonly admitted by almost all philosophers"; VI 5,24: p. 392,22–23; Compend. Tim. Plat. 2 a: p. 38,3–5 Kraus-Walzer). The precise role of this axiom in Galen's thought has been well explored by Hankinson, Galen, On the therapeutic method, pp. 141–143, who points out that its validity, in Galen's eyes, depended largely on its having an empirical basis. Its importance here is that it is firmly believed in by everybody, i.e. it corresponds intellectually to the empirical evidence just noted. It confirms him in his view that these actions cannot take place without some cause or other, and helps to provide a link between the substance of the faculties and the soul. Those who held a strongly physicalist view of the natural faculties might reply that there was no further need to posit a soul, as all the activities which Galen claims provide empirical evidence for the soul could have a merely physical explanation. But Galen might legitimately say that a consideration of causation suggests that more than a mechanism is required in even so physical activity as walking (why do we walk rather than run? or even decide to walk at all or at a particular mo-

1 A counter-example of this phrase without a further connective is at In Hipp. Epid. I comm. II 56: CMG V 10,1, p. 78,7 (if the text is correct).

ment?), and that this consideration helps to support the universal belief in the existence of the soul, even if there remains considerable debate about precisely how these activities and actions are caused, or about the links in the chain of causation. A consideration of certain activities indicates the participation of the soul without revealing the means by which that participation is effected. The rest of this book is taken up with Galen's own answer to this problem, and with finding a place for soul in what others might prefer to see as a largely mechanical process.

P. 110,15: ἀλλὰ is here not adversative, but progressive and connective, reinforced by καὶ, a common usage among medical writers; see J. D. Denniston, The Greek particles, 2nd ed., Oxford, 1954, pp. 21–22. The following participle θέμενοι (line 18) continues the construction θεώμενοι μὲν (line 6) ... ἐννοοῦντες δὲ (lines 10–11).

P. 110,17 ὄνομα – 21: In the Greek manuscripts and editions, neither θεμένων nor εἶναι fits into the sentence structure, which, I have argued above (p. 203, the note to p. 110,4–21), has been disrupted by the loss of its main clause. In order to make a main verb, Niccolò turned ἀλλὰ καὶ – ποιητικήν (lines 15–21) into a new main clause, changing the participle θεμένων into the main verb, "imposuerunt", linking the sentence to ὥσπερ by opening with "ita et". He seems not to have read εἶναι, introducing a participle "dicentes" to give clarity to a sentence which, unusually for him, departed some way from the Greek: "uirtutem dicentes eorum que fiunt uniuscuiusque factiuam".

Cornarius, following Nic., emended θεμένων to ἔθεντο, an emendation which creates an unacceptable double hiatus, before and after the verb, and still leaves the rest of the sentence without an apparent connection to what has preceded it. Goulston in the notes in his exemplar of the Basileensis and in the margin of his printed edition read θέμενοι in parallel with the participles at lines 6 and 10. The hiatus after θέμενοι is within the degrees of permissibility listed by De Lacy, in: CMG V 4,1,2, pp. 53–55. Goulston in his notes found a main verb by adding λέγομεν after εἶναι, perhaps following Nic.'s "dicentes". But since Galen is talking about men in general, and goes on immediately to describe what they believe, one expects the third person of the verb, not the first.

Ph. De Lacy, in a letter to me, suggests a further emendation: to delete εἶναι as an intrusion made by a scribe who failed to see that δύναμιν ... ποιητικὴν was in apposition to ὄνομα. The word may also have been introduced as a result of an expansion of a dittography of the last two letters of δύναμιν.

P. 110,19 δύναμιν: Both here, and still more so, at De fac. nat. I 4: Scr. min. III 107,14–16 Helmr. = II 9,13–14 K., Galen emphasises that his use of the word δύναμις is only a provisional way of referring to a cause whose essence is as yet unknown. Cf. also pp. 62,10 and 112,21 and the notes ad loc.

P. 110,21 οὕτω – 24: Galen refers to scammony, an extract of the root of Convolvulus scammonia, and the medlar for their own properties and as ingredients in other drugs; for scammony see e.g. Thrasyb. 42: Scr. min. III 91,21–22 Helmr. = V 887,10 K.; Meth. med. XIV 8: X 971,9–11 K.; for medlar, e.g. De simpl. med. temp. et fac. VII 12: XII 72,4–5 K.; De comp. med. sec. loc. IX 5: XIII 289,14 K.; in general, see R. J. Durling, A Dictionary of medical terms in Galen,

Leiden, New York, Köln, 1993 (Studies in ancient medicine 5), pp. 291; 234, respectively, and, for a wider discussion of their identification, J. André, Les noms de plantes dans la Rome antique, Paris, 1985, pp. 228; 160. Scammony in particular remained long in standard medical use. The British Pharmaceutical Codex of 1907 devoted three pages to its use as a strong purgative, pp. 1003–1005, warning against adulteration and confusion with jalap resin.

The Latin translation of τὸ μέσπιλον, "zaroli", derives from a common variant of the Arabic *zaʿrūr;* see A. Dietrich, Dioscurides triumphans. Ein anonymer arabischer Kommentar (Ende 12. Jahrh. n. Chr.) zur Materia medica. Arabischer Text nebst kommentierter deutscher Übersetzung, ed., part 2, Abh. d. Akademie d. Wiss. in Göttingen, philol.-hist. Kl., ser. 3, 173, Göttingen, 1988, pp. 181–182. Vernacular versions of the word can be found in Spanish and Portuguese and, particularly, in Italian, from which derives the English form of the word "azarole"; see The Oxford English Dictionary, 2nd ed., 1989, p. 842. P. A. Mattioli, Commentarii in VI libros Pedacii Dioscoridis, Venice, 1583, pp. 228–232, reporting the Arabic form of the word as *zaror*, *zarur* and *alzurur*, notes that a type of medlar grew thickly in the Naples region, where it was commonly called "azarolo". Mattioli's refusal to identify the plant with the common medlar, Mespilus Germanicus, led many subsequent botanists to equate Dioscorides' plant with the Neapolitan medlar, Crataegus azarolus, or some other variety.[1] The form of the Latin word, and, according to Mattioli, the common usage of the vernacular form in the Naples region would support an Italian origin for the translation, but the presence of identical forms also in Spanish and Portuguese advises caution.

P. 110,24 οἱ – 13: Having established the overall truth of his observations about the potentialities of the two drugs by appealing first to 'what everyone says they have', Galen then contrasts this unanimity with the variety of explanations for these actions given by the experts, 'those who have worked on the so-called theory of nature'. Röhr's discussion of ancient explanations for the working of drugs (pp. 96–133), shows conclusively that the debate was not confined to medical men or to those whom we might term philosophers, but was already a standard feature of the so-called Problem literature, expositions of particular scientific and non-scientific problems aimed at a literate audience. Galen's description also makes it clear that, in his view at least, these opinions were held by respectable theorists, not magicians, sorcerers, theurgists and the like, some of whose explanations for their magic come close to what Galen offers here.

P. 112,1 ἄλλος – 2 ἑαυτούς: The idiomatic use of the singular ἄλλος ἄλλο followed by the plural πείσαντες ἑαυτούς, the reading of L, is supported by Nic. ("alius aliud suadentes sibi ipsis") and perhaps also by the Arabo-Latin version, "unusquisque" (p. 110,24). It is also easier to see why the singular ἄλλος ἄλλο should have been turned to the plural ἄλλως ἄλλοι than the reverse. For other examples, cf. Gal., In Hipp. Epid. VI comm. I 5; III 25: CMG V 10,2,2, pp. 19,29; 162,19–20. At III 20: CMG V 10,2,2, p. 154,20, Galen uses

1 Cf. for an earlier discussion of the identity of the plant, G. Manardus, Epistulae medicinales, X 1, Lyons, 1549, pp. 304–305.

this idiom with a singular verb, followed immediately by a plural participle connected with ἅπαντες. See also R. Kühner and B. Gerth, Ausführliche Grammatik der griechischen Sprache. Satzlehre, 4th ed., Hanover, 1955, Erster Teil, pp. 286–288; E. Wenkebach, Beiträge zur Textgeschichte der Epidemienkommentare Galens II, Abh. d. Preuß. Akademie d. Wiss., phil.-hist. Kl. 9, Berlin, 1928, pp. 4–5.

P. 112,2 οἱ – 5 οὐσίαις: That some drugs worked through incorporeal properties dwelling in their sensible substances was not a belief that Galen himself shared. It was at times one that came close to magic; cf. the texts assembled by E. R. Dodds, The Greeks and the irrational, Berkeley, Los Angeles, London, 1951, pp. 292–294, but it was attractive to those who believed that qualities are incorporeal; cf. the pseudo-Galenic treatise Quod qualitates incorporeae sint: XIX 463–484 K.; new edition by M. Giusta, Turin, 1976.

P. 112,5 οἱ – 13: The second category of explanation, and one that Galen himself follows in his own writings, is material: it is "the substances themselves" that "act according to their own particular nature". The list that follows presents a series of possibilities, exemplifying the type of material explanation offered and itself subdivided into the theory of the four elements, on the one hand, and that of (various) primary bodies, on the other. Although retaining the manuscript reading ἑκάστην in the text of his edition, i.e. "each individual nature", Goulston suggested in the margin the alternative and better ἑκάστης, "the individual nature of each substance".

P. 112,9 ἢ – 13: Galen frequently lists the alternative explanations offered for the ultimate portions of matter (see the testimonia). Although elsewhere Galen strongly attacks the Epicurean and Democritean notions of atoms and the Asclepiadean ἄναρμα, especially at De elem. ex Hipp. sent. 2,9: CMG V 1,2, p. 60,1–3; De diff. morb. 2: VI 839,16–840,5 K.; and In Hipp. De nat. hom. comm. I 6: CMG V 9,1, p. 21,11–18, largely because their explanations fail to explain phenomena such as pain, he is prepared to allow them here, if only because the persistence of these alternatives confirms him in his belief that these problems cannot, as yet, be satisfactorily answered, negatively or positively. His own view, expressed most clearly in the treatises De elementis ex Hippocratis sententia and De temperamentis, and associated by him with Hippocrates, Plato, Aristotle, and the Stoics, is that the properties of drugs, for instance, are the result of the mixing together of the four elements with their four primary qualities.

P. 112,11 ἄτομα: For atoms, posited by Democritus, Leucippus, and Epicurus and his school, see e.g. R. Löbl, Demokrits Atome. Eine Untersuchung zur Überlieferung und zu einigen wichtigen Lehrstücken in Demokrits Physik, Bonn, 1976 (Habelts Dissertationsdrucke, Reihe Klassische Philologie 24); Kirk, Raven, Schofield, pp. 413–428; Long and Sedley, vol. 1, pp. 37–44. Stückelberger, esp. pp. 89–123, offers a speculative exposition of the opinions of Erasistratus, Asclepiades, and Galen on the Democritean atoms.

ἄναρμα: This term[1] was used in particular by Asclepiades and his fol-

[1] In the Arabo-Latin version the word is translated positively ("possint continuari"): in what follows, the negative expression ἀμερῆ is correctly translated as "non possint diuidi", which raises the possibility that "non" has dropped out here.

lowers (cf. Vallance, pp. 7–43) and Galen may be referring also to Heraclides of Pontus, who believed in ἄναρμοι ὄγκοι (see H. B. Gottschalk, Heraclides of Pontus, Oxford, 1980, pp. 37–57; Stückelberger, pp. 89–113). At De elem. ex Hipp. sent. 2,7: CMG V 1,2, p. 58,21–22, Galen ascribes a belief in ἄναρμα to 'some of the same group as Epicurus and Democritus', which implies that he saw some connection between the theories of Asclepiades and those of Epicurus.

P. 112,12 ἀμερῆ: Simplicius (In Arist. Phys. comm.: CAG X, p. 925,13–17) claims that Leucippus and Democritus described their primary bodies as partless, ἀμερές (cf. Stob., Anth. I 14,1: I 143,4 Wachsmuth-Hense), and Galen (De elem. ex Hipp. sent. 2,17: CMG V 1,2, p. 62,6–7) reports that Diodorus and Leucippus believed that the primary bodies were indivisible (ἀδιαίρετα) because of their smallness.[1] But earlier in that treatise (2,6–7: CMG V 1,2, p. 58,19–22) he had specifically denied that Epicurus and Democritus had called their primary bodies ἀμερῆ; that was done by 'others of the same school'. He may thus be aligning himself with those who believed that this name came into use for the Democritean atoms only in Hellenistic times, perhaps with Diodorus Cronus (d. c. 284 B.C.). Cf. S. Luria, Democritea, Leningrad, 1970, p. 51, no. 124; D. Sedley, Diodorus Cronus and Hellenistic philosophy, Proceedings of the Cambridge Philological Society, n. s. 23, 1977, pp. 85–89.

ὁμοιομερῆ: This theory was favoured by Anaxagoras and Archelaus among the Presocratic philosophers. Galen (De elem. ex Hipp. sent. 9,11: CMG V 1,2, p. 130,8–9) mentions Anaxagoras in the context of ὁμοιομέρειαι, "homoeomeries", "the things with like parts", as the ultimate building blocks of matter, Anaxagoras himself does not appear to have used neither word and may instead have called them "seeds" (cf. Kirk, Raven, Schofield, p. 377; G. B. Kerferd, Anaxagoras and the concept of matter before Aristotle, Bulletin of the John Rylands Library 52, 1969, pp. 129–143; W. G. Mann, Anaxagoras and the homoiomere, Phronesis 25, 1980, pp. 228–249). But when Galen used the word in an anatomical sense to describe body tissues, he did not mention Anaxagoras, but took Aristotle as his starting-point (see e.g. De plac. Hipp. et Plat. VIII 4,9: CMG V 4,1,2, p. 500,8; In Hipp. De nat. hom. comm. I prooem.: CMG V 9,1, p. 6,14–15, and the comment by G. Strohmaier, Galeni De partium homoeomerium differentia libelli versio Arabica, ed., transl., and comm., CMG Suppl. Or. III, Berlin, 1970, pp. 87–91). For the later development of this theory, see J. M. Forrester, The homoeomerous parts and their replacement by Bichat's tissues, Medical History 38, 1994, pp. 444–458.

The Arabo-Latin version adds a negative ("non possint similium partium esse", lines 12–13), as if the word were originally ἀνομοιομερῆ.

P. 112,14 τὴν – 16 εἶναι: The view that the soul was something incorporeal was held by the Platonists, who took their cue from the Timaeus (69 c), e.g. by Alcinous, whose Didascalicus provides a neat exposition of Platonic doctrine in the time of Galen (see esp. 23–25: pp. 45–51 Whittaker). Where the Platonists differed among themselves was over the extent to which any part of the tripartite soul could be thought of as possessing body, and many

[1] Sorabji, p. 356, misleadingly attributes this view to Democritus.

drew a distinction between the rational part, located in the brain and incorporeal, and the other two parts, which, if not themselves corporeal, were strongly influenced by the composition of the body in which they were set. For the third part, located in the liver, see De Lacy, pp. 42–63.[1]

P. 112,16 τινὲς δὲ πνεῦμα: Galen is referring here to the Stoics (cf. Long and Sedley, vol. 1, pp. 313–323). It was a view that he himself was not prepared to accept, for a variety of reasons. In his opinion, *pneuma* was only the instrument of the soul, not the soul itself (see De plac. Hipp. et Plat. VII 3,19–22: CMG V 4,1,2, pp. 442,36–444,11).

P. 112,16 καθάπερ – 114,5: Who these "others" are is not easy to determine, although Aristotle in De anima I 5: 409 b 18–410 b 22 had included such materialists in his survey of earlier views on the soul. The Epicureans certainly held a materialist view of the soul, and linked certain patterns of the soul to the arrangement of atoms from which they assumed it was made up (see Usener, Epicurea, fr. 310–316: pp. 216,22–219,28) but none of their formulations corresponds precisely to what Galen says here. On the other hand, at De fac. nat. I 12: Scr. min. III 120,21–25 Helmr. = II 27,14–28,2 K., Galen had the Epicureans and also Asclepiades in mind, when he associated this view of the soul with those who believed that substance was unchangable and unalterable, subdivided into fine particles separated by void.[2] There is also a case for seeing some Peripatetics as Galen's target here, for in one of his last writings he interpreted Aristotle's opinion that the soul was the form of the body to mean that the soul was identical to the mixture of the four primary qualities or the four primary elements that make up the body. The faculties of the soul, like its activities, thus depended on its essence, i.e. on its physical make-up.[3] This was a view to which Galen was increasingly sympathetic, for he rebuked Andronicus the Peripatetic for declaring that the soul was either a mixture or a faculty dependent on mixture. Had he not mentioned faculty, Galen would have been satisfied.[4] But Galen's point here does

1 The sixth-century epigram of Agathias, Anth. Pal. XI 354, attacking Nicostratus, "the second Aristotle and Plato's peer" for his agnosticism in refusing to say whether the soul was mortal and corporeal, or the reverse, shows how commonplace this debate became later.

2 If Vallance (pp. 8–43) is right, unlike the Epicureans, Asclepiades did not believe that his particles themselves were unalterable, for they could be 'crushed' and reassembled into different shapes.

3 See Gal., Quod animi mores corp. temp. sequ. 3: Scr. min. II 37,17–26 Müller = IV 774, 7–18 K. Müller excluded the last sentence as a later addition, and H. Schöne, Verbesserungen zum Galentext, SB d. Preuß. Akademie d. Wiss., phil.- hist. Kl. 1924, 15, Berlin, 1924, p. 97, transferred it to follow p. 33,9 Müller. But transposition is unlikely, and the sentence was certainly in its present position when the Arabic translation was made in the ninth century (see p. 43 Biesterfeldt).

4 See Gal., Quod animi mores corp. temp. sequ. 4: Scr. min. II 44,12–20 Müller = IV 782, 14–783, 2 K. For the textual problem involved in the identification, see Moraux, Der Aristotelismus, vol. I, p. 134 n. 9; Gottschalk, p. 1113. Unknown to Moraux, the name of Andronicus appears in the Arabic version of this text (see p. 49 Biesterfeldt), and presumably in the (lost) manuscript used by the Aldine printers. For later Peripatetic views, cf. Moraux, Der Aristotelismus, vol. II, pp. 741–742.

not depend on the identification of this or that thinker, or this or that group. He intends to show merely that these views can be and are held in ways that do not allow for proof or disproof. Indeed, the very existence of these divergent views proves his point.

P. 112,20 ὧν ποιεῖν πέφυκε: This phrase repeated in a slightly different wording at p. 114, 5 emphasises Galen's commitment to an explanation in terms of natural activity. Faculties, or capacities, are there so that whatever natural activities are necessary for life may be carried out, and as he argues in the opening section of De fac. nat. I 4: Scr. min. III 107,10–16 Helmr. = II 9, 9–14 K., each activity must have a cause, and that cause, at least provisionally until a more precise explanation is available, can be termed a faculty. It is not there by chance, but is the result of the benevolent workings of Nature, who has organised the human body efficiently and purposefully.

P. 112,21 οὐκ – 114,5: In two clauses each with a genitive absolute, Galen now qualifies his presentation of the theory that the soul has no independent existence and that faculties are merely the result of the particular makeup of the body. In the first, he warns his readers that faculties do not take on the individual nature of various substances; in the second, he stresses that they are merely the properties of the operating substance which is the cause of the perceptible effects. Exactly what he means by this is made clearer at De fac. nat. I 4: Scr. min. III 107,12–20 Helmr. = II 9,11–10,1 K., where Galen emphasises that his use of the word "faculty" is merely provisional until the true essence of the operating cause is known. This definition of a faculty and its relationship to the operating cause leaves the way open for a vitalist interpretation of Man without necessarily excluding a materialist one.

P. 112,22 οὐσιῶν: As it stands, οὐσῶν, the reading of the Greek manuscripts, of Nic. ("existentibus"), and of all the editions, makes sense neither logically nor grammatically, while the Arabo-Latin version appears to have followed a very different, and equally unlikely, text. An anonymous annotator of the sixteenth century in the Basle edition now in the Cambridge University Library, classmark Path. a 72, made the excellent suggestion οὐσιῶν, which gives point to the sentence by emphasising that faculties do not take on the specific nature of various (τινων) substances.

P. 114,13 βέλτιον – 19: Goulston in his Dublin notes suggested that ἔοικεν had fallen out after ὡς (line 15), but this is not necessary, as ὡς is here used consecutively. Galen's point is that he wished he had enough sound knowledge to pronounce about these matters in as definite a manner as others had done, but he cannot convince himself that he has.

P. 114,17 βεβαίαν – 19: For knowledge as the result of proper, sound demonstration, see above pp. 164–167 the notes to pp. 80,15–82,5. In cases like this, according to Galen, merely to acknowledge the absence of a firm demonstration is one step on the right road.

P. 114,20 ὅσα – 27 φιλοσοφίαν: A complicated sentence is not helped by Galen's repetitions and strings of participles, and translators have offered various interpretations of the Greek. The Arabo-Latin version takes διὰ – ἀκριβῶς closely with ἐπεκόσμησεν, and appears not to have translated τὰ . . . ἀποτελούμενα at all. Niccolò, on the other hand, translated ἀποτελούμενα as if it were ἀποτελουμένων: "quia ea que cognoscuntur . . . efficiunt". The difficulty that lies behind all these faulty versions is that of linking the various clauses together and of understanding the precise connotations of ἀποτελούμενα. Galen does not possess as yet certainty of knowledge in some matters pertaining to health and morality, but if they were known for certain, they would give added lustre to what is already being achieved (reading τὰ with A) as a result of careful understanding in actual practice and moral philosophy. διὰ – ἀκριβῶς thus goes with ἀποτελούμενα.[1] The sentence means that something worthwhile can be achieved even without certain knowledge in more theoretical matters. But one should still regard this knowledge as inessential; it is useful, but not necessary, an added bonus rather than a cornerstone of medicine.

P. 114,27 ἣν: Galen uses the singular relative referring to moral philosophy only, since medicine, it goes without saying, is in Galen's eyes both useful and capable of being learned by those who put their minds to it.

P. 116,1–2 βιβλία: Galen's choice of words leaves the identification of the two books irritatingly vague. He himself, at De libris propr. 12 (13): Scr. min. II 121,7–122,6 Müller = XIX 45,9–46,10 K., listed together 23 works on ethical themes, at the head of which he placed De affectuum et peccatorum dignotione (CMG V 4,1,1, pp. 3–68). Another book of relevance is De moribus, of which only an Arabic epitome survives (pp. 1–51 Kraus; English translation, by Mattock, pp. 235–260). A third possibility is Quod animi mores corporis temperamenta sequantur (Scr. min. II 32–79 Müller = IV 767–822 K.), but this is not included by Galen himself among his ethical treatises.

P. 116,5 Ὅτι – 12: As necessary knowledge, i.e. things that Galen knows with certainty and that he regards as essential for medicine, Galen adds to the theory of the four elements that he has explained earlier (pp. 62,19–64,4) the idea that the elements are mixed together, not, as Empedocles had suggested, "crushed together" or pulverised into a mass of juxtaposed tiny fragments (although given the fact that Galen describes the process elsewhere with a variety of terms, one should be careful about attributing the actual word καταθραύεσθαι to Empedocles).[2] The reason why Galen can reject so confidently the view of Empedocles is because, in his view, it does not explain adequately the genesis of pain (see e.g. De elem. ex Hipp. sent. 9,11: CMG V 1,2, pp. 128,24–130,10).[3]

1 Hankinson, Galen's anatomy of the soul, p. 206, translates "they . . . bring both medicine and ethical philosophy to completion", and compares De plac. Hipp. et Plat. IX 9,9: CMG V 4,1,2, p. 600,10–18. But the parallel is not exact, and the voice of the verb is passive, not middle.

2 This fragment, Empedocl., A 43: I, p. 291,25–26 D.-K., is not discussed or cited in M. R. Wright, Empedocles: the extant fragments, New Haven and London, 1981, although the other Galenic parallels are, pp. 37–40. J. Longrigg reminds me that the words θραύεσθαι and θραύσματα are found in Theophr., De sensu 11 = Empedocl., A 86: I p. 302,29 D.-K., and in Aet. I 13,1 = Empedocl., A 43: I, p. 291,19 D.-K., in connection with Empedocles' theories. Cf. J. Longrigg, 'Roots', Classical Review, n. s. 17, 1967, pp. 1–4.

3 For Empedocles' physicalist explanation of pain, see Empedocl., A 86; 95: I, pp. 302,18; 303,38; 307,21–28 D.-K., references I owe to J. Longrigg.

P. 116,12 εἴτε – 17: The debate about mixtures was one between the Peripatetics on the one hand, who believed that the mixture was one of qualities only, and Zeno of Citium and the Stoics on the other, who declared it to be a complete mingling of substances as well.[1] At De elem. ex Hipp. sent. 9, 33: CMG V 1,2, p. 136,15–18 (where Galen uses almost identical language) and at Meth. med. I 2: X 16,12–15 K., Galen ascribes the first view to Aristotle, perhaps an inference from De generat. et corrupt. I 10: 328 a 18–b 22, but here he gives no name (cf. De Lacy, in: CMG V 1,2, p. 200, the note to p. 136, 15–20). That this was a live debate in Galen's day is clear above all from the writings of his younger contemporary, Alexander of Aphrodisias, and his school, notably in De mixtione and in the Quaestiones (II 3: pp. 47,28–50,25 Bruns); cf. R. B. Todd, Alexander of Aphrodisias on Stoic physics. A study of the De mixtione with preliminary essays, text, translation and commentary, Leiden, 1976 (Philosophia Antiqua 28).

P. 116,17 πιθανώτερον – 19: Galen shows again his impatience with metaphysics for going beyond what he understands as proof. His view in general is that there is no doubt that there can be a complete alteration of substance as a result of some form of mixture, and that this alteration is qualitatively perceptible, and hence is most likely to have involved at least a mixing together of qualities (cf. De fac. nat. I 2: Scr. min. III 104,2–20 Helmr. = II 5, 3–6,1 K.).

P. 116,20 τήν – 26: Cf. above, pp. 140–141; 142–144, the notes to pp. 58,22–60,6; 60,3–6. Galen returns once again to his definition of the soul, refusing to give his assent either to those who believe that it is something immortal but temporarily mixing with the substances of the body in the same way as the elements are mixed together or to those who deny all existence to the soul itself qua individual essence. His refusal to commit himself is based on what he sees as the proper basis for certainty, logical proof, and he then goes on to point to an empirical observation (note σαφῶς, line 27) directed against those who believe in the totally independent existence of soul.

P. 116,26 ἐκεῖνο – 118,5: For the notion of the soul taking up residence within the body, cf. Gal., In Plat. Tim. comm. III 2: CMG Suppl. I, p. 11,21–36. Galen's description of the soul as 'enslaved' to the body suggests that he considered that even the rational part of the soul might be subject to the direct effects of bodily changes. The same imagery, with its implication of a strong determinism, is also found at Quod animi mores corp. temp. sequ. 3. 5: Scr. min. II 41,15–18; 48,5–8 Müller = IV 779,11–13; 787,6–9 K., although elsewhere in that book Galen rejects such a straightforward physical explanation of moral actions, and, as Hankinson, Galen's anatomy of the soul, p. 204, points out, he nowhere explains the nature of the soul's dependence on the body. In the Arabic epitome of De moribus (2: pp. 49–50 Kraus = p. 248 Mattock) Galen offers a slightly different interpretation, arguing that man's soul

1 For the former, in the pre-Galenic period, cf. J. Mansfeld, Zeno and Aristotle on mixture, Mnemosyne 36, 1983, pp. 306–310; Moraux, Der Aristotelismus, vol. I, pp. 282–283; for the Stoics, cf. S. Sambursky, Physics of the Stoics, London, 1959; Long and Sedley, vol. 1, pp. 290–294.

could not only continue to remain in existence after removal from the body, but also survive the loss of its two irrational parts if they perished along with the body. But the provisionality of the argument here is also apparent, and the Arabic epitomator may not always have been as accurate in his rendering as one would have liked; cf. Walzer, New light, p. 92 (repr. in: Walzer, Greek into Arabic, p. 157). However, such an opinion was certainly, in Galen's eyes, held by Plato, and Galen himself was willing to concede that the two lower parts of the soul were destroyed at death along with the liver and the heart, even if he was not prepared to say that the remaining, rational, part of the soul was or was not immortal (see Quod animi mores corp. temp. sequ. 3: Scr. min. II 36,12–19 Müller = IV 772,18–773,6 K.; cf. Lloyd, Scholarship, pp. 14–19). But these disputes were secondary to the main point at issue, namely that Plato, Hippocrates, and Aristotle were in agreement that the soul was at times dependent on the body, and that this was something that could be 'clearly seen', i.e. empirically demonstrated.

P. 118,3 disposita – 5 quod: The translator does not preserve the striking metaphor δουλεύει (line 1), which may already have fallen out within the Arabic tradition; one would also expect "disposita" and "generate secundum quod" instead of the readings "dispositio" and "generatio eius quod" (α), unless these are also the result of some corruption within the Arabic. But these are easy mistakes to make in resolving a heavily abbreviated text, and I have emended accordingly.

P. 118,8 τῆς – 9 μετεμψυχώσεως: Galen signals by καλουμένης that he is here using a technical term. According to LSJ, both ἐμψύχωσις and its corresponding verb are not found until the time of Galen, and indeed this passage provides the earliest evidence for the noun, which reappears in Plot., Enn. IV 3,9, and in the pseudo-Galenic treatise Ad Gaurum quomodo animetur fetus 2,4; 11,1. 2. 3: pp. 35,25; 48,14. 21; 49,20 Kalbfleisch.[1] The context of these non-Galenic references is securely neo-Platonic, and Galen may well be attesting to a development within contemporary Platonism that does not appear in our surviving philosophical sources for another generation or so. μετεμψύχωσις, the transmigration of souls, is a term favoured by the (neo-)Pythagoreans and later the neo-Platonists. Whether Galen knew of it directly through links with Pythagoreans in Rome is impossible to say, although he was familiar with the so-called Carmen aureum of Pythagoras (see De animi cuiusl. pecc. dign. et cur. 5,10; 6,10: CMG V 4,1,1, pp. 18,22–25; 21,8–10). His contacts with Jews and Christians might also have introduced him to similar debates on the soul within those communities. The Arabo-Latin version paraphrases, "modum quo currit dispositio uite", almost certainly to avoid giving offence to Muslim and Christian readers; cf. for other examples in Ḥunayn's translations, G. Strohmaier, Die griechischen Götter in einer christlich-arabi-

[1] I exclude Anth. Pal. IX 774, by Glaucus of Athens, which appears in a block of early Byzantine epigrams, and is thus unlikely to have been written by the Hellenistic epigrammatist of that name; see K. v. Radinger, art. "Glaukos" (no. 38), in: RE VII, 1910, col. 1420. A reference nearly contemporary with the use of this word in our text is Alexander of Aphrodisias, In Arist. Top. comm.: CAG II 2, p. 137,28.

schen Übersetzung. Zum Traumbuch des Artemidor in der Version des Ḥunain ibn Isḥāḳ, in: F. Altheim and R. Stiehl, Die Araber in der Alten Welt, vol. 5,1, Berlin, 1968, pp. 141–142 (repr. in: Strohmaier, Von Demokrit bis Dante, pp. 241–242).

P. 118,10 ἐπιτήδειόν – 29: Galen repeats here his argument and examples from Quod animi mores corporis temperamenta sequantur to show that certain physical changes in the body inevitably result in death and the departure of the soul, and thus that the soul resides in the body only so long as the body is in a healthy state. They are not included, as they were there, in order to pose a problem for those who think of the soul as something totally incorporeal, or to help distinguish between the material and non-material view of the soul. Rather they explain why Galen does not need to investigate the precise way in which the soul enters the body. If, as Galen is convinced, the body must first be in the right condition to receive the soul and if, when the body is altered seriously for the worse, the soul will inevitably depart, then the preparation of the healthy body is a prerequisite for the arrival and residence of the soul, and hence for life, not the other way round.

The omission of πάντως – σῶμα (lines 28–29) is likely to have taken place before the Latin translation was made, since there are no obvious traces in the Latin Mss. of any dislocation.

P. 120,8 καθάπερ – 12 / 120,5 neque – 12: Galen now expands his description of moral philosophy to include practical philosophy and politics, which for him are near equivalents. It does not matter which word one chooses to use, provided that one distinguishes any or all from speculative philosophy. He makes a similar point in his exaltation of practical philosophy at De plac. Hipp. et Plat. IX 7,9–12: CMG V 4,1,2, p. 588,7–22. The Arabo-Latin version differs in several ways from the Greek. It repeats ἠθικὴν φιλοσοφίαν, and translates the alternatives, πρακτικήν τε καὶ πολιτικήν, as if they were alternative explanations of why one should refer to the "aptatio morum" as "moralis". Finally, instead of making a distinction between this and "theoretical philosophy", the translator distinguishes "it" ("ipsam"), apparently the "particula *sc.* moralis" from "opus pratice". How and when these changes occurred is difficult to determine, but such misunderstanding is untypical of Ḥunayn and his school. Although it is tempting to emend the Latin to read "consuetudinem siue que docet bene operari", this is not adequate, as the translator may well have been working from an already faulty text.

P. 120,15 ὁπόσαι – 16 ὁποῖαι / 120,15 quot – 16 sint: The agreement of A and Nic. ("quot sunt et"), who usually agrees with L, indicates that εἰσι should come after τε, not after ὁποῖαι, where L and the editions have it. The Arabo-Latin version offers an interesting divergence within the manuscripts: all agree on writing the first interrogative as "quod" (in error for "quot"), but differ on the second. C γ have "quid", which corresponds to the original Greek, ε has "quot", which would be correct if the Arabic had inverted the order of the interrogatives. Alternatively, the reading of ε represents an intelligent attempt by a scribe to improve the text.

P. 120,16–17 κατὰ ἀκολουθίαν: Unlike πᾶν τὸ ἀκόλουθον (p. 104,7–8), where the emphasis is on the need to investigate the logical consequences of any statement carefully, the phrase here appears to emphasise the chronological order of the questions. Galen now returns to the question of sensation and the natural faculties that he had broken off at p. 114,5.

P. 120,19 ἀδύνατον – 25 / 120,21 et impossibile – 25: Although προγνωρίσαι (instead of πρὶν γνωρίσαι), the reading of the oldest manuscript L and the version of Niccolò ("precognoscere"), makes a stylistically elegant variation with the following γνωρίζειν (line 24) Galen is not complaining that it is impossible to tell in advance what is suitable or unsuitable or to attract the one and reject the other. Rather, his point is that it appears to be the case that without knowing first what is suitable one cannot attract it, and hence that attraction demands some form of preliminary sense perception. The reading of A and of Goulston's Codex Adelphi (see his edition, p. 214, and the note ad loc.) is thus to be followed, as it makes clear the temporal priority of sensation. The unusually vague way in which Galen sets out the argument, twice using φαίνεται and an infinitive, is deliberate, for he is setting out the premisses of a syllogistic argument in which he himself does not believe in quite the same way as some of his (and Plato's) audience. The Arabo-Latin version does not include πρὶν – ἀλλότριον, an error which through similarity of wording could have occurred at any point in the transmission.

P. 122,1 Διὰ τοῦτο – 7: The misunderstanding consists in Plato's audience thinking that there was a general faculty of recognition within plants. Galen argues that Plato was referring to something very specific, the recognition of things appropriate and inappropriate, which is brought about through (very basic) feelings of pleasure and pain. By using the phrase ἄλλαις . . . αἰσθήσεσιν (Tim. 77 a), Plato was indicating clearly that he was not using the word with all its normal connotations of the five senses, sight, hearing, smell, taste and touch (cf. earlier, 65 e, where he understands sense perception in the normal way).

P. 122,1 Et – 5: The Arabo-Latin version ends in textual confusion in the middle of the sentence after the Platonic quotation, and is followed by an equally mutilated sentence (line 6). There are two minor textual problems: "igitur", the reading of the manuscripts, makes little sense, and, given the very abbreviated and badly written archetype of this Arabo-Latin version, is best explained as a miscopying of "genus". D^2 E^2 inserted above the line after "aliud" the words "de uirtute sensitiua". Although these might be seen as a reference to what follows in Galen and has once formed part of the translation, they are far more likely to represent a guess at the meaning of "aliud".

P. 122,3 ἕτερον – 4 φυτοῖς: Although editors have printed these words as if they were those of Plato (Tim.77 a/b) they are, at best, an amalgam of what Plato says there: plants have some form of perception, as a result of possessing what Plato terms the third part of the soul, and they are a "different sort of living creature", mixed with other forms and sense perceptions. As Schröder (in: CMG Suppl. I, p. 43, the note to p. 11,19–20) noted, the infinitive εἶναι in A is preferable to the indicative ἐστι in L, unless the allusion is to be prefaced by ὡς, an addition suggested by Goulston, p. 214 (cf. the app. crit.).

P. 122,6 magnum – 124,12: Einarson, pp. 258–259, performed the difficult task of identifying the source of this passage as the pseudo-Aristotelian De pomo (pp. 58,4–59,2 Plezia) but he left it to others to draw further conclusions. The text of the fragment in the manuscripts of De sententiis is sufficiently close to that of the Manfredian version of De pomo to rule out the possibility that the fragment was already present in the codex from which the translator made his own version.[1] In other words, the translation of De sententiis and that of De pomo are independent of one another, and the collocation of the two texts in the common source of the surviving manuscripts was made at some point between 1260 and 1350. Although it is tempting to think that a copyist deliberately added the section from De pomo as a neat way of resolving many of Galen's doubts and uncertainties, the fact that De sententiis is mutilated at the end and De pomo at the beginning (and the end) indicates rather that there has been some mechanical loss of a leaf or quire in the process of transmission.

P. 122,7 τούτων – 14: Plato (Tim. 77 b) declares that the third part of the soul has a share in sensation (ᾧ . . . μέτεστιν . . . αἰσθήσεως), both pleasant and painful, and in appetite, and Galen follows him closely here and below (p. 124,13–16) in associating what is appropriate or inappropriate with pleasure and pain. But at this point he makes two significant additions. Firstly, he calls the third part of the soul the "vegetative soul", a term that Aristotle had used (Eth. Nic. I 13: 1102 a 32; b 29) and which Galen frequently equated with Plato's third part of the soul (e.g. De plac. Hipp. et Plat. VI 3,7: CMG V 4,1,1, p. 374,9–17); discussion by De Lacy, pp. 43–57, and Lloyd, Scholarship, pp. 15–16. But at De anima II 3: 414 a 32–b 16, Aristotle had expressly denied that plants possess any form of sense perception, allowing them only the nutritive faculty, and, equally, confining pleasure and pain, and all forms of desire, to sense perception, and hence to animals.[2] Thus although one need not criticise Galen too harshly for employing an Aristotelian term for the third part of the soul, and even for claiming that Plato's sensation was something specific and differed from what might generally be understood by that term, on his own definition of what Plato had meant he was wrong to associate Aristotle, even by implication, with that view. Cf. above, p. 192, the note to p. 102,18–19.

Galen's second addition is an expansion of pleasure and pain to include similar or analogous affections. The definite article τὰ in L derives from dittography after ἀνάλογα and before παθήματα.

P. 124,1 πρὸς – 2 οὐσίας: The Aldine editors amalgamated the readings of the L tradition (πρὸς τὰς οἰκείας τοῖς τρεφομένοις οὐσίας) and of A (πρὸς τὸ οἰκεῖον τοῖς τρεφομένοις) to produce an ugly and impossible text:

1 Plezia records in his apparatus criticus variants from only seven of the more than 70 manuscripts of De pomo, and hence speculation on the significance of particular variants is otiose.

2 Mansfeld, Doxography, pp. 3188–3190, citing Clement, Strom. VIII 10,3–4; Theodoret, Graec. aff. cur. V 24–25, and Aetius, Plac. V 26, shows that a knowledge of these divergent views was commonplace. Aristotle, De anima III 11: 433 b 31–434 a 3, had allowed imperfect animals with perception by touch to have pleasure and pain, and hence desires, but there is no suggestion that he considered plants to be in this category.

πρὸς τὸ οἰκεῖον τοῖς τρεφομένοις οὐσίας. This was emended to ... τῆς τρεφομένης ... by Cornarius in his Jena notes, by Chartier in his edition, and by Goulston in his Dublin notes. Goulston had been preceded in this by Caius, who had first made the emendation himself in his exemplar of the Basle edition, and later added: "ita etiam cast. in adelphi", a reading of the Codex Adelphi more likely to be the record of a conjecture than a true manuscript reading. But none of these scholars knew the right reading of L and Nic. ("ad proprias eis que nutriuntur substantias").

P. 124,8 μηδὲ – 9: Plato (Tim. 77 c) declared that plants had no self-motion (τῆς ὑφ' ἑαυτοῦ κινήσεως) and hence remained fixed and stationary in the ground. Here Galen is using κίνησις in a different sense, that of motion as activity which arises from within the individual (ἐξ ἑαυτῶν), and which he declares is a distinguishing mark of all living things. As he put it at In Plat. Tim. comm. III 2: CMG Suppl. I, p. 11,9–12, if it is proposed that the soul is the origin of movement, and if it is agreed that plants have this source of movement within themselves, then they will be properly called "ensouled"; and all men call a body with soul a living creature (or an animal). Not all would have accepted this argument. Aristotle was prepared to allow that plants had a soul, but not that they were living creatures; the Stoics denied both that they had a soul and that they were living creatures. They willingly conceded that plants had movement ἐξ ἑαυτῶν, but distinguished it from movement ἀφ' ἑαυτῶν: the former was produced naturally, by nature, the latter by the soul (see Chrys., fr. 988: SVF II, pp. 287,33–288,35). Cf. also the similar formulation in Aet., Plac. V 26,3: Diels, Doxographi Graeci, p. 438,15–20, as well as Schröder, in: CMG Suppl. I, p. 41, the note to p. 11,11; and, for a general survey of the debate, Self-motion. From Aristotle to Newton, ed. M. L. Gill and J. G. Lennox, Princeton, 1994.

P. 124,8 μηδὲ: Goulston in his Dublin notes gives μηδὲ, the reading of A, for the μήτε of L and the early editions, probably as a result of a conjecture.

P. 124,9 ἀλλὰ – 22: Just as Galen had earlier declared (p. 120,4–10) that a philosophical question, the nature of the soul, was irrelevant to medicine, so he now argues that a physical problem, how (and why) plants attract nutriment, is of only slight value for medicine, and, a fortiori, of no use whatsoever to philosophy.

P. 124,20 ἔτι δὲ: Goulston reports in the notes to his edition that the codex Adelphi read ἔστι δὲ, although he was not prepared to change his text; he also wondered whether the word αὐτῆς (line 22) should not be αὐτοῦ, but the feminine αὐτῆς refers back to γνῶσις and should be retained.

P. 124,22: The ending of this book is for a student of Galen profoundly unsatisfactory; repetitive, rambling, uncertain, and concluding with what amounts to a footnote to a discussion in which he himself has apparently no or little interest. In explicating Plato, Galen seems to have lost the thread of his general argument, and to have moved from outlining his major theories as a guide to authenticity to defending another's paradox. There is no summing up, such as one finds at the end of De usu partium or De praecognitione, but, as in De placitis Hippocratis et Platonis, Galen simply comes to a stop, even if more might have been said. Galen's tendency, usually kept within bounds, to wander off the immediate point to offer brief observations on a related topic, finally triumphs. The old man's powers to control the overall structure of his investigation are noticeably weaker, his judgment less forceful, his criticisms less vigorous. Whether death, or simply reaching the end of his secretary's bookroll, caused Galen to break off here is a matter only for sad conjecture.

INDICES

* = exempla; → = vide

A. Index nominum Graecorum

Ἀριστοτέλης -ους ἢ Θεοφράστου, τὰ μὲν τοῖς πολλοῖς γεγραφότων, τὰς δὲ ἀκροάσεις τοῖς ἑταίροις 106,3

(Γαληνός) ἐγώ 94,4 108,11. 23 114,6. 27 116, 27 120,3 124,3 ἡμεῖς 70,23 104,4 (e corr.) νέος μὲν γὰρ ὢν ... προϊὼν δὲ κατὰ τὴν ἡλικίαν ... 90,23–27 τὴν ψυχήν, εἰ μὲν ἀθάνατος οὖσα ταῖς σωματικαῖς οὐσίαις κεραννυμένη τὰ ζῷα διοικεῖ, γιγνώσκειν βεβαίως οὐκ ἐπαγγέλλομαι, καθάπερ οὐδὲ εἰ μηδεμία καθ' ἑαυτὴν ἔστιν οὐσία ψυχῆς 116,20–26 ἐγὼ ... δι' ἑτέρων ὑπομνημάτων ἐδήλωσα 106,24–27 item 120,12–14 ἐν τοῖς Περὶ <τῆς> τῶν ἁπλῶν φαρμάκων δυνάμεως 84,12sq. ἐν τῷ Περὶ χρείας σφυγμῶν ... γράμματι 90, 10sq. γέγραπταί μοι περὶ τούτου (sc. περὶ ἠθικῆς φιλοσοφίας) δύο βιβλία 116,1sq.

Ἐμπεδοκλῆς ὡς ὁ Ἐ. ἡγεῖτο, κατὰ σμικρὰ μόρια καταθραυομένων (sc. τῶν στοιχείων) 116,10

Θεόφραστος Ἀριστοτέλους ἢ -ου, τὰ μὲν τοῖς πολλοῖς γεγραφότων, τὰς δὲ ἀκροάσεις τοῖς ἑταίροις 106,4

παλαιός οἱ -οί 72,9

Πλάτων 106,22 108,22 124,22 Π. αὐτὸς ἔμψυχα μὲν ἀεὶ λέγει τὰ ζῷα, τοὺς λίθους δὲ καὶ τὰς πόας καὶ τὰ ξύλα καὶ ... τὰ φυτὰ πάντα τῶν ἀψύχων σωμάτων εἶναί φησιν 104,15 τὸν -ωνα καὶ ζῷα καλοῦντα τὰ φυτὰ καὶ μετέχειν αἰσθήσεως μόνης φάσκοντα τῆς τῶν οἰκείων τε καὶ ἀλλοτρίων διαγνωστικῆς 124,14 item 122,3 124,4

Τίμαιος ἐν -ῳ ... εἰς ὅλον τὸν κόσμον ἐκτετάσθαι λέγῃ (sc. Πλάτων) τὴν ψυχὴν αὐτοῦ 104,20 (tit.)

B. Index verborum Graecorum

ἀγγεῖον pl. (κατὰ τὴν μήτραν) 92,5
ἄγνοια (ἐμψυχώσεώς τε καὶ μετεμψυχώσεως) 118,8
ἄδηκτος (τὸ ἔμφυτον θερμόν) 66,10
ἀδύνατος -όν ἐστι c. inf. 120,19 c. acc. c. inf. 92,2 120,3
ἀεί 104,16
ἀηδής (τὸ ἐπίκτητον θερμόν) 66,9
ἀθάνατος (ψυχή) 116,20
αἷμα 92,2. 4. 7 98,23 118,16
αἱμάτωσις pl. (καθ' ἧπαρ) 86,18
αἰσθάνεσθαι 72,24. 25 110,9 (τινός) 76, 10
αἴσθησις 106,8 108,12 124,4 (διαγνωστική) 124,14 (ἰσχυρά) 76,17 (ναρκώδης) 76,3 (πρόχειρος) 104,13 (τῶν οἰκείων τε καὶ ἀλλοτρίων) 108,7 (γένος) 122,4 (δύναμις) 72,13 88,20
αἰσθητικός 112,4 (f. l.) (διαγνώσεις) 122, 12 (δύναμις) 120,24 (μόριον) 72,7. 17 74,10 – comp. (μόρια) 72,21 (νεῦρα) 74,6
αἰσθητός (οὐσίαι) 112,4
αἰτία (ἔργων) 110,17 – pl. (ἔργων) 110,12
ἄκαιρος adv. 106,9 108,8
ἀκμάζειν οἱ -οντες 64,23 66,1
ἀκολουθεῖν (τινί) 74,17
ἀκολουθία 120,17 124,12
ἀκόλουθος τὸ -ον 104,8
ἀκούειν 64,20 106,21 οἱ -οντες 106,11 122,5
ἀκουστός (ποιότητες) 122,15
ἀκριβής (γνῶσις) 124,21 – adv. 114,25 124, 16 – comp. adv. 104,7

ἀκρόασις pl. 106,6
ἀκροατής pl. 104,22
ἄκων 74,24
ἀλήϑεια 114,10
ἀληϑής 108,7 (λόγος) 92,1
ἀλλά* 92,7 104,20 μηδὲ ..., ἀ. 112,18 οὐ(κ) ..., ἀ. 108,17 114,1 οὐ γὰρ ..., ἀ. 64,20 οὐδὲ γὰρ ..., ἀ. 108,2 → μόνος
ἀλλήλων 116,14
ἀλλοιοῦν 88,2 – pass. 118,24 (μεγάλην ἀλλοίωσιν) 118,12
ἀλλοίωσις (μεγάλη ἐν τῇ κράσει) 118,13 (ἐκ τῆς δυνάμεως) 72,19 (κατὰ τὸ σῶμα) 118,29
ἀλλοιωτικός (δύναμις) 108,17
ἄλλος 98,26 104,10 114,8. 16 122,12 ἄ. -ο 112,1sq. οὐδὲν -ο 124,17 οἱ μὲν ..., τινὲς δὲ ..., καϑάπερ -οι 112,17 τἄλλα 94,11
ἀλλότριος τὸ -ον 88,1 120,19. 22 124,20 τὰ -α 122,7 124,15 (αἴσϑησις) 108,6 124,6 (ἀπόκρισις) 120,23
ἄλυπος (τὸ ἔμφυτον ϑερμόν) 66,10
ἅμα ἅ. καί 84,17. 18 τε ἅ. καί 114,28 τε ἅ. ... τε 88,9
ἀμερής (πρῶτα σώματα) 112,12
ἄμετρος adv. 118,19
ἀμυδρός (ὀδύνη) 76,6
ἄν[I] c. coni. praes. 66,6 88,15 120,11 – c. opt. praes. 70,20 c. inf. aor. 124,7 – c. imperf. 106,23 c. ind. aor. 114,24
ἄν[II] 88,16 124,15 κἄν 116,27
ἀναγκαῖος (γνῶσις) 114,21 124,10 -όν (ἐστι) c. inf. 116,15 120,5 ὅταν -όν μοι γένηται c. inf. 108,23
ἀνάγκη ἐξ -ης 98,25
ἀναίτιος adv. 110,14
ἀνάλογος (παϑήματα, τινί) 122,11
ἀναπείϑειν 114,16
ἀναπνοή 118,27
ἄναρμος (πρῶτα σώματα) 112,11
ἀναφανδόν 106,21
ἀνήρ τἀνδρός 106,1 τἀνδρί 108,25 – pl. (ἀξιόλογοι) 90,23
ἀνϑρώπινος (σώματα) 88,24
ἄνϑρωπος pl. 88,26 110,6
ἀνία 122,9
ἄντικρυς 108,24
ἀξιόλογος (ἄνδρες) 90,24 (διαφωνία) 104,4 (ὀδύνη) 76,8
ἀξίωμα (πιστόν) 110,13
ἀπαγγέλλειν pass. 116,23 (f. l.)
ἅπας 90,25 110,22 ἅπασα αἴσϑησις 106,7 item 86,22 ἅπαντα τὰ σώματα 116,6 αἱ ἅπασαι φλέβες 92,25 τὰ τοιαῦτα ἅπαντα 114,20
ἁπλοῦς (φάρμακα) 84,13 (tit.) – adv. 86,2 106,20 114,9
ἀπό 72,11 90,3 106,25 ὄνομα τίϑεσϑαι ἀ. τινος 110,18
ἀποβλάστημα pl. (τοῦ πρώτου τῶν αἰσϑητικῶν μορίων) 74,11
ἀπόδειξις 106,9 (βεβαία) 114,18 (μακρά) 106,14
ἀποκρίνειν (τὸ ἀλλότριον) 88,2 120,18 124,20
ἀπόκρισις (τῶν ἀλλοτρίων) 120,23
ἀποκριτικός (δύναμις) 108,15
ἀπόλαυσις 124,18
ἀπορεῖν 108,27
ἀποτελεῖν (αἰσϑητικὸν αὐτό) 72,18 – pass. 114,26
ἀποφαίνειν med. 108,1 114,15 116,17 (τὴν ϑερμὴν καὶ ὑγρὰν κρᾶσιν ἀρίστην) 68,5 (περί τινος) 104,12 106,12 114,8 c. acc. c. inf. 112,3
ἀποχωρεῖν 104,24 (f. l.)
ἀποχωρίζειν (τινός) 104,24 (e corr.)
ἀπτός (ποιότητες) 122,16
ἀρετή pl. (ψυχῆς ἠϑικαί) 114,23
ἄριστος (κρᾶσις) 68,5. 7
ἀρκεῖν -εῖ c. inf. (πρός τι) 124,19 – med. c. part. 104,14 c. inf. 124,11
ἀρτηρία pl. 94,8 (κίνησις) 90,1
ἄρτι 108,15 114,12
ἀρχή *initium* 116,3 – *principium* 74,15 (κινήσεως) 108,5
ἀσκεῖν 114,29
ἀσώματος (δυνάμεις) 112,3 (οὐσία) 112,15
ἄτομος (πρῶτα σώματα) 112,11
ἄτοπος comp. (λόγος) 94,3
αὐαίνειν pass. 88,17
αὐξάνειν 88,9 98,16
αὔξησις pl. (καϑ' ἕκαστον μόριον) 86,20
αὐτός* 66,15 70,16 72,18 74,14 – -ὰ τὰ σώματα 70,18 item 74,27 94,6 ἡ ψυχὴ -ή 112,14 Πλάτων αὐ. 104,15 αὐ. ἐκεῖνος 106,29 108,9
αὑτοῦ → ἑαυτοῦ
ἀφικνεῖσϑαι (εἴς τι) 72,17 92,26 (ἐπί τι) 92,9 106,15. 26
ἄχρηστος (γνῶσις) 124,21
ἄχρι c. gen. 104,8 108,2. 26 114,12 124,12
ἄψυχος (σώματα) 104,19

βαδίζειν 110,8
βέβαιος (ἀπόδειξις) 114,18 (γνῶσις) <104, 8> 114,17 – adv. 114,24 116,7. 23
βελτίων 114,13
βιβλίον pl. 116,2
βλάπτειν pass. 98,20 108,20 118,7
βοήθεια (σμικρά) 90,9
βούλεσθαι 120,11 (v. l.) c. inf. 114,19. 29
βραχύς (ὠφέλεια) 86,6 κατὰ -ύ 106,13

γάρ* 66,8 καὶ γ. τοι 112,13 μὲν γ. 70,18 72,7 90,23 οὐ γ. 64,18 οὐδὲ γ. 106,29
γαστήρ 110,24 αἱ ἐν τῇ -τρὶ πέψεις 86, 18
γε [66,11] 72,17 92,24 98,11 γε μήν 116,20 εἴ γε 74,12 ἤτοι γε 112,7 καὶ ... γε 118,5 οὐ μὴν ... γε 88,18 90,4 ὥσπερ γε καί 66,2
γένεσις 92,6 (sc. αἵματος) 98,26
γεννᾶν pass. 66,13 92,3
γένος (αἰσθήσεως) 122,4 (τῶν ἡδέων τε καὶ οὐχ ἡδέων) 124,16 (φαρμάκων) 84,19 – pl. (πρῶτα πυρετῶν) 66,14
γέρων pl. (ἡλικία) 70,14
γευστός (ποιότητες) 122,16
γί(γ)νεσθαι* (βοήθεια ἐκ τῶν σφυγμῶν) 90,9 item 88,22 92,25 110,14. 20 sim. 122,11 (τὰ μόρια αἰσθητικώτερα) 72,21 item 108,24 (τὰ ἔργα ὑπὸ μιᾶς ἢ δύο ποιοτήτων) 86,15 item 98,24 120,16
γι(γ)νώσκειν (περί τινος) 114,14 (ὅτι) 116,8 (ὡς) 104,6 εἰ ..., γ. 116,23 item 110, 16 116,16 c. acc. c. inf. 120,3 – pass. 114,24 τὰ -όμενα 114,25
γνωρίζειν 120,24 (ὁποῖον) 120,20
γνώρισμα (ὀδύνης) 76,7
γνωριστικός (δύναμις τῶν οἰκείων) 122,6
γνῶσις 114,21 124,10 (ἀκριβής) 124,21 (βεβαία) <104,9> 114,17
γοῦν 72,11 86,8 104,15 110,21
γράμμα ἐν τῷ Περὶ χρείας σφυγμῶν -τι 90,11
γράφειν 106,5 – pass. (περί τινος) 116,1 120,13

δακνώδης (τὸ ἐπίκτητον θερμόν) 66,9
δέ* 72,14 δὲ καί 64,17 δ' οὖν 106,24 → μέν
δεικνύναι, -ύειν (τοιαῦτα τὰ καθαίροντα) 84,22 c. acc. c. inf. 66,14 72,8 – pass. 90,11 (ὅπως) 64,17 c. part. 84,12 c. acc. c. inf. 64,21
δεῖν med. (τινός) 88,6 106,9
δέχεσθαι 72,20 118,11
δηλητήριος (sc. φάρμακα) 84,23 86,3
δηλονότι 124,6
δηλοῦν c. acc. c. inf. 76,12. 14 (ἀφ' ὧν κινούμενος ἐπὶ τὴν δόξαν ἀφίκετο) 106,27
διά* c. gen. 72,11. 23. 24 τὰ δ. τοῦ σώματος ἐνεργούμενα 110,7 sim. 114,3. 25 δ. μακρᾶς ἀποδείξεως 106,13 δι' ἑτέρων ὑπομνημάτων 106,26 – c. acc. 74,7 110,15 118,7 δ. τοῦτο 72,21 120,4 122,1
διάγνωσις (τῶν οἰκείων τε καὶ ἀλλοτρίων) 122,8 (ποιοτήτων) 122,17 – pl. (αἰσθητικαί) 122,12
διαγνωστικός (αἴσθησις τῶν οἰκείων) 124,15
διαιρεῖν 76,4
δίαιτα (ὑγιεινή) 98,14
διακόπτειν 74,19. 23. 25
διαμένειν 88,23 90,7 (ἔν τινι) 88,7 90,3
διαπλάττειν 94,7. 11. 16 – pass. 90,25 92,23 94,5
διασῴζειν 86,27 88,15
διατείνειν med. 106,28
διατέμνειν 74,12
διαφέρειν (τινός τινι) 86,1 οὐ -οίσει c. inf. 72,16
διαφωνεῖν pass. τὰ -ούμενα 110,2
διαφωνία 104,27 (ἀξιόλογος) 104,3 (φαντασία) 70,15
διέρχεσθαι *explanare* 114,12
διήκειν (διά τινος) 106,19
διοικεῖν 86,23 116,22
διότι 74,10 76,17
δόγμα 106,8 – pl. 114,8
δοκεῖν τινί c. inf. 124,4 -ῶ μοι c. inf. 120,3 -εῖ τινι c. inf. 72,9 c. acc. c. inf. 104,3 τὰ -οῦντα (τινί) 104,25
δόξα 98,20 106,25
δουλεύειν (τινί) 118,1
δρᾶν 114,5
δύναμις 72,16. 19. 23 88,16 (αἰσθητικῆς ἔργον) 120,25 (γνωριστική) 122,6 (καθαρτική) 110,22 (ποιητική) 110,19 (αἰσθήσεώς τε καὶ κινήσεως) 72,13 88,20 (κινήσεως) 90,2 (φαρμάκων) 84,13 (tit.) – pl. 88,10 108,14 112,21 114,4 (ἀσώματοι) 112,4 (φυσικαί) 86,25 90,5 120,14 (ἑστία καὶ πηγὴ φυσικῶν) 88,12
δύνασθαι c. inf. 74,22 104,23 110,18 122, 19bis 124,2
δυνατός (φιλοσοφία) 114,28 -όν (sc. ἐστί) c. inf. 124,17
δύο 86,11. 15 116,2

ἐάν 70,16 74,22 108,11 ἐάν τε ... ἐάν τε 98, 21/22 → ἄν[II]
ἑαυτοῦ, αὑτοῦ 86,23. 27 88,3. 16 106,2 108,5 112,2 116,25 122,20 124,8. 17
ἐγγίνεσϑαι (τινί) 124,18
ἐγκέφαλος 88,19
ἐγώ → ind. nom. (Γαληνός)
ἔδεσμα pl. (φλεγματικὰ ἢ χολοποιά) 98, 16
ἐϑέλειν 120,11
εἰ c. ind. praes. 86,27 c. ind. aor. εἰ γάρ 106,20 – c. opt. praes. εἴ ποτε 88,10 c. opt. aor. εἴ γε 74,12 – *num* 116,20. 24
εἰδέναι 114,9. 11
εἰκός εἰ. (sc. ἐστί) c. acc. c. inf. 92,22 τὸ εἰ. 108,3
εἶναι* 64,22 66,8 90,23 ὅταν σφοδρῶς ᾖ τὸ περιέχον ψυχρόν 118,18 τὰ νεῦρα τῆς ψυχροτέρας εἶναι κράσεως 70,24 τὰ φυτὰ πάντα τῶν ἀψύχων σωμάτων εἶναι 104,20 item 124,16 ἔσϑ' ὅτε 86,5 110,8 (f. l.) – *existere* 70,15 116,25 122,3
εἰπεῖν 106,22 108,14 (περί τινος) 114,19 c. acc. c. inf. 122,3 124,17
εἴπερ c. ind. plusquamperf. 114,14 – c. ind. aor. 114,24
εἰς* 72,16 92,9 94,13 εἰς τὸ διαμένειν βοήϑεια 90,7 item 98,19 106,9
εἷς 86,11. 15 ἓν μὲν ... ἕτερον δὲ ... καὶ τρίτον 66,15
εἰσοικίζειν med. (τινί) 116,27
εἰσπνοή pl. (φλογός) 118,21
εἴτε εἴ. ... εἴ. 116,12/14
ἐκ, ἐξ* 88,19 ἡ ἐξ ἑαυτῶν κίνησις 124,8 γίνεσϑαι βοήϑειαν ἐκ τῶν σφυγμῶν 90,9 item 108,18 ἡ ἐκ τῶν κατὰ τὸ χόριον ἁπασῶν φλεβῶν γενομένη φλέψ 92,24 ἐξ οὗ (sc. αἵματος) τὴν γένεσιν ἔχει τὸ κυούμενον 92,6 ἐκ τῆς κράσεως γενομένην sc. φύσιν 112,7 item 116,5 δηλοῦν ἔκ τινος 76,11. 13 sim. 110,12 ἡ ἐκ τῆς δυνάμεως ἀλλοίωσις 72,18 ἐξ ἀνάγκης 98,25
ἕκαστος 72,17 86,19. 23 112,6 120,11 -ον τῶν μορίων 88,21 item 88,4 110,20
ἐκεῖνος 72,11 112,22 116,26 → αὐτός
ἐκκρίνειν pass. 98,12
ἐκπονεῖν (ϑεωρίαν) 112,1
ἐκτείνειν pass. (εἴς τι) 104,26
ἑκτικός (sc. πυρετοί) 66,16
ἐκφεύγειν (αἴσϑησιν) 106,7
ἐλάττων (τὸ ἔμφυτον ϑερμόν) 66,6
ἕλκειν (τὸ οἰκεῖον) 88,1 120,17 124,17. 19 (πρὸς ἑαυτήν) 122,20 – pass. τὰ ἑλχϑέντα 88,4
ἑλκτικός (δύναμις) 108,15
ἐμαυτοῦ 114,7. 16
ἔμπροσϑεν 76,14
ἐμφύειν med. (εἴς τι) 92,10
ἔμφυτος (δυνάμεις) 90,5 (ϑερμασία) 66,12 (τὸ ϑερμόν) 64,21 66,4. 8. 10
ἔμψυχος (ζῷα) 104,15
ἐμψύχωσις (ἄγνοια) 118,8
ἐν* 88,22. 23 108,5 118,13 120,2 ἐν ταῖς κενώσεσι 118,15 item 118,17 122,1 ἐν τῷ Περὶ χρείας σφυγμῶν γράμματι 90,10 item 84,12 ὅπως μὴ πλεονάσαντες ἐν φλεγματικοῖς ἐδέσμασιν αὐξήσωμεν 98,15 ἐν παρέργῳ 104,11 κἀν 70,22 74,24
ἐναντίος τἀναντία 106,2
ἐναργής adv. 110,6
ἐνέργεια pl. 86,21
ἐνεργεῖν 84,16. 21 86,12 112,5 114,1 – pass. 110,7
ἐνϑένδε 116,3
ἔνιοι -α μὲν ..., -α δέ 86,15/16 item 84,12/16 ἔ. μὲν ..., τινὲς δέ 94,12 item 86,11 τινὰ μὲν ... περὶ τινῶν δὲ ..., καϑάπερ ἐπ' -ων 108,27
ἐνίοτε 74,19. 25 86,7
ἐννοεῖν c. acc. c. inf. 110,10
ἐνοικεῖν (τινί) 112,4
ἐνταῦϑα κἀνταῦϑα 118,28
ἐξιέναι (-ειμι) 118,14
ἐξομοιοῦν (τινί) 124,17 (πρός τι) 88,3
ἐπαγγέλλειν med. c. inf. 116,23
ἐπαινεῖν 108,24 124,13
ἐπειδάν κἀπειδάν 118,27
ἐπεξέρχεσϑαι 104,7
ἕπεσϑαι 74,13 (τινί) 74,8 90,23 98,25
ἐπί* c. gen. ἐπ' ἄλλων 114,15 item 108,27 110,2 – c. dat. ἐ. τῇ φλεγμονῇ 76,6. 16 ἐ. σήψει χυμῶν sc. πυρετοί 66,17 – c. acc. 72,12 92,8 106,14 ἐ. πλέον 120,12
ἐπιγίνεσϑαι 76,4
ἐπιδεικνύναι pass. (ὁπόσαι) 120,15
ἐπικοσμεῖν 114,23
ἐπικουρία 88,6
ἐπίκτητος (τὸ ϑερμόν) 66,1. 9
ἐπιπέμπειν 88,8
ἐπιρρεῖν 90,2 (ἐπί τι) 72,11
ἐπίστασϑαι (τὴν οὐσίαν, ἥτις ἐστίν) 120, 7 (ὅτι) 110,5 (ὡς) 124,19
ἐπιστημονικός (λόγοι) 104,23
ἐπίτασις (ποιότητος) 64,19

ἐπιτείνειν pass. (τινί) 74,26
ἐπιτήδειος (σῶμα) 118,10 (τροφή) 88,9
ἐπιφέρειν (κινδύνους) 74,9
ἐργάζεσθαι 76,1 (αἰσθανόμενα sc. τὰ νεῦρα) 72,26
ἔργον (δυνάμεως) 120,25 – pl. (τέχνης) 98,19 (φύσεως) 86,14 (αἰτίαι) 110,11. 17
ἐρεῖν pass. (ὅτι) 72,14
ἐρέσθαι (τί) 108,11
ἑστία (δυνάμεων) 88,11
ἑταῖρος pl. 106,6
ἕτερος 84,19 106,26 114,17 120,13 122,3 τὸ -ον αὐτῶν 110,3 -όν τι 94,15 ἓν μὲν ... -ον δὲ ... καὶ τρίτον 66,16
ἔτι 86,19 94,7 apud comp. 94,3 124,20
ἕτοιμος comp. adv. 72,19
εὐαίσθητος comp. (θερμὸν σῶμα) 70,25
εὔδηλος -όν ἐστι (ὅτι) 98,17
εὐκρασία (φυσική) 120,1 (οὐσίας) 90,7
εὔλογος -όν ἐστιν c. acc. c. inf. 94,9
ἐφεκτικός (δύναμις γαστρός) 110,24
ἐφήμερος (sc. πυρετοί) 66,16
ἔχειν 88,23 92,6 108,5 110,1. 5. 23 112,21 114,1. 4. 17. 18 122,17 124,5 (πλέον τὸ ἔμφυτον θερμόν) 66,4 item 86,25 98,18 114,21

ζητεῖν 104,8
ζήτησις 120,16
ζῷον 86,26 (μόριον) 86,22 (σῶμα) 66,7 – pl. 88,25 104,5. 16 108,12 116,22 124,7. 14 (νεκρά) 106,19

ἤ* 72,15 84,18 86,11 ἢ ... ἢ 120,22/23 ἢ ... ἢ ... ἢ 84,14sq. ἤτοι γε ... ἢ 112,9 τε ... καὶ ... ἢ 118,22 – μᾶλλον ἢ 108,9 οὐδὲν ἄλλο ... ἢ 124,18
ἡγεῖσθαι 108,23 116,11 c. acc. c. inf. 90,24 94,12 118,7
ἡγεμονικός τὸ -όν (ψυχῆς) 72,10
ἡδονή 122,9 124,18
ἡδύς γένος τῶν -έων τε καὶ οὐχ -έων 124,16
ἠθικός (ἀρεταί) 114,23 (φιλοσοφία) 108,20. 21 114,27 120,8 124,21
ἥκειν (ἄχρι τινός) <104,9>
ἡλικία 90,27 (γερόντων) 70,14
ἡμεῖς 86,4. 10 110,14 116,7 ἡ ψυχὴ -ῶν 112,14 → ind. nom. (Γαληνός)
ἧπαρ 86,19 88,8 92,9. 22. 26 94,10
ἤπερ 94,1
ἤτοι ἤ. γε ... ἢ 112,7

θανάσιμος (sc. φάρμακα) 86,2. 4
θεᾶσθαι 110,6
θεῖος comp. (τὸ) -ότερον 94,15
θερμαίνειν 84,14. 17 – pass. 118,20
θερμασία (τροπὴ ἐμφύτου) 66,13
θερμός (ζῷα) 104,5 (κρᾶσις) 68,4 (σῶμα) 72,1 τὸ -όν (ἔμφυτον) 64,22 66,4. 8. 11 (πρὸς τὴν αἴσθησιν) 104,13 – comp. (μόρια) 72,20 (παῖδες) 64,22
θεωρητικός (sc. φιλοσοφία) 120,12
θεωρία (φυσική) 104,21 108,2 112,1
θρέψις pl. (καθ' ἕκαστον μόριον) 86,20

ἴασις pl. (νοσημάτων) 120,6
ἰατρικός (τέχνη) 108,19 118,6 (φιλοσοφία) 124,11 (ἡ) -ή 114,26 124,19
ἰατρός pl. 68,6 74,6. 16
ἴδιος (ὕπαρξις) 112,18 (φύσις) 112,6. 22
ἰδιότης (οὐσίας) 84,20 86,13 112,19
ἰέναι 72,23 116,14
ἰσχυρός (αἴσθησις) 76,17
ἴσως 104,3

καθαίρειν 84,23
καθάπερ 86,26 108,27 112,16 114,15 κ. οὐδέ 116,24 120,8
καθαρτικός (δύναμις) 110,23
καθεκτικός (δύναμις) 108,16
καθόλου κ. φάναι 104,18
καί* 66,5. 10. 17 κ. γάρ τοι κ. 112,13 κ. μέντοι κ. 74,15sq. 86,13sq. δὲ κ. 64,17 ὥσπερ γε κ. 66,2 κ. ... κ. 124,14 κ. ... κ. ... κ. 104,17sq. 122,20sq. κἂν 70,22 74,24 κἀνταῦθα 118,28 κἀπειδάν 118,27 → μόνος, οὕτω(ς), τε
καίτοι c. part. 122,2
καλεῖν 124,14 – pass. τὰ δηλητήρια -ούμενα 86,1 item 118,8
κάμνειν 88,10 ὁ -ων 74,21
καρδία 90,3. 25 92,8 94,2. 5. 7
κατά* c. gen. τὸ μέρος, καθ' οὗ συμβάλλουσιν αἱ ῥίζαι 88,13 – c. acc. κ. τὸ τοῦ ζῴου σῶμα 66,7 item 74,14 86,19bis 92,5 τὰ ἀποτελούμενα κ. ἰατρικὴν 114,26 sim. 98,13 κ. σμικρὰ μόρια καταθραύεσθαι 116,11 κ. τὰς τῶν νεύρων φλεγμονάς 76,9 item 66,11 74,27 118,20 κ. τὴν ἰδιότητα τῆς οὐσίας ἐνεργεῖν sc. φάρμακα 84,20 item 64,19 70,18. 20 86,11. 16. 24 βλαβήσεσθαι κατ' οὐδετέραν δόξαν 98,20 κ. βραχύ 106,13 κ. πρῶτον λόγον 98,24 καθ' ὁρμὴν (κίνησις) 72,14 108,13 καθ' ὁρμὴν ἢ προαίρεσιν 72,15 κ. συζυγίαν 84,16 κ. φύ-

σιν 88,7 μηδεμία καθ' ἑαυτὴν οὐσία 116,25 κ. τοῦτο 118,5 124,6
καταβάλλειν pass. (εἴς τι) 94,12
καταγινώσκειν (τινός) 106,23
καταθραύειν pass. (κατά τι) 116,12
κατακαίειν pass. 106,18
κατακολουθεῖν (λόγοις) 104,22
κατέχειν 122,20
κένωσις pl. (αἵματος) 118,16
κεραννύναι pass. (τινί) 116,22 (δι' ὅλων) 116,9
κίνδυνος 74,13 – pl. 74,8. 18
κινεῖν pass. 106,25
κίνησις (καθ' ὁρμήν) 108,13 (ἐξ ἑαυτῶν) 124,9 (ἀρχή) 108,5 (δύναμις) 88,20 (ἀρτηριῶν δύναμις) 90,2 δύναμις τῆς καθ' ὁρμὴν -εως 72,14
κλάδος pl. 88,17
κοινός (πρός τι) 86,25
κόσμος 104,25 (ψυχή) 106,19
κρᾶσις 118,13 (θερμὴ καὶ ὑγρά) 68,4 (ψυχροτέρα) 70,25 (στοιχείων) 112,8 116,6 118,4 (σωμάτων) 70,19 118,25 – pl. 116,19
κυεῖν pass. 94,6 τὸ -ούμενον 92,6 τὰ -ούμενα 94,16

λαμβάνειν pass. (sc. φάρμακα) 86,6
λανθάνειν 74,22 (τινά) 74,21
λέγειν 72,15 106,2 108,8. 13. 23 (στοιχειώδεις τοὺς χυμούς) 98,22 item 104,13. 16 c. acc. c. inf. 70,17 104,4. 26 124,4 – pass. 64,17 106,10 (τὰ φυτὰ ζῷα) 124,7 item 70,20 c. inf. 112,21 114,4
λίθος pl. 104,17 106,16
λογίζεσθαι c. inf. 76,4
λόγος 90,27 94,3 122,1 (συμπέρασμα) 106,15 κατὰ πρῶτον -ον 98,24 – pl. 106,8 (ἐπιστημονικοί) 104,23

μακρός (ἀπόδειξις) 106,13
μάλα comp. μᾶλλον αἰσθανόμενα 72,25 μᾶλλον ἤ 108,9 ἔτι δὲ μᾶλλον 124,20 οὐδὲν μᾶλλον 76,1
μέγας (ἀλλοίωσις) 118,12
μέν* μὲν ... δ' 64,21 70,18. 23 76,11 98,23 μὲν γάρ 72,7 μὲν (...), οὐ μήν 92,1 114,13 ὁ μέν τις ..., ὁ δέ 70,16 οἱ μὲν ..., τινὲς δέ 112,14 τινὲς μὲν ..., τινὲς δὲ ..., τινὲς δὲ ..., τινὲς δέ 112,11
μένειν (ἔμφυτοι) 90,5
μέντοι 108,4 116,26 118,15 120,21 (f. l.) καὶ μ. καί 74,16 86,14
μέρος 88,13 (ἠθικῆς φιλοσοφίας φυσικόν) 108,22
μέσος (τάξις) 114,7
μέσπιλον 110,23
μετά c. gen. 86,6 μ. τοῦ ἐστερῆσθαι 124,8
μεταβάλλειν 88,2 (πρός τι) 122,21
μετεμψύχωσις (ἄγνοια) 118,9
μετέχειν (τινός) 122,13 124,14
μέτριος adv. 76,13
μέτρον 64,20
μέχρι μ. ... ἄν 88,15
μή 74,21 76,2 98,14 104,6 106,27 110,16 122,18 124,2
μηδέ 76,17 112,17 124,8. 9
μηδείς 76,8 110,14 116,25 -ὲν ... μήτε ... μήτε 108,18
μηδέποτε 86,3
μηκέτι 74,14
μήκων (ὀπός) 86,8
μήν γε μ. 116,20 οὐ μ. ... γε 88,18 90,3 οὐ μ. οὐδέ 92,22 μὲν (...), οὐ μ. 92,1 114,16
μήτε μηδὲν ... μ. ... μ. 108,19
μήτρα τὰ κατὰ τὴν -αν ἀγγεῖα 92,5 – pl. 94,13
μικρός → σμικρός
μίξις (χρησίμων τινῶν) 86,6
μνημονεύειν (τινός) 124,22
μόνος 98,23 116,15 122,8 124,14. 19 – adv. -ον 122,17 124,12 οὐ -ον ..., ἀλλὰ καί 118,24
μόριον 72,8. 17 (σαρκῶδες) 74,23 (ζῴου) 86,22 αἱ καθ' ἕκαστον -ον αὐξήσεις τε καὶ θρέψεις 86,20 – pl. 88,21 (θερμότερα) 72,20 (κυούμενα) 94,6 (σμικρά) 116,11 (σώματος) 72,13 (οὐσίαι) 90,6 τοῦ πρώτου τῶν αἰσθητικῶν -ων ἀποβλαστήματα 74,11

ναρκώδης (αἴσθησις) 76,3 τὸ -ες 76,5
νεκρός (ζῷα) 106,19
νέος 90,23
νεῦρον 74,13. 20 76,5 (τριχοειδές) 74,25 – pl. 70,23 72,12. 23. 25 74,7 (φλεγμοναί) 74,19 76,6. 9. 16
νοεῖν c. acc. c. inf. 110,15
νομίζειν c. acc. c. inf. 94,17 106,1 108,7 112,15 114,13 116,18 – pass. c. acc. c. inf. 74,5
νόσημα pl. (ἰάσεις) 120,6
νῦν 116,2 (v. l.)
νυνί 116,2
νύττειν pass. 74,20

ξηραίνειν 84,15. 19
ξηρός (ἡλικία) 70,17. 20
ξύλον pl. 104,18

ὁ* ὁ Πλάτων 106,22 122,3 124,14. 21 item 116,10 τὸ «πλεῖστον» 64,18 τὰ τῆς φυσικῆς θεωρίας 108,1 ἐν τοῖς Περὶ <τῆς> τῶν ἁπλῶν φαρμάκων δυνάμεως 84,12 item 90,10 τὸ ναρκῶδες 76,5 item 86,27 88,1 98,11 οἱ παλαιοί 72,9 item 104,24 106,4 τὸ διαπλάττον 94,16 item 92,6 οἱ οἰόμενοι 94,4 item 106,10 114,29 τὰ κυούμενα 94,16 item 84,22 τὸ σπασθῆναι 76,11 item 76,13 84,14. 17 88,7 124,8 τὸ τὰ δηλητήρια μηδέποτ' ὠφελεῖν 86,3 item 90,7 τὸ ἕτερον 110,2 τὰ τοιαῦτα 106,11 108,8 124,21 τὰ τοιαῦτα ἅπαντα 114,20 ὁ μέν τις ..., ὁ δέ 70,16/17 οἱ μὲν ..., οἱ δέ 112, 2/5 οἱ μὲν ..., τινὲς δὲ ..., καθάπερ ἄλλοι 112,14 δόγματα, τὰ μὲν ..., τὰ δέ 114,9/10 τἆλλα 94,11 τἀνδρός 106,1 τἀνδρί 108,25 τἀναντία 106,2
ὀδυνᾶν med. 76,14
ὀδύνη 76,1 (ἀμυδρᾶς γνώρισμα) 76,6 (ἀξιόλογος) 76,8 (σφοδρά) 76,15
ὅθεν 124,21
οἴεσθαι c. acc. c. inf. 94,4 122,5
οἰκεῖος (οὐσίαι) 124,1 τὸ -ον 88,1 120,18. 21 124,17. 19 τὰ -α 122,7 124,15 (αἴσθησις) 108,6 124,5 (ὁλκή) 120,22
οἱονεί 72,23
οἷος adv. 88,11
ὀλίγος sup. ὀλίγιστος (ἀκροαταί) 104,21
ὁλκή (τῶν οἰκείων) 120,22
ὅλος 116,13 -η ἡ οὐσία 86,13. 17 item 74,12. 19 104,25 ἡ -η οὐσία 84,21 δι' -ων κεράννυσθαι 116,9
ὁμοιομερής (πρῶτα σώματα) 112,12
ὅμοιος adv. (τινί) 88,18
ὁμολογεῖν pass. 98,18
ὄνομα 110,17 – pl. (sc. πυρετῶν) 66,15
ὀνομάζειν 112,15 (f. l.) 120,10 (τὰς δυνάμεις φυσικάς) 108,18 – pass. αἱ φυσικαὶ -όμεναι δυνάμεις 86,24 90,4 item 86,2 110, 25
ὁποῖος -όν τι 108,22 120,20. 21 ὁπόσαι τε καὶ -αι 120,16
ὀπός (μήκωνος) 86,9
ὁπόσος -αι τε καὶ ὁποῖαι 120,15
ὅπως 64,17 120,17 – fin. c. coni. ὅ. μή 98,14
ὁρᾶν c. acc. c. part. 108,21 118,26
ὁρατός (ποιότητες) 122,14
ὄργανον 94,14
ὀρθός adv. 70,19 124,4
ὁρμή καθ' -ήν 72,15 ἡ καθ' -ὴν κίνησις 72, 14 108,13
ὅς* 66,14 72,9 74,9 86,25 114,11 ἀφ' ὧν κινούμενος ἐπὶ τὴν δόξαν ἀφίκετο 106,25 ἣν (sc. φιλοσοφίαν) ἐγώ φημι χρησίμην εἶναι 114,27
ὅσος 88,25 114,20
ὅσοσπερ τοσούτῳ χείρονα ..., -ῳπερ ἂν ἔλαττον 66,6
ὅσπερ 94,12 116,2 118,2 ὅ. καί 124,20
ὅστις 110,16 120,5 124,15
ὄστρακον pl. 106,17
ὀσφραντός (ποιότητες) 122,15
ὅταν 104,6. 9. 20 106,6 108,21 118,18
ὅτε ἔσθ' ὅ. 86,5 110,8 (f. l.)
ὅτι 72,14 110,4 116,5. 27 ὅ. γάρ 98,11 ὅ. μέντοι 108,4
οὐ, οὐκ, οὐχ* 68,6 72,15. 26 116,10 124,16 οὐ (σ)μικρός 76,12 90,8 οὐ γάρ 64,18 οὐκ ..., καθάπερ οὐδέ 116,23 → μήν, μόνος, οὐδέ
οὐδέ 106,16 οὐ. γάρ 106,29 οὐκ ..., καθάπερ οὐ. 116,24 οὐκ ... οὔτε ... οὔτε ..., καθάπερ οὐ. 120,8 ὅθεν οὐ. 124,21 οὐ μὴν οὐ. 92,22 ὥσπερ οὐ. 106,3
οὐδείς 74,13 110,1 114,11 -ὲν ἄλλο 124,17 -ὲν μᾶλλον 76,1 -ὲν βλαβήσεσθαι 98,19 118,6
οὐδέτερος 98,20
οὔκουν 106,11
οὖν 98,18 106,24 114,19 120,1 122,1
οὐσία 86,17 114,2 (ἀσώματος) 112,15 (σαρκώδης) 72,26 (ψυχῆς) 116,25 120,4 (εὐκρασία sc. μορίων) 90,8 (ἰδιότης) 84,21 86,13 (ἰδιότης σώματος) 112,19 – pl. 112,6 (αἰσθηταί) 112,5 (οἰκεῖαι) 124,2 (σωματικαί) 116,13. 21 (μορίων) 90,6 (φύσις) 112,22 (e corr.)
οὔτε οὔτ' ... οὔ. 116,15/16 οὔ. quinquies 122,14–16 οὐκ ... οὔ. ... οὔ. ... καθάπερ οὐδέ 120,6/7
οὗτος* 88,15. 19. 23 94,10. 14 98,18 104,11 αὕτη ἡ δύναμις 72,16 item 92,7 αἱ ἐνέργειαι αὗται 86,22 item 92,4 98,17 106,26 ταῦτα μόνα 122,7 item 124,19 διὰ τοῦτο 72,21 120,4 122,1 κατὰ τοῦτο 118,5 124,7
οὕτω(ς) 108,1 118,24 ἁπλῶς οὔ. 106,20 οὔ. γοῦν καί 86,7 οὔ. γοῦν καὶ ..., ὥσπερ 110,21 οὔ. δὲ καί 74,23 90,1 οὔ. καί 70,22 ὥσπερ ..., οὔ. καί 94,11 ἐγνώκειν οὔ. ... ὡς ἀποφαίνεσθαι 114,14

ὀχετός pl. 72,24

πάθημα pl. 122,11
παῖς pl. 64,23 66,2
παλαίειν 110,9
παλαιός → ind. nom.
παντάπασιν 110,1
πάντως 118,28
παρά c. dat. 116,7
παραγίνεσθαι 92,4 (e coni.)
παρακοή 122,2
παραπλήσιος (παθήματα, τινί) 122,10
παραχρῆμα 118,14
παρεῖναι οἱ -όντες 106,23
πάρεργον ἐν -ῳ 104,11
πᾶς πᾶν τὸ ἀκόλουθον 104,7 ὁ λόγος πᾶς 106,15 πάντες οἱ ἄνθρωποι 110,5 item 72, 12 114,29 οἱ παρόντες πάντες 106,24 item 104,19 πάντες ἡμεῖς 110,13
πείθειν 112,2
περί* c. gen. π. τινος σκοπεῖσθαι 104,10 item 90,10 (tit.) 104,11 106,11 120,12
περιέχειν 118,19
περιττός τὸ -όν (χολῶν καὶ φλέγματος) 98,11
περίττωμα pl. (κρᾶσις ὑγρῶν) 70,21
πέττειν 122,21
πέψις pl. (ἐν τῇ γαστρί) 86,18
πηγή (δυνάμεων) 88,11
πιθανός (λόγος) 92,1 τὸ -όν 108,2. 26 114, 12 124,13 – comp. 110,3 -ώτερόν ἐστι c. acc. c. inf. 116,17
πιστός (ἀξίωμα) 110,13
πιστοῦν pass. 110,13 (f. l.)
πλεονάζειν 98,14
πλεονεκτεῖν (τῶν φυτῶν τὰ ζῷα) 108,11
πνεῦμα 112,16
πόη pl. 104,17
ποιεῖν 110,19bis 112,20 (αἰσθανόμενα τὰ νεῦρα) 72,24 – med. (ἀρχήν) 116,4 item 120,24
ποιητικός δύναμις τῶν γινομένων ἑκάστου -ή 110,20
ποιός 112,9 118,4
ποιότης (ἐπίτασις) 64,19 – pl. 86,11. 16 116,15. 18 (ὁρατῶν, ἀκουστῶν, ὀσφραντῶν, γευστῶν, ἁπτῶν διάγνωσις) 122,17
πολιτικός (φιλοσοφία) 120,10
πολλάκις 86,9
πολυειδής adv. 110,10
πολύς 74,5 76,8 106,8 πολλοὶ τῶν ἰατρῶν 68,5 74,16 οἱ πολλοί 104,24 106,5. 22 – comp. 64,20 (τὸ ἔμφυτον θερμόν) 66,4 ἐπὶ πλέον 120,12 – sup. 64,18
πόρρω (τινός) 88,25
πόσις pl. (φαρμάκων) 118,17. 23
ποτέ εἴ π. 88,10
πρᾶγμα 104,10
πρακτικός (φιλοσοφία) 120,9
πράττειν 116,3 (f. l.)
πρέμνον 88,14
πρίν c. inf. 120,20 – c. gen. 106,12
πρό c. gen. 94,8
προαίρεσις κατὰ -ιν 72,15
προγνωρίζειν 120,20 (f. l.)
προέρχεσθαι (ἄχρι τοῦ πιθανοῦ) 108,3. 26 114,13 124,13
προϊέναι (-ειμι) (κατὰ τὴν ἡλικίαν) 90,26
προνοεῖν med. c. acc. c. inf. 98,13
πρός c. acc. 122,20 124,1 ἐξομοιοῦν π. τι 88,3 γνῶσις οὐκ ἀναγκαία π. ὑγείαν 114,22 item 88,7 114,3 118,5 124,19 π. τὴν αἴσθησιν 104,12 ἃς (sc. δυνάμεις) κοινὰς ἔχει π. τὰ φυτά 86,26
προσάγειν 116,3
προσέτι 116,9
προσηκόντως 124,7
προσιέναι (-ίημι) med. 124,3
προσκρούειν (τοῖς ἀκούουσιν) 106,10
πρότερος 92,23 – adv. 92,9 94,1
πρόχειρος (αἴσθησις) 104,12
πρῶτος 90,25 98,24 (τὸ αἰσθητικόν) 72,7 item 74,10 (γένη) 66,15 (σώματα) 112,10
πυρέσσειν οἱ -οντες 66,3
πυρετός 66,5 – pl. 66,13 118,21

ῥίζα pl. 88,14. 16
ῥοπή 110,1

σαρκώδης (μόριον) 74,22 (οὐσία) 72,26
σάρξ pl. 74,7
σαφής adv. 92,24 116,27 120,20 122,2
σήπειν pass. 106,18
σῆψις (χυμῶν) 66,17
σκαμμωνία 110,21
σκοπεῖν 124,16 – med. (περί τινος) 104,10
(σ)μικρός (βοήθεια) 90,8 (μόρια) 116,11 (φλεγμονή) 76,12 – adv. -ὸν ὕστερον 76, 10
σπᾶν pass. 76,11bis
σπέρμα 94,14
σπλάγχνον 92,3
στερεῖν pass. (τινός) 118,27 124,9
στερεός (σώματα) 70,19

στοιχεῖον pl. (τεττάρων κρᾶσις) 112,8 116,6 118,3
στοιχειώδης (χυμοί) 98,21
συζυγία κατὰ -αν 84,16
συμβάλλειν (αἱ ῥίζαι τῷ πρέμνῳ) 88,14
συμπάσχειν (τινί) 74,15
συμπέρασμα (λόγου) 106,14
σύν 94,10
συναποφαίνεσθαι (τινί) 106,27 108,25
σύνθεσις (πρώτων σωμάτων) 112,9
σφοδρός (ὀδύνη) 76,15 – adv. 118,15. 18
σφυγμός pl. 90,9 (χρεία) 90,10 (tit.)
σῴζειν pass. 88,17
σῶμα 110,7 118,11. 29 120,2 (θερμόν) 72,1 (ζῴου) 66,7 (κρᾶσις) 118,25 (μόρια) 72,12 (οὐσία) 112,19 (ὑγεία) 114,22 – pl. 116,7 118,1 (ἀνθρώπινα) 88,24 (ἄψυχα) 104,19 (σύνθεσις πρώτων) 112,10 (στερεῶν κρᾶσις) 70,19
σωματικός (οὐσίαι) 116,13. 21

τάξις (μέση) 114,7
τάττειν (εἰς μέσην τάξιν ἐμαυτόν) 114,7
τε* 86,21 τε ... τε 88,24/25 τε ... ἔτι τε 86, 18/19 τε ἅμα ... τε 88,8/10 τε ἅμα καί 114,28 ἐάν τε ... ἐάν τε 98,21/22 τε ..., ἔτι δέ 94,7 τε ... τε ... τε 122,9sq. τε (...) καί 66,9 68,6 72,13 84,23 124,16 τε καὶ ... καί 88,2 τε ... καὶ ... καὶ ... τε καί 108, 15/16 τε ... καὶ ... ἤ 118,20 καὶ ... καὶ ... τε 110,10
τέμνειν pass. 74,26 76,2
τέσσαρες, -ττ-, δ' (στοιχεῖα) 112,8 116, 5 118,3 (χυμοί) 98,21
τέχνη (ἰατρική) 108,19 118,6 (ἔργα sc. ἰατρικῆς) 98,19
τηρεῖν pass. 118,29
τιθέναι med. (ὄνομα ἀπό τινος) 110,18
τίς subst. 108,11
τις* 104,3. 7 108,11 118,7 τις τῶν χυμῶν 98,16 ῥιζῶν τι 88,17 ὁ μέν τις ..., ὁ δέ 70,16 τινὰ μὲν ... περὶ τινῶν δὲ ..., καθάπερ ἐπ' ἐνίων 108,24/25 τινὲς μὲν ..., τινὲς δὲ ..., τινὲς δὲ ..., τινὲς δέ 112,10–12 ἔνια μὲν ..., τινὰ δέ 86,12 item 94,14 οἱ μὲν ..., τινὲς δὲ ..., καθάπερ ἄλλοι 112,16 αἰτίαι τινές 110,12 item 86,7 112,17 120,16 122,2 τις φαντασία 70,15 item 74,23 86,26 88,11 106,7 τι ἄλλο πρᾶγμα 104,10 ἕτερόν τι θειότερον 94,15 ὁποῖός τις 108,22 120,21 (e corr.). 21 τι τοιοῦτον 106,22
τοι καὶ γάρ τοι καί 112,13
τοίνυν 114,6
τοιοῦτος 84,22 τι -ον 106,22 τὰ -αῦτα 106,12 108,8 124,21 τὰ -αῦτα ἅπαντα, ὅσα 114,20 ἡ -αύτη γνῶσις 124,10
τομή 74,27
τοσοῦτος -ῳ χείρονα ..., ὅσῳπερ ἂν ἔλαττον 66,5
τρεῖς 66,14 98,26
τρέφειν 122,18bis. 19 124,3 – pass. 124,1. 20
τρέχειν 110,8
τρίτος 66,17
τριχοειδής (νεῦρον) 74,25
τροπή (θερμασίας) 66,12
τροφή (ἐπιτήδειος) 88,9

ὑγεία (σώματος) 114,22 (φυλακή) 120,7
ὑγιαίνειν οἱ -οντες 66,3
ὑγιεινός (δίαιτα) 98,13
ὑγραίνειν 84,15. 18
ὑγρός (ἡλικία) 70,17. 22 (κρᾶσις) 68,4 (περιττώματα) 70,21
ὕπαρξις 88,22 (ἰδία) 112,18
ὑπάρχειν 66,6 94,15 110,12 (τινί) 86,21 88, 21
ὑπερθερμαίνειν 118,22
ὑπισχνεῖσθαι 116,2
ὑπό c. gen. νομίζεσθαι ὑ. τινος 74,5 item 86,15 94,5 98,23 114,4
ὑπόμνημα pl. 106,27 120,13
ὑποπτεύειν (τὸν λόγον ὡς πιθανόν) 90, 27
ὕστερος adv. 76,2. 10

φαίνειν med. (ἐκεῖνο ... ὅτι) 116,26 c. inf. 94,4 120,25 ἀδύνατον εἶναι -εται 120,19 c. part. 92,7. 23 124,16
φάναι c. inf. 116,8 c. acc. c. inf. 104,20 108, 4 110,22 112,13 114,28 116,16 120,17 καθόλου φ. 104,18 ὡς ἔφην 118,3 124,19
φαντασία (διαφωνίας) 70,15
φάρμακον pl. 86,10 (ἁπλῶν δύναμις) 84,13 (tit.) (γένος) 84,20 (πόσεις) 118,18. 23
φάσκειν c. acc. c. inf. 70,23 124,15
φέρειν (ὠφέλειαν) 86,5
φιλοσοφία (ἠθική) 108,20 114,27 120,9 124,20 (ἠθικῆς φυσικὸν μέρος) 108,21 (ἰατρική) 124,11
φιλόσοφος οἱ -οι 68,6
φλεβοτομία pl. 74,24
φλέγμα (τὸ περιττόν) 98,12
φλεγμαίνειν 74,20
φλεγματικός (ἐδέσματα) 98,15

φλεγμονή 74,14 76,13 (νεύρων) 76,7. 16 – pl. (νεύρων) 74,18 76,9 item 74,8
φλέψ 74,27 92,8. 26 – pl. 94,9 (κατὰ τὸ χόριον) 92,25
φλόξ (εἰσπνοαί) 118,22
φοβεῖσθαι 74,17
φύειν med. πεφυκέναι c. inf. 112,20 114,5 124,20 (f. l.)
φυλακή (ὑγείας) 120,7
φυλάττειν med. c. inf. 108,9
φυσικός 110,13 (f. l.) 122,13 (f. l.) (δυνάμεις) 86,24 88,12 90,4 108,17 120,14 (εὐκρασία) 120,1 (θεωρία) 104,21 108,1 110,25 (ἠθικῆς φιλοσοφίας μέρος) 108,22
φύσις 88,4. 26 98,23 (ἰδία) 112,7 114,1 (ἔργα) 86,14 -ει 72,22 110,13 τὸ κατὰ -ιν 88,8 – pl. (sc. σωμάτων) 118,2
φυτικός (ψυχή) 122,13
φυτόν 88,18 – pl. 86,26 88,13 104,6. 18 108, 4. 12 122,4 124,5. 14

χείρων (πυρετός) 66,5
χολή pl. (τὸ περιττόν) 98,12
χολοποιός (ἐδέσματα) 98,15
χορηγεῖν pass. 88,19
χόριον αἱ κατὰ τὸ -ον φλέβες 92,25
χρεία (σφυγμῶν) 90,10 (tit.)
χρῆναι χρή 108,2 (f. l.) c. inf. 64,21 98,11 104,<9>. 27 106,11 c. acc. c. inf. 118,10
χρῆσθαι (τινί) 86,9
χρήσιμος (φιλοσοφία) 114,28 (τὰ) -α (μίξις) 86,7
χυμός pl. 98,17. 26 (τέσσαρες) 98,22 (σῆψις) 66,17
χωρίζειν (τινός) 120,11 – pass. (τινός) 118, 26 120,2
χωρίς c. gen. 92,2

ψάμμος 106,17
ψύχειν 84,15. 18 118,17 – pass. 118,15
ψυχή 110,4 112,14 116,20. 22 (f. l.) 118,11. 14. 26 120,2 (φυτική) 122,13 (κόσμου) 104,26 106,20 (ἀρεταί) 114,23 (τὸ ἡγεμονικόν) 72,10 (οὐσία) 116,26
ψυχικός (δυνάμεις) 108,17
ψυχρός (φυτά) 104,5 τὸ -όν 104,13 118,19 – comp. (κρᾶσις) 70,24 (μόρια) 72,22 (σῶμα) 72,1

ὡς ὡς ... δέδεικται 90,10 item 72,8 86,17 116,10 118,3 120,11 124,18 ὑπώπτευσα τὸν λόγον ὡς πιθανόν 92,1 – γινώσκειν, ὡς 104,6 item 124,19 sim. 110,2 114,9. 11 – consec. 74,12 οὕτω ... ὡς 114,15
ὥσπερ 88,13 106,2 110,4 114,17 ὥ. γε καί 66,2 ὥ. ..., οὕτω 94,9 οὕτω ..., ὥ. 110, 23
ὥστε c. ind. 124,3
ὠφέλεια (βραχεῖα) 86,5
ὠφελεῖν 86,4. 10

C. Index nominum Latinorum

antiquus *subst.* -i 56,5 (sententia) 72,10 multi -orum famosi 90,24
Archistrates 80,2 (*f. l.*)
Aristotiles potes eam (*sc.* uirtutem naturalem) nominare animam sicut nominauerunt eam Plato et A. 102,19 sermones -is et Theopha contradicunt eis adinuicem qui composuerunt libros ad opus multorum in aliquibus rebus et libros ad opus discipulorum suorum 106,3 respondit A.: qui ... uult esse sapiens legat ... VIII primos libros quos agregaui quousque perueniat ad librum De anima 122,11 ([Arist.])
Asclepiades → Fisedis

Berthenis (= Parthenius) *poeta* 54,10. 17 56, 6 (sermo) 56,5 B. uersificator 54,5. 9. 14
Boelius (= Lycus) *commentator Hippocratis* 64,11

Chrasis, Chrosis (= Chrysippus) *Stoicus* 82,15 (liber) 80,6
Chrysippus → Chrasis

Elumerephilis (= Herophilei) E. dicens quod sit (*sc.* spiritus) in unaquaque parte partium membri radicalis 80,4
Empedocles E., qui ea (*sc.* elementa) diuisit in minimas particulas 116,13
Erasistratus 80,2

Fisedis (= Asclepiades) F. ... dicens neruum esse minime sensibilem 76,20

Galienus 54,5 – ego 54,5. 19 56,6. 10bis 78,

10 96,8 106,26 108,7. 8. 19. 22 114,21 116,9. 21. 26 118,6 egoipse 58,16 78,12 nos 72,7 quod curauerit (*sc.* deus) me semel de una infirmitate 58,9sq. dico quod non habeo scientiam utrum mundus sit generatus et utrum aliquid sit extra uel non aliquid sit extra 56,12–14 ego dico quod nulla scientia est in me de substantia *sc.* deitatum 58,2–4 ego dico quod in plantis est principium motus et uirtutis regitiue 62,3 de corporibus celestibus recuso me habere scientiam 62,18sq. me non habere scientiam substantie anime que sit, et utrum sit mortalis aut immortalis ... 76,25–78,3 *item* 60,5sq. 80,7sq. 116,23–118,1 ego scio ... quod regimen animalium ... completur a tribus principiis 90,16sq. ego nescio que est illa uirtus ... que format embrionem ... et que substantia sit 90,18sq. ego demonstraui in aliis libris 106,24 *item* 120, 12sq. in libro meo De colera nigra 100,2sq. *item* 100,4 ego posui probationem ... in meo libro De elementis secundum sententiam Ypocratis et in commento libri sui De humana natura in tribus dictionibus 64,1–3 *item* 94,18–21 in libro meo De generibus complexionum et De elementis secundum sententiam Ypocratis 66,1–3 in meo libro Complexionum 66,20 *item* 68,3 declaraui in libro meo De iuuamento membrorum quia in iuuentute mea ... cum perueni ad perfectam etatem ... 90, 22–92,3 scripsi ... unam dictionem De medicinis purgatiuis 96,9sq. egoipse monstraui in prima dictione mei libri De regimento sanitatis 78,17 ego composui in Sententiis Ypocratis et Platonis librum uolens quod esset michi defensio et memoria in senectute 60,8sq. *item* 60,13 in septima dictione libri De sententiis Ypocratis et Platonis et in aliis libris 80,10sq. ego demonstraui in libro meo De simplici medicina 84,12sq. ego nominaui uirtutes que sunt in hac anima naturam in libro De uirtutibus naturalibus 62,15sq. in tribus dictionibus (*sc.* libri De uirtutibus naturalibus) 62,4 in libro meo De uirtutibus naturalibus et in alio meo libro De medicinis purgantibus 100,22sq. in meo libro Febrium 66,19 in Iuuamento pulsuum 90,10sq. quod composui de meis libris 56,7 in dictione quam scripsi de formatione embrionis 62,12 in uno librorum et in dictione in qua reprobaui Boelium 64,10sq. in dictione per quam reprobaui dictionem libri Chrasis 80,6 in una dictione in qua reprobaui quendam philosophum de secta reubach 84,4sq. ego compilaui de hiis (*sc.* de philosophia morali) duas dictiones 114,29

Grecus (lingua) 86,1

Herophilei → Elumerephilis

Hippocrates → Ypocras

Lycus → Boelius

Parthenius → Berthenis

Pictagoras (= Protagoras) *sophista* P. recusando se de ipsis (*sc.* deis) scire 58,1

Plato 106,21. 25. 29 108,10 (sententia) 108,23 (sententie) 60,8 *(tit.)* 80,11 *(tit.)* *sim.* 60,13 *(tit.)* in senectute, que est domina obliuionis, sicut ait P. 60,10 socii -nis philosophi 62,13 demonstrauit P. in libro suo (*sc.* Republica), quod anima habet tres species 82,10 potes eam (*sc.* uirtutem naturalem) nominare animam sicut nominauerunt eam P. et Aristotiles 102,19 *item* 62,14 -nem dicentem ... de animalibus quod sint animata, et dicit de lapidibus et lignis et omnibus plantis quod sint corpora non habentia animam 104,15 P. dixerit ... quod in plantis est aliud genus sensus 122,2

Protagoras → Pictagoras

reuac, reubach 62,14 philosophus de secta r. 84,5

Socrates 58,19

Theopha (= Theophrastus) sermones Aristotilis et Th. contradicunt eis adinuicem qui composuerunt libros ad opus multorum in aliquibus rebus et libros ad opus discipulorum suorum 106,4

Thimeus in libro suo qui nominatur Th. in quo locutus fuit (*sc.* Plato) de scientia naturali 82,13 *(tit.)* in libro suo -o de scientia naturali ... dixit quod anima mundi expansa est per totum mundum 104,21 *(tit.)*

Ypocras (sententia) 96,2 (sententie) 60,8 *(tit.)* 80,11 *(tit.)* *item* 60,13 *(tit.)* secundum sententiam -tis 64,2 *(tit.)* 66,3 *(tit.)* 94,21 *(tit.)* Y. fuit primus qui iudicauit quod hec (*sc.* corpora) sint creata ex temperamento ignis terre aque et aeris 62,19 -ti in libro Amphorismorum dicenti: „Que – et cetera" (*Hipp. Aphor. I 14: IV 466,8 L.*) 64,11–13 liber -tis De humana natura 94,20 *item* 64,2sq. 98,5 Y. in secunda dictione libri sui Epidimiarum 70,1 dicens in principio secunde dictionis eiusdem libri sui Elguefete ... hoc dictum: „fuerunt – estate" (*Hipp. Epid. II 1,1: V 72,3sq. L.*) 70,5–7 dixit in secunda dictione hoc dictum: „Et – uentis" (*Hipp. Epid. III 2: I 224,7 Kw. = III 66,14 L.*) 70,7sq. in tertia dictione eiusdem libri (*sc.* Epidimiarum) 70,3sq.

D. Index verborum Latinorum

a, ab* 60,12ter. 16 62,2 78,8bis. 10 regimen completur a tribus principiis 90,17 *item* 94,3 *sim.* 56,23 58,5 accidit a paucitate caloris 102,22 *sim.* 120,25 superhabundat (*sc.* cor) a calore 60,19 multum a sanguine 118,17 alter ab alqa re 102,22 *item* 64,8
ac non accidit maior dolor ac si 74,27
accendere (caliditatem) 102,14 – *pass.* (calor) 62,2
accidere 66,18. 22. 23 70,9 74,13. 18. 26 76,11. 12. 15. 18 110,13 116,17 118,16. 20. 21 122,1 (alcui, alcui rei) 54,5bis. 19 74,7. 14 76,6. 8. 9. 24 82,8 84,8 -it (quod) 102,22
accipere 58,19 98,19
acquisitus (calor) 66,6. 11
actio 100,19 (*f. l.*)
actiuus (qualitates) 84,9 (substantia) 84,11 potentia -a istarum operationum 110,19
acus 74,3
acutus (corpus) 74,2
ad* 54,6 72,13. 16 92,6 uenire ad complementum 56,1 *sim.* 92,1 est necessaria ad sanitatem 114,22 *item* 114,23 paratus ad alqam rem 80,14 *sim.* 118,11. 12 sunt potentes ad intelligendum 104,23 *item* 110,17 composui librum ad exercitandum eos 82,3 membra indigent ad hoc quod remaneant 88,6 *item* 90,6 106,11 ad opus 104,22 106,6 comparatio ad estatem 68,21 *item* 68,21 104,2 subtilis ad modum capilli 74,25 reuertitur usque ad uentrem sinistrum cordis 92,17 *item* 102,2
addiscere 56,2 82,17
additio 114,25
adimplere pass. 86,18
adinuicem 106,1. 5 116,16
adiutorium (epatis) 88,8 90,8
adiuuamen 82,17 (*v. l.*) (caloris) 62,1 (*v. l.*)
admirari 106,22
aduentus (anime) 78,6. 8 (corporis) 78,6. 8
ae- → e-
aer 118,18 (dispositiones) 70,6 temperamentum ignis terre aque et -is 62,20
affirmare 80,17 (super alqam rem) 80,18
agere *pass.* 92,12 (in alqa re) 78,2 (*v. l.*)
agregare (libros) 122,14 ([Arist.])
aiere 54,16 60,10 (quia) 54,5
aliquando 74,14 76,23 84,2bis 86,5 102,1
aliquis* 54,7 56,13 64,18 80,18 non -id 56,14 in -o ipsorum (*sc.* librorum) 60,10 *item* 68,1 74,22 92,19 a. ... alius 70,15 -i ... quidam ... quidam ... quidam 112,9 -i ... quidam ... quidam alii 112,15 – *adi.* 62,1. 9 74,2bis. 20 non habeo -am notitiam 114,11 -a alia dispositio 98,28
alius* 62,11 68,6 84,20 86,7 90,26 -e due commixtiones 96,6 aliqua -a dispositio 98,28 omnia -a membra 94,8 *item* 96,1 98,24 – *subst.* 64,8 68,14 82,16 110,5 quidam -i 112,17 aliquis ... a. 70,17 unum ... -ud 78,8
alter (ab alqa re) 102,22 *i. q.* alius 68,2 – *subst.* unus ..., a. 54,10 unus ... a. ... tertius 82,10. 15
alterare 84,14. 17. 21 86,11. 13 88,3 (alteratione debili) 96,13 – *pass.* 118,13 (in frigiditatem) 78,18
alteratio 62,22 84,8 96,14 (debilis) 96,13 (uehemens) 118,14 (caloris) 66,14 (*sc.* corporis) 118,15 (uirtutis) 72,19
altercari (de alqa re) 54,8
altus *comp.* (gradus) 124,9 ([Arist.])
amator (ueritatis) 80,16
amphorismus *pl.* (liber) 64,12 (*tit.*)
anhelitus → hanelitus
anima 58,22. 23 60,3. 10 62,14. 15 78,1. 13. 20. 23 80,13 82,8. 11. 14 102,19 104,20 110,6 112,14. 18 114,17 116,24 118,11. 14. 25. 27 122,15 (*tit.*) ([Arist.]) (instrumenta rationalis) 80,12 (mundi) 104,25 106,18 (aduentus) 78,6. 8

(bonitates) 82,6 (nobilitas) 114,23 (partes) 72,12 82,17 (sedes) 122,17 ([Arist.]) (spiritus) 80,2. 11 (substantia) 60,4 76,25 78,9. 13 80,1. 8 120,3
animal 104,6 (membrum) 74,1 – *pl.* 86,27 88,23 96,16 102,9. 10. 20 104,17 108,13 116,25 (corpora) 70,13 80,2 100,14 102,15 104,2 (genus) 64,10 96,17 (membrum) 86,22 (oculi) 124,2 ([Arist.]) (regimen) 58,6 90,15. 16
animalis (spiritus) 80,10 (uirtus) 108,19
animatus (animalia) 104,17
annus [70,15] (constitutio) 70,8 (Hipp.) (conuersio) 70,4 (dispositiones) 70,9 (hore) 70, 3 (tempora) 68,20 70,13
ante 56,10 114,12 paulo a. 80,9 108,15 – *c. acc.* 116,7
antequam *c. ind. perf.* 102,8 *c. coni. praes.* 100,13
antiquus (anima) 122,19 ([Arist.]) (medici et philosophi) 104,4 → *ind. nom.*
apostema (nerui) 74,18 76,18 *item* 74,13 76, 15 – *pl.* 74,7. 8 76,6. 9. 13 (infirmitas) 76,24
apparere 58,9 84,1 90,21 98,27
appetitiuus (uirtus) 62,10 108,16
appropriare *pass.* (sanguis corpori) 98,9
appropriatus (natura *sc.* corpori) 112,22 (sanguis nature) 94,23
aptatio (morum) 120,5
apud *c. acc.* 76,4 78,22
aqua 72,24 96,23 98,2 temperamentum ignis terre -e et aeris 62,20
aquosus (humiditas) 96,22
arbor 74,11 88,11
arefactio (membri) 76,12
arena *pl.* 106,19
arguere 106,13
ars (gramatice) 56,1 (medicine) 108,20 118,7 *item* 56,2 (medicine et philosophie) 54,20
arteria 106,2 *(f. l.)* – *pl.* 60,19
assimilare *pass.* 98,9 108,6 (alcui rei) 88,1 *(v. l.)*. 5
attractio (flamme) 118,22 (hora humoris) 96,12
attractiuus (uirtus) 120,17
attrahere 62,5. 6 86,27 88,3 96,4. 5. 7bis. 11. 13. 15bis. 20 100,1 102,2. 5 120,18. 22
audere *c. inf.* 106,28
audire 78,4 †80,18 *c. acc. c. inf.* 54,13 *c. acc. c. part.* 80,18 -entes 106,13
augmentum 62,8
auris 78,4
australis (constitutio anni) 70,8 (Hipp.)
aut* 92,11 96,8 100,14 aut ... aut ... uel ... uel 66,24 aut ... aut ... aut ... aut 66,23 → utrum
autem 54,10 60,4. 11 62,7 68,21 70,11 78,7. 10 80,7 82,12 90,4. 16. 19 110,4

bis 96,9
bonitas *pl.* (inuentiones anime) 82,6
bonus *adv.* 72,4bis 120,8
branca *pl.* (radicis) 88,14
briga (contraria) 58,8

cadauer *pl.* 106,20
cadere 110,1
caelestis → celestis
caliditas 64,5 68,13. 23. 24 70,3. 4 84,10. 15. 18 102,14 104,2 118,20 (fortis) 70,7 (Hipp.) (innata) 102,12 (naturalis) 102,11 (genus) 102,15
calidus 68,9. 9 *(f. l.)* 104,12 (animal) 104,6 (complexio) 68,3. 10. 13. 15 100,15 (corpora) 68,17 72,3 (elementum) 66,23. 24bis (medicine) 118,23 (natura) 68,18 (sensus) 102,22 – *subst.* -um 70,13 – *comp.* (receptio) 72,19 (uer) 68,22
calor 64,14 98,27 102,21. 22 (acquisitus) 66,5. 11 (innatus) 64,12 (Hipp.). 13 (Hipp.) 66,4 (naturalis) 60,19 64,9 66,8. 10 (alteratio naturalis) 66,14 (paucitas naturalis) 104,1 (principium naturalis) 102,20 (substantia naturalis) 64,15 (iuuamen) 62,2
canon *pl.* 98,20 *(f. l.)*
capillus 74,25
carnosus (membrum) 74,21 76,22
caro 72,27 74,7 76,19 (punctura) 74,3
cauda (spine) 92,15
causa 98,7 118,25 – *pl.* (rerum) 84,2
celare <124,1> ([Arist.])
celestis (corpora) 62,18
cerebrum 60,12 74,11 82,9. 15 88,16. 20 (corpus) 80,13 (uentriculi) 80,12
certitudo (*sc.* sententiarum) 114,9
certus 116,27 (dictum) 92,3 (occasiones) 110,12 – *adv.* 102,7
ceterus 90,18 – *subst.* et -a 64,13
cholera → colera
cibarius *subst.* -a (fleumatica et generantia coleram) 98,15
cibus 100,23
circa *c. acc.* 92,14
citrinus (colera) 94,18 98,1. 7
clamare 74,3

claritas (intellectus) 122,10 ([Arist.])
cogere *c. inf.* 106,25
cognoscere 122,16 ([Arist.]) 124,5 ([Arist.])
colera 96,14 98,16 (citrina) 94,18 98,7 (euacuatio citrine) 98,1 (nigra) 98,7 100,3 *(tit.)*. 13. 15. 16 102,1 *item* 100,5 (significatio nigre) 100,12 – *pl.* (superhabundantia duarum) 98,12
colligere *pass.* (sillogismus) 106,16
color 98,27 *(f. l.)*
comburere *pass.* 106,20
commentum (libri sui [*sc.* Ypocratis] De humana natura) 64,2 *item* 94,19
commiscere *pass.* (de alqa re) 64,6
committere *f. l.* 82,11. 17. 18
commixtio 78,5 96,5 112,8 *(f. l.)* 116,23 (elementorum) 112,6 116,8. 10 118,5 (medicinarum) 86,7 (cum alqa re) 116,25 – *pl.* 96,4. 6 (elementorum) 78,6 (generatio) 96,1
communicare 62,16 102,16bis
comparatio (ad alqam rem) 68,20. 21 104,2
compilare (dictiones) 114,29
complementum 56,1
complere *pass.* 90,13. 17
complexio 68,4. 13. 24 118,13 (calida) 68,10 (calida et humida) 68,3. 12. 15 (frigida) 68, 11 72,1. 22 (humida) 68,11 (mala calida et sicca) 100,15 (naturalis) 118,29 (pessima) 70,1 (sensibilis) 78,16 (sicca) 68,11 70,17. 20 (corporis) 78,18 (etatis) 70,16 (humorum) 70,21 (membrorum) 70,19 72,1 (temperamentum substantie) 90,7 (ueris) 68,22 70, 13 – *pl.* 72,5 (genera) 66,2 *(tit.)* (liber) 66, 20 *(tit.)* (modi) 66,20. 25. 26 68,7. 8. 15 70,12 (modi simplicium) 66,22
componere 56,7 (libros) 56,3. 4 60,8 82,3 106,5 *item* 54,9 – *pass.* 92,14
compositio (corporis) 90,21 (primorum) 112,8 – *pl.* 94,18 (quatuor) 94,21
compositus (complexiones) 66,21 (modi complexionum) 66,23
concauitas *pl.* 80,3
confirmare *pass.* 106,16 *(f. l.)*
congregare *pass.* 84,2
congregatio (uenarum) 92,25
coniungere *pass.* 92,15
consentire (quod) 96,12
conseruare 88,12 98,14
conseruatio (sanitatis) 120,4
considerare *pass.* 68,22
consiliari 106,16 *(f. l.)*
consistere 118,29 -entes (*opp.* pueri) 66,5. 6
constipatiuus (potentia) 110,22
constitutio (anni) 70,8 (Hipp.)
constructio *f. l.* 78,16. 18
consuetudo 120,7 de -ine est *c. inf.* 64,8
consumere *pass.* 76,11
contexere *pass.* (sillogismus) 100,7
continere 118,18 – *pass.* 80,2
contingere (ut) 68,12
continuare 100,9 – *pass.* 112,10 (cum alqa re) 92,7. 10
continuus *adv.* 88,21
contradicere 82,2 106,4
contrahere 100,1 *(f. l.)*
contrarius 88,2 (alcui rei) 54,12 108,7 120, 20 (Boelius Ypocrati) 64,11 (briga) 58,8 (modus) 54,10 98,1 (res) 120,23 – *subst.* -um 106,2 *(e coni.)* (qualitates) 64,6 per -um 98,2 -a (alcui rei) 62,6
conturbatio (sanguinis) 100,17
conuenibilis 78,2
conueniens (alcui rei) 120,19. 22 (ad alqam rem) 118,11 c. est *c. inf.* 116,21 – *subst.* -tia 100,10 (alcui rei) 62,5 – *adv.* 78,3
conuenire 104,24 106,1 (alcui rei) 86,24 -it 68,12 *(f. l.)* (quod) 106,14 118,10
conuersio (anni) 70,4 (hore) 70,2
conuertere (in alqam rem) 96,8 – *pass.* (in alqam rem) 100,19
conuocare (in testimonium) 56,6bis
cor 60,12. 18 62,2 82,10. 15 90,3 92,11. 20 94,2. 4. 5 102,14. 21 (embrionis) 92,13 (generatio) 92,23 (informatio) 90,25 (uentres) 92,18
corporeus (anima) 60,11 (substantia) 78,24 116,16. 26 – *subst.* -um 56,18
corpus 66,10 72,18 78,1. 2. 14. 16. 21 80,9 84,8. 15. 21 86,12 98,6. 7. 9. 10. 17. 22 100,23 102,16. 21. [22] 110,8 118,10. 25. 28bis 122,17 ([Arist.]). 20 ([Arist.]) 124,3 ([Arist.]) (acutum) 74,2 (humanum) 88,22 (animalium) 100,14 (cerebri) 80,13 (aduentus) 78,7 (aduentus sensibilis) 78,8 (complexio) 78,18 (compositio) 90,21 (forma) 78,10 (generatio) 78,5 (humor) 96,7 (locus) 82,12 (membra) 72,14 82,16 102,12 (pars) 74,2 (proprietas) 112,20 (sanitas) 114,23 (significatio) 80,9 – *pl.* 62,18 68,16. 18 104,19 118,3 (calida) 72,2 (celestia) 62,18 (frigida) 72,3 (sana, non sana) 94,22 (animalium) 70,12 80,2 102,15 104,2 (mortuorum et plantarum) 68,17 (*sc.* senum) 70,22 (elementa) 62,22 (generatio) 116,7. 11 (natura) 68,19 (regimen) 90,13

corruptio (*sc.* splenis) 98,28
coruscatio (dispositio) 82,19
creare 94,7 – *pass.* 62,20 122,20 ([Arist.])
creator 56,23 124,5 ([Arist.]) (rerum) 56,17
credere 80,15 (quod) 76,2 *c. inf.* 58,13
crescere 64,12 (Hipp.)
cum^I* *c. ind.* cum *temporale* 54,9 92,1 cum ..., tunc 78,19 *vi conditionali* 62,13. 14 68, 10. 12 74,17 cum *causale* 64,13 72,15 – quod cum 70,2. 4 – *c. coni.* cum *narrativum* 54,7 cum *causale* 54,16 120,14 cum *concessivum* 78,12 *vi conditionali* 56,9. 15 68,9. 18 cum *temporale* 54,13. 15 92,13
cum^II* aduentus anime est cum aduentu corporis 78,6 *item* 66,25 78,14 84,1. 2 92,19 94,7 misceri cum alqa re 68,2 *item* 116,26 communicare cum alqo, alqa re 62,16 102, 17 per uenas continuatas cum matrice 92,7 *item* 92,10 cum commixtione aliarum medicinarum 86,7 pungere cum alqa re 74, 2bis medicine alterant cum duabus qualitatibus 84,17 *item* 84,18. 19 86,12. 13bis. 18 cum difficultate 56,2 *item* 98,3 secum 96,12 108,25
cura 114,24 *(f. l.)*
curare (alqem de alqa re) 58,10
curatio (morborum) 120,3 – *pl.* (egritudinum) 82,8
currere 72,25 †86,23 88,20 102,1 118,8
cursus 72,25
custodire 78,16 86,25

dare 88,16 102,21 – *pass.* 96,23 114,24 (medicina) 96,21 98,2
de* attrahere de uena sanguinem 102,3 haberi iuuamen de alqa re 86,3. 4 curare de infirmitate 58,10 prohibere de alqa re 82, 5 timere de alqa re 74,17 quod attrahit (*sc.* planta) de nutrimento 62,6 *item* 76,22 84,5 96,4. 5. 6 commisceri de qualitatibus 64,6 reprobare de alqa re 64,11 *sim.* 78,15 generatio febrium est de alteratione caloris 66,13 *item* 74,27 122,1 altercari de alqa re 54,8 *item* 56,7. 17 58,2. 3 62,16 *(tit.)* 64,1 *(tit.)*. 2 *(tit.)* de anima uideo quod est 58,22 *item* 58,7 102,10 114,6 sentire de certitudine 114,9 *item* 56,8 116,27 de consuetudine 64,8 de natura est *c. inf.* 88,19
debere 56,17 *(f. l.)* *c. inf.* 56,10 58,18 60,5. 14 64,18 *(f. l.)*. 20 78,3 82,6 94,5 98,19 104,8 -et *c. inf.* 106,18 *c. acc. c. inf.* 100,5
debilis (alteratio) 96,13. 14
decere 98,17 *(f. l.)*
declarare 80,7 124,9 ([Arist.]) (quia) 90,22 – *pass.* 56,3
declinare 124,7 ([Arist.]) (in alqam rem) 98,28
defectus (hanelitus) 118,26 (intellectus) 56, 2 (studentium) 54,19
defensio 60,9
deferre *pass.* 62,2
deficere 78,21bis
definitio → diffinitio
deitas 56,20 58,21 (substantia) 58,17 (uirtus) 56,20
demonstrare 60,12 64,10 72,5 90,10 94,18 100,4 (quia) 84,12 (quod) 60,14 62,19 64,3. 5 66,1. 14. 20 80,6. 10 82,10 86,15 98,5 100,2. 22 (quot) 64,17 *item* 106,24 – *pass.* (quod) 96,19 (quot) 120,14
demonstratio 64,10 *(f. l.)* (manifesta) 96,19 – *pl.* 60,13 (manerierum) 60,14
denominare (occasionem animam) 60,2 – *pass.* (istud humor) 100,18
describere 62,12 *(f. l.)*
desiccare *pass.* 78,19 88,14
desiderare *c. inf.* 100,9
destruere *pass.* 54,16
deterior (febris) 66,11
determinare (utrum ... uel) 62,9
deuenire (ad alqam rem) 104,8
deus 56,23 (omnipotens) 94,15 (operationes) 58,8
dexter *subst.* ad -am 124,7 ([Arist.])
diafragma 92,13. 20. 26
dicere* 54,16 58,1bis 64,12. 13 68,10. 12. 20 70,1 72,6 78,9. 10 80,9 (dictum) 70,5. 7 (iudicium) 106,28 (de alqa re) 80,8 108,1 (dictum de alqa re) 112,13 (quod) 56,9. 12. 15 58,3 62,3. 22 68,14bis 70,16 (de alqa re quod) 62,13 100,20 102,14 104,16. 17 *c. acc. c. inf.* 54,11 76,20 – *pass.* 70,20 84,14 114,3 (quod) 54,5. 6 92,20 98,8 106,18 (de alqa re quod) 112,20 *c. inf.* 64,18
dictio 62,12 64,10 80,6 84,4 (libri) 80,6 (prima libri De regimento sanitatis) 78,17 (secunda libri Epidimiarum) 70,2 *item* 70,7 (principium secunde libri Elguefete) 70,5 (septima libri De sententiis Ypocratis et Platonis) 80,10 (tertia libri *sc.* Epidimiarum) 70,3 una d. De medicinis purgatiuis 96,9 – *pl.* 62,4 64,3 114,29
dictum 70,6. 7 90,12 92,2 116,22 (*sc.* Berthenis) 54,13 (pars *sc.* Platonis) 108,25 – *pl.* 64,21 72,5 78,1 100,3 (uera) 104,23

differentia (inter sermonem meum et sermonem Berthenis) 56,5 *item* 86,2 120,10
differre (animalia plantis) 108,12
difficultas 56,2
diffinitio (rei) 106,9
digerere 62,6
digestio 86,19
digestiuus (uirtus) 62,6. 7. 11 108,17
dignus *comp.* (complexio) 66,22 68,6. 8. 15 (modus complexionum) 66,26 70,12
diligere 80,17
diminutio (infirmitatis) 96,3 (inflationis) 96,22
dimittere 118,14 *c. inf.* 100,6
directus *subst.* in -o pectoris 92,17
discere 122,13 ([Arist.])
discipulus *pl.* ad opus -orum 106,7
discooperire 74,1 82,1
disponere *pass.* 118,3 *(e corr.)*
dispositio 118,3 *(f. l.)* (mala) 98,28 (-num aeris) 70,6 (eundi) 110,8 *item* 110,9 (tonitrui) 82,19 (uirtutis) 88,15. 18 (uite) 118,9 – *pl.* (*sc.* corporis) 78,3 (d. aeris) 70,6 -nes -num anni 70,9
dissentire 104,23
diu 100,14
diuersificare *pass.* 98,8
diuersitas 110,1 (in temporibus senectutis) 70,14 (inter medicos et philosophos) 104,4
diuersus 110,24 (ab alqa re) 64,8 (motus) 82,7 (res) 110,10 -o modo 84,10
diuidere 88,2 (in alqam rem) 116,14 – *pass.* 84,2 86,16 88,15 112,12 (ab alqa re) 112,19 (in alqam rem) 80,3
diuinare 110,15 *(f. l.)*
diuinatio *pl.* 58,6
docere 124,12 ([Arist.]) *c. inf.* 120,8
dolor 76,14 (maior) 74,27 (paucitas) 76,14 (sensus) 74,4 76,10 (species) 76,8
domina (obliuionis) 60,9
dominium (elementi) 66,22 68,1 (frigiditatis) 66,25 (frigidi et humidi) 66,23
donec 78,16
dorsum 92,16
ducere 108,3
dum 122,15 ([Arist.])
dummodo 120,10
duo 54,7 64,8. 16 70,9 72,5 78,1 96,6 98,20 100,3. 12 114,29 (colere) 98,12 (qualitates) 84,9. 17 86,13. 17 (spatule) 92,17 (uentres cordis) 92,18
duplex (alteratio) 84,9
e → ex
efficere *pass.* (membrum sensibile) 72,17
effimerus (*sc.* febris) 66,16
ego 54,13 124,9 ([Arist.]) → *ind. nom.* Galienus
egoipse → *ind. nom.* Galienus
egritudo 76,5 e. elchatir 74,17 – *pl.* 78,22 (mortales) 70,9 (curationes) 82,8
elchadir 76,2. 5 *(def.)*
elchatir 74,8 76,18 egritudo e. 74,17
elementum 64,7 (dominium calidi, frigidi, sicci, humidi) 66,22 – *pl.* 64,2 *(tit.)*. 6 66,2 *(tit.)* 78,7 94,20 *(tit.)* 98,24 (corporum) 62,22 (commixtiones) 78,6 112,7 116,9. 10 118,6 (dominium) 68,1
elguefete secunda dictio libri E. 70,5 *(tit.)*
embrio 62,8 90,19 92,6 (cor) 92,13 (formatio) 62,12 (formator) 94,13 (generatio) 90, 15 92,8 (mater) 92,19
enim 74,4 88,10 92,4
ens 112,18
epar 60,12 82,10. 15 86,21 88,9 92,10 94,1. 6 100,13 102,3. 12. 18. 20 (adiutorium) 88,8 90, 8 (generatio) 92,24
ephem- → effim-
epidimia *pl.* secunda dictio libri -arum 70,2 *(tit.)*
equalis (complexio) 66,21 – *adv.* 96,8
equiuocatio 70,11
ergo 56,23 68,18 78,7 102,1 110,11
errare 54,12 90,12 – *pass.* 64,19
error 122,2
eruptio 98,28
esse* 54,16. 17. 20 56,1. 3. 4. 10 60,3. 15. 17 64,16 78,6 de natura uirtutis est currere 88,20 substantia non est existens 78,9 *item* 78,16 94,9 hoc est 64,22 68,11 78,13 96,3 100,17 id est 62,10 84,8 86,2. 10 98,20 *i. q.* existere 56,14bis. 23 58,4 100,7. 9
estas 68,21 70,3. 7 (Hipp.)
et* 54,7. 12. 15. 19 60,4. 17 102,6 ignis terre aque et aeris 62,20 *item* 62,11 non ..., et non 102,5 sed et 102,4. 7 et ... et 58,18/19 66,21 86,20/21 94,6 104,18 et ... et ... et 62,5sq. 68,23 88,1–3 106,19 et *septies* 82, 19sq.
etas (perfecta) 92,1 (complexio) 70,16
ethicus (*sc.* febris) 66,17
etiam 60,18 62,15 64,16. 17 78,21 84,7 86,15. 25 98,27 100,4. 9. 18 112,14 116,10 et sicut ..., ita e. 78,23
etsi 78,1 → si

euacuare 96,21 98,11 – *pass.* 96,23 118,16
euacuatio 98,4 (colere) 98,1
euacuatiuus (medicina) 96,21
euentus *pl.* 124,4 ([Arist.])
euidens *comp. adv.* 120,13
euomere 98,4 *(f. l.)*
ex* ex quibus (*sc.* propositionibus) contexitur sillogismus 100,7 generatio est ex quatuor elementis 78,7 *item* 92,7 nutriri ex alqa re 102,6 *item* 102,10 accidere ex alqa re 66,18. 22. 23. 24 74,13 *sim.* 62,20 78,5 in aliquibus ex ipsis 114,10 ex necessitate 98,7
excedere 68,14
excitare *pass.* 82,3 *(f. l.)*
excusare *c. acc. c. inf.* 76,25
exemplum 74,22
exercitare ad -andum (in alqa re) 82,3 – *pass.* 56,1 (in alqa re) 54,20 56,4 110,23
exercitium (primum) 56,4
exire (a semita recta) 124,11 ([Arist.]) (ab alqa re) 124,2 ([Arist.]) (extra alqam rem) 106,8
existentia (naturalis *sc.* corporum) 68,16
existere 76,16 96,20 98,6 116,7 (per se) 78, 9 112,18 118,1
expandere *pass.* 80,3 92,16 104,25
expellere 80,19 (contraria) 62,5 *item* 88,1 120,19
expergere *pass.* 72,16
experiri 58,15
exponere (narrationem) 56,10 (uersus) 54, 8. 14 *item* 54,10. 11
expositio 54,11 (sententia) 54,12 – *pl.* 114,14
expulsiuus (uirtus) 62,11 108,17 120,19
extendere *pass.* 94,1 102,2
extinctio (*sc.* anime) 78,22
extinguere *pass.* 78,21
extra 56,14bis 60,18 – *c. acc.* 96,1 106,9
extremitas (radicis spine) 92,15

facere 62,7 94,9. 19 116,3 ad -iendum 110,17 *c. acc. c. inf.* 76,6 – *pass.* 68,20. 21 74,20 76,1
faex → fex
falsus (sententie) 82,1
familiaris *subst.* -es 54,17 56,6
famosus *subst.* -i (antiquorum) 90,24
febricitare -antes 66,9
febris 66,9 – *pl.* 72,5 *(f. l.)* 118,21 (generatio) 66,13 (genera) 66,15. 19 (liber) 66,19 *(tit.)*
festinare 102,1
fex 100,17 *(f. l.)* (in uino et in oleo) 100,18
fieri 86,19 100,13. 14 (alteratio debilis) 96,14
figere *pass.* 88,22 90,3. 21
finire *pass.* <124,3> ([Arist.])
finis (scientie) 108,2 (senii) 78,19 in -e 56,11 76,1
firmiter 58,13 114,15
firmus (notitia) 104,9 (alcuius rei) 56,10 – *comp. adv.* 58,20
flamma (attractio ignis) 118,22
fleubothomare *pass.* 74,26
fleubothomia (hora) 74,23
fleuma 70,23 94,18 98,7 (superhabundantia) 98,13
fleumaticus (cibarii) 98,15 (potus) 100,20
fluere 72,12 88,20
forma (corporis) 78,10
formare 62,8 90,18 – *pass.* 82,1
formatio 94,12 *(f. l.)* (embrionis) 62,12
formator (embrionis) 94,12
fortasse 102,4. 7
fortis 64,22 106,10 *(f. l.)* (caliditas) 70,7 (Hipp.) (calor) 64,14 – *comp.* (sanguis) 98, 10
frigiditas 68,23. 24 78,18 84,10. 15. 19 118,15 (dominium) 66,25 (ultimitas) 78,19
frigidus 104,12 (aer) 118,19 (complexio) 68, 11 72,2. 23 (corpora) 72,3 (elementum) 66, 23 (humor) 70,24 (planta) 104,7 – *subst.* -um (dominium) 66,24
fulgor (dispositio) 82,19
fulguratio (dispositio) 82,19 *(v. l.)*

generare 90,20 94,5 98,8. 15 – *pass.* 56,13 90,17 92,5. 20. 25 94,4. 22 98,6. 22 100,2. 13 112,6 118,5
generatio 64,15 118,5 *(f. l.)* (*sc.* anime) 78,7 (commixtionum) 94,23 (cordis) 92,22 (corporis) 78,5 116,6. 11 (embrionis) 90,15 92,8 (epatis) 92,23 (febrium) 66,13 (humorum) 98,25 (sanguinis) 86,20 98,25
genus (animalium) 64,9 96,17 (caliditatis) 102,15 (medicinarum) 84,20 (sensus) 122,4 *(e coni.)* in -ere 82,7 84,8 – *pl.* (complexionum) 66,1 *(tit.)* (febrium) 66,19 (prima febrium) 66,15
gradus (altior) 124,9 ([Arist.]) (magnus) 122,7 ([Arist.]) 124,8 ([Arist.]) (mediocris) 114,6
gramaticus *subst.* -a (ars) 56,1 -i 54,7
grando (dispositio) 84,1

gratia uerbi g. 84,22 96,21
guibentirie medicine que nominantur in Greca lingua g. id est uenena 86,1

habere* 58,11 72,22 76,21. 22bis (scientiam) 56,12. 15. 17 62,19 76,25 *item* 56,9 114,11. 12 res ita non se -et 102,7 *c. inf.* 112,20 *i. q.* scire (de alqa re) 58,21 – *pass.* 86,4. 5
habitare 78,1 80,13 82,12
habitudo (naturalis *sc.* corporum) 68,18
hanelitus (defectus) 118,26
harena → arena
hepar → epar
hic* 54,19 58,15. 18. 20 62,1. 11. 20 64,16 112,14 in hiis in quibus iudicauit 106,27 *item* 56,8 110,1 114,12. 25 probatio huius 96,2 *item* 116,3 hec omnia 84,3 post hoc 70,8 78,21 96,9 propter hoc 76,2 102,14 104,3 propter hoc idem 104,1 secundum hoc 102,17 hoc est 64,21 68,11 100,17 hic mundus 56,22 *item* 60,13. 16 62,15. 16 in hoc tempore nostro 116,1 hec duo 64,16
hiems → hyems
homo 100,10 108,3 110,17 122,7 ([Arist.]) (natura) 88,24 – *pl.* 58,16 60,2 76,4
hora (attractionis) 96,12 (fleubothomie) 74, 23 (ire) 62,2 conuersio -e -arum anni 70,2 – *pl.* h. -arum anni 70,3
humanus (corpus) 88,22 (natura) 64,2 *(tit.)* 94,20 *(tit.)* 98,5 *(tit.)*
humiditas 68,13. 23. 24 70,3. 5 84,10. 16. 18 (quantitas aquose) 96,22
humidus 68,9. 9 *(f. l.)* 70,20 *(f. l.)* (complexio) 68,3. 11. 13. 15 70,16 (corpora) 68,17 (elementum) 66,23 (humor) 70,25 (membra) 70,23 (natura) 68,19 – *subst.* -um 70, 13 (dominium) 66,24bis – *comp.* (uer) 68,21
humor 96,11. 18 98,3 100,13 102,5. 7. 8. 10 (frigidus et humidus) 70,24 (significatio melancholici) 100,11 (niger) 100,1. 16. 17. 18 (attractio) 96,13 – *pl.* 68,1 *(f. l.)* 96,7. 16. 20 98,10. 17. 21 (corporis) 96,7 (complexio) 70, 21 (generatio) 98,25 (putredo) 66,18
hyems 68,21
hypo- → ypo

iam 124,9 ([Arist.])
iarcan 96,23 98,2
ibi 104,2
idem 54,13 78,2 106,27 propter hoc idem 104,1 eadem sententia 64,4 *item* 68,3 70,4. 5 eodem modo 68,12. 20 70,14. 25 in isto eodem libro 60,14 ex aliqua commixtione eadem commixtionibus 78,6
ideo 72,20
igitur 56,16 98,11 116,18 122,4 *(f. l.)* *in initio enuntiati* 56,12 78,15 96,19 106,14 116,5
ignis (flamma) 118,22 (temperamentum) 62, 20
ignorantia (obscuritas) 122,8 ([Arist.])
illaudabilis (modi complexionum) 66,26
ille* 54,15 56,21 68,4. 13 80,19 90,27 per terram -orum 54,7 i. qui 54,11 84,3 90,12 94,9 *item* 56,4 58,12 62,22 90,20 -ud quod 56,7. 9 58,19 62,6 -a incisio 74,20. 27 *item* 54,12 80,18 96,14 -a egritudo que 76,5 *item* 88,23 90,18 92,18 106,9
imaginatio → ymaginatio
immo 108,2
immortalis (anima) 60,11 78,1. 13. 23 116,24 (substantia anime) 76,26
impossibilis -e est (quod) 78,7 92,3 102,2. 4 118,27 120,21
in* *c. acc.* 102,21 declinans in corruptionem 98,28 conuocare in testimonium 56,6. 7 *item* 54,17 conuersio anni in caliditatem 70,4 *item* 78,18 96,8bis 100,19 *sim.* 80,3 116,14 – *c. abl.* 54,7 56,18. 19. 22 58,3 conuersio hore anni in caliditate 70,3 in libro Ypocratis et Platonis 60,13 *item* 60,14 62, 4bis. 12 64,3bis operationes dei in nobis 58,8 augmentum in puero 62,8 *item* 64,9 66,4. 5. 6. 7bis. 8 in diuinationibus et in sompniis 58,6sq. *sim.* 68,13. 24 70,6. 9 studere in arte medicine 54,20 *item* 56,1. 4 62,22 ea que sunt in scientia loyce 60,15 *item* 84,3 composui in Sententiis Ypocratis et Platonis librum 60,8 superhabundare in substantia 64,14. 23 *item* 64,19. 22 70,14 in uita sua 54, 6 *item* 60,9 62,2 70,13 74,23 si consideretur complexio ueris in seipsa 68,22 *item* 76,19 96,15 in comparatione 104,2 in directo 92,17 in fine 56,11 76,1 *item* 78,19 in genere 82,7 84,8 in parte 108,27 in primis 92,9. 14 in similitudine 98,10 in ueritate 80,16 in ultimo 56,3 *item* 118,23 commentum libri De humana natura in tribus dictionibus 64,3 in Greca lingua 86,1 in parua quantitate sumitur 86,6 *item* 98,3
incarcerare *pass.* 122,18 ([Arist.])
incidere 74,24 – *pass.* 74,15 76,3
incipere *c. inf.* 54,10
incisio 74,19. 20. 27
incorporare 116,16

incorporeus (anima) 60,11 78,1. 13 (substantia) 78,24 112,16 (uirtutes) 112,2 – *subst.* -um 56,19
indagare (de alqa re quid) 80,8
inde 102,4 106,16
indigere (alqa re) 62,1 88,6 90,8 106,10 *c. inf.* 54,16 56,6
indiuisibilis (prima) 112,9
inducere (in testimonium) 54,17
inficere *pass.* 54,16
infirmitas 58,10 74,10 (apostematum) 76,23 (*sc.* corporis) 98,6 (diminutio) 98,1
infirmus *subst.* 74,21 (neruus) 74,19
inflatio (diminutio) 96,22
influere 72,23
informare 90,20
informatio (cordis) 90,25 (membrorum) 90,26
infra *c. acc.* 92,17
infrigidare *pass.* 78,19
initium (motus et sensus) 108,5 *(v. l.)*
innatus (caliditas) 102,12 (calor) 64,12 (Hipp.). 13 (Hipp.) 66,4
inquirere 98,13 100,6 104,8. 10
insanus (Plato) 106,23
instrumentum 94,12 – *pl.* (anime) 80,12
intactus (radix) 88,13
intellectus (claritas) 122,10 ([Arist.]) (defectus) 56,2
intelligere 54,9 64,20 72,4bis 90,12. 14 100,9 122,11 ([Arist.]) (quia) 78,10 (quid) 68,9 *item* 122,16 ([Arist.]) ad -endum 104,23 – *pass.* 68,10. 12 100,11. 12
intentio 90,21
inter *c. acc.* 70,11 uer i. tempora anni 68,20 *item* 90,18 96,15. 16 differentia i. sermonem meum et sermonem Berthenis 56,5 *item* 86,2 104,4 120,11 temperata i. caliditatem et frigiditatem et siccitatem et humiditatem 68,23
interrogare *pass.* (quid) 108,11
intra *c. acc.* 96,20
inuenire 54,7 68,16 74,22 80,19 118,4 (multos medicorum paratos) 80,14 *item* 110,23 (quod) 74,3 *c. acc. c. inf.* 76,21 *c. acc. c. part.* 78,14 104,15 110,19 – *pass.* 58,6 62,4 78,9 114,19 (uer humidius) 68,21 *item* 68, 22. 23
inuentio (rei) 80,17 (sillogismorum) 82,5 – *pl.* (bonitatum) 82,6
inuicem 106,5 *(v. l.)*
ipse* 56,23 78,21 80,6 88,9 96,8. 15 112,6 in seipsa 68,22 -a radix 88,15 *item* 96,23 98, 27bis *i. q.* is 54,11bis 56,2 58,2. 4. 5. 22 60,10 62,3. 20 64,3 rami -ius 88,14 *item* 114,9 *i. q.* hic 66,21 92,8 116,21 120,11 -i uersus 54,14 → *ind. nom.* Galienus
ira (hora) 62,2
ire 124,6 ([Arist.]) eundi 110,8
iris → yris
is* 54,9 62,4. 5. 14bis. 15 76,13 dictum eius 54, 13 *item* 58,5 78,7 88,12 118,12 is qui 60,15 80,15 112,4 eo quod 76,16 92,24 100,18 106,8 110,6 id est 56,20 62,10 84,8. 10 86,2. 10 ea natura 112,22
iste* 58,20 64,20 74,1 86,3. 4 88,21 100,18 unum -orum 68,12 *item* 88,3. 4 -i familiares 54,17 *item* 56,11. 15. 17 62,10 64,7 66,25 68, 19 in -o eodem libro 60,14
ita 70,18 102,7 ita (...) quod 60,17 80,5 secundum quod ..., ita 76,19 80,9 sicut ..., ita etiam 78,23
item 100,12
iudicare 106,26. 27 108,25. 26 (de alqa re) 62,21bis 68,18 104,11 114,15. 16 (quod) 62,19 78,24 82,14 112,1. 3 (iudicio naturali quod) 114,7 (de alqa re quod) 68,4 (de alqa re utrum) 60,10 *item* 80,8 *(v. l.)* – *pass.* 80,15 106,14
iudicium 76,20 102,1 106,29 108,1 (naturale) 114,8 (de alqa re) 116,20 – *pl.* 80, 15
iustus non est -um (quod) 104,27
iuuamen 82,17. 19 86,4. 6 (caloris) 62,1
iuuamentum 82,17 *(v. l.)*. 19 *(v. l.)* 86,4 *(v. l.)* 98,4 (membrorum) 90,22 *(tit.)* (pulsuum) 90,10 *(tit.)*
iuuare 86,8 114,27
iuuentus 90,23

lac (papaueris) 86,9
lapis *pl.* 104,18 106,19
latus in -ere 74,26
laudare 108,24
laxatiuus (medicine) 84,23 96,4 (potentia) 110,21
legere 122,13 ([Arist.])
lex 58,18
liber 60,8 82,3. 11 96,3bis (Complexionum) 66,20 *item* 68,3 (De colera nigra) 100,2 *item* 100,4 (De elementis secundum sententiam Ypocratis) 64,1 94,20 (De generibus complexionum et De elementis secundum sententiam Ypocratis) 66,1 (De iuua-

mento membrorum) 90,22 (De medicinis purgantibus) 100,22 (prima dictio De regimento sanitatis) 78,17 (septima dictio De sententiis Ypocratis et Platonis) 80,10 *item* 60,13. 14 (De simplici medicina) 84,12 (De uirtutibus naturalibus) 62,16 100,22 *item* 62,16 (Febrium) 66,19 (De anima *sc.* Aristotilis) 122,15 ([Arist.]) (Chrasis) 80,6 (Thimeus *sc.* Platonis) 104,20 *item* 82,12 (Amphorismorum *sc.* Ypocratis) 64,11 (Ypocratis De humana natura) 94,19 98,5 (secunda dictio Elguefete *sc.* Ypocratis) 70,5 (secunda dictio Epidimiarum *sc.* Ypocratis) 70,2 *item* 70,4 (pars) 80,7 commentum -bri (*sc.* Ypocratis) De humana natura 64,2 – *pl.* 56,3. 4. 7 64,3. 10 80,11 106,5. 7. 24 120,13 122,13 ([Arist.])

liberare 58,11 (*f. l.*) – *pass.* 58,14

liberatio 58,11 (*e coni.*)

licet *c. coni.* 66,5 88,13 92,11

licitus est -um alcui *c. inf.* 120,9

lignum *pl.* 104,18

lingua 78,4 (Greca) 86,1

listilia 98,2 → stillea

locare *pass.* 56,20

locus 56,19 62,9 90,12. 12 (*f. l.*) 104,16 116,4 (proprius) 108,9 (corporis) 82,12 (scolarum) 54,7 -o instrumenti 94,12 *item* 102,14. 20 in -o sanguinis 96,18 *item* 98,23 102,12 – *pl.* 82,14 106,12

logica → loyca

longinquus *comp.* 92,12 (*f. l.*)

longitudo (spine) 92,16

longus (tempus) 80,19 – *comp.* (uia) 92,12

loqui 78,5 120,12. 13 (de alqa re) 66,19 68,3 82,13 (super alqa re) 96,9

loyca (scientia) 60,16

luctari -andi 110,10

luna 84,2

lux (scientie) 122,9 ([Arist.])

magis †58,8 72,2. 27 74,3 m. sensibilis 72,21 74,6 76,19. 23 *item* 62,11 64,14 68,17bis 88,13 96,16 110,2 116,21 plus m. proprius 96,16 quanto m. 60,5 quanto m. minus 66,9 – *sup.* 100,10

magnus (gradus) 122,6 ([Arist.]) (quantitas) 96,22 98,3 (uiolentia) 98,3 – *comp.* (dolor) 74,27 (sol) 80,16 – *sup.* (gradus) 124,8 ([Arist.])

malus (complexio) 100,14 (dispositio) 98,28 – *comp.* 100,5 – *sup.* (complexio) 70,1

manere 78,14

maneries *pl.* (demonstrationes rationis et memorie) 60,15

manifestare 80,1 100,3 (quod) 72,7 (utrum) 80,1 – *pass.* 56,3

manifestus 100,4 118,2 (demonstratio) 96, 19 (sensus) 104,13 (significatio) 58,14 -um est (quod) 56,16 76,4 – *adv.* 110,7 122,3 – *comp.* 96,14

mare 58,11 84,1 (*f. l.*)

mater (embrionis) 92,19

materia 78,11bis – *pl.* 118,4 (*f. l.*). 18 (*f. l.*)

matrix 62,9 90,15. 19 92,7. 11. 13. 15 (*f. l.*). 19 (*f. l.*) 94,10. 13

mediare 78,15 114,4

medicamentum (purgatiuum) 102,5

medicare in -ando 78,22

medicina 114,26 (ars) 54,20 108,20 118,8 (opus) 98,18 100,1 *i. q.* medicamentum 96, 20 (*f. l.*) 98,3 (euacuatiua) 96,21 (purgatiua) 96,12 98,2 (simplex) 84,13 (*tit.*) (natura) 96, 7 – *pl.* 84,13. 23 86,10 118,18 (laxatiue) 84, 22 (laxatiue et uomice) 96,4 (mortifere) 86,3. 5 (purgatiue) 96,10 (*tit.*). 10 *item* 100,23 (*tit.*) (natura purgatiuarum) 96,20 (commixtio) 86,8 (genus) 84,20 (potio calidarum) 118,23

medicus 78,22 98,8 (*f. l.*) – *pl.* 68,5. 14 74,5. 16. 23 76,3 80,14 84,5. 7 (antiqui) 104,5 (populares) 62,17

mediocris (gradus) 114,7

medius *subst.* sine -o 78,12

melanc(h)olicus (humor) 100,11 (potus) 100,21

melancolia 94,18 (*f. l.*)

membrum 60,16 72,10. 12. 17 74,12. 14 76,11 88,17 92,4 (carnosum) 74,21 76,22 (primum sensibilium) 72,8 (partes radicalis) 80,5 (animalis) 74,1 (nutritio animalium) 86,22 (corporis) 82,16 102,12 (arefactio) 76,12 (complexio) 72,1 (substantia) 90,7 – *pl.* 60,16 72,24 74,8 76,23 86,23 88,6 94,4. 8 102,8 (radicalia) 80,3 (complexio radicalium senum) 70,19 (corporis) 72,13 (*sc.* senum) 70,22 (informatio) 90,26 (iuuamentum) 90,22 (*tit.*) (substantia) 90,5

memoria 60,9 (maneries) 60,15

mensura (potentie) 110,25

merito 98,8

metheorus *subst.* -a (scientia) 84,3

meus* 54,16. 17 56,5. 7 60,13 64,1 66,1. 20 90, 21. 23 94,19bis 114,17

ministrare (neruis sensum) 72,25 *item* 72,26 92,18. 21
minutus (partes) 80,4
mirabilis (uirtus) 58,15
mirus *adv.* 84,2bis
miscere *pass.* 68,2
mittere †58,8 88,8
mixtio 116,23 *(f. l.)*
modicus (adiutorium) 90,9 (occasio) 100,19
modo 54,15 120,13. 16
modus 118,8 (dignior) 70,12 (dignior complexionum) 66,26 aliquo -o 78,11 contrario -o 54,10 98,1 diuerso -o 84,11 eodem -o 68,12. 20 70,14. 25 ad -um capilli 74,25 secundum hunc -um 102,16 secundum -um sufficientie 114,13 – *pl.* 64,18 120,17 (complexionum) 66,20. 22. 25 68,7. 8. 15 70,12
monstrare 96,3 114,21 (quod) 78,12. 17 94,21 96,10
moralis (particula) 120,7 (philosophia) 108,21 114,26
morbus *pl.* (curatio) 120,3
mordicatiuus (calor) 66,12
moriri 78,16
mortalis 116,24 *(f. l.)* (anima) 60,6. 10 78,23 (egritudines) 70,10 (substantia anime) 76,26
mortiferus (medicine) 86,3. 5
mortuus *subst.* -i (corpora) 68,17
mos *pl.* (aptatio) 120,5
motiuus (uirtus) 72,15
motus 88,17 90,21 102,22 *(f. l.)* (uoluntarius) 60,16 108,14 (occasio uoluntarii) 60,3 (dispositio terre) 84,1 (principium) 62,3 108,5 (principium operationis) 60,18 – *pl.* (diuersi) 82,7 (principium) 60,12 82,9
mouere 90,1 – *pass.* 74,12
mulier 92,21
multotiens 86,9
multus 70,6 (Hipp.) 76,13 80,14 90,23 102,9 106,10 (sensibilitas) 76,17 – *subst.* -um 118,17 -i 54,20 76,8 100,9 104,24 (opus) 106,6 -i medicorum et philosophorum 80,14 *item* 68,5 74,5. 16 84,7 – *adv.* 68,3 70,24 82,2 84,7 118,19 – *comp. adv.* 66,4. 6. 8 74,4 108,9 plus magis 96,16 – *sup.* 64,18. 21 (calor) 64,12 (Hipp.). 13 (Hipp.)
mundus 56,13. 18. 22 104,26 (anima) 104,25 106,18
mutare †82,18 – *pass.* 88,24 *(v. l.)*

nam 60,1 68,9
narrare 54,15 56,11 62,4. 11 70,2. 4 82,16 108,8. 15. 22 114,12 116,2. 8 (quod) 70,8 – *pass.* 106,12
narratio 106,13 (rerum) 56,10
nasci 62,8 *(f. l.)* (apostemata) 74,9 76,6
natura 62,15. 16 88,5. 7. [25bis] 94,23 96,8 112,22 (humana) 64,3 *(tit.)* 94,20 *(tit.)* 98,5 *(tit.)* (propria) 112,5 (anime) 122,18 ([Arist.]) (animalium) 88,23 96,18 (corporum) 68,19 (hominis) 88,24 (medicine) 96,6. 20 (uirtutis) 90,3 extra -am 96,1 de -a uirtutis est currere 88,19 n. sua est ut conuertatur 100,18 – *pl.* 118,4
naturalis (caliditas) 102,11 (calor) 60,19 64,9. 15 66,8. 10. 14 102,20 104,1 (complexio) 118,29 (existentia) 68,16 (habitudo) 68,18 (iudicium) 114,8 (operationes) 78,15 86,16 (pars philosophie) 108,24 (scientia) 82,13 104,21 108,2 110,23 (uirtutes) 62,16 *(tit.)* 86,24 88,10 90,4 100,22 *(tit.)* 102,17. 18 120,15 – *adv.* 72,22 120,24
naufragium 58,12
ne 98,16
nec non ... nec 80,17 116,27
necessarius 78,12 (notitia ad sanitatem) 114,22 (scientia) 116,20 alcui *c. inf.* 84,3 est -um (quod) 108,22 *c. inf.* 120,1 – *adv.* -o 98,26 100,5
necessitas ex -te 98,7
negligere 84,8
neque non ... n. 114,23 non ... n. ... n. 120,4/5
neruus 74,15 76,3. 16. 19. 20. 21. 22. 23 (apostema) 76,19 (apostema infirmi) 74,18 (pars) 74,24 (punctura) 74,4 (sensibilitas) 76,17 – *pl.* 72,13. 25. 27 74,6. 10 76,7. 9 (partis corporis) 74,2
nescire 58,17 110,14 118,8 (quod) 104,7 (que) 90,18
nichil 110,12
niger (colera) 98,7 100,3 *(tit.)*. 12. 13. 15. 16 102,1 (humor) 100,1. 16. 17. 18 (sanguis) 102,3 – *subst.* -um (purum) 100,19
nisi non ... n. 56,23 64,16 68,16 112,5 116,17 120,24 numquam ... n. 100,8
nix (dispositio) 84,1
nobilis *comp.* (expositiones) 114,14 – *subst.* -ius 94,14
nobilitas (anime) 114,23
nocere 58,16 98,17 100,1 108,20 118,7
nocitiuus (calor) 66,12
nolle *c. inf.* 54,13. 15 100,9

nomen 100,10 *(f. l.)* (caliditatis) 64,5

nominare 62,14 80,8. 10 82,4. 11 102,19 108, 14 110,15 120,9 (uirtutes naturam) 62,15 *item* 62,13. 15 64,9 66,16 102,17. 18 120,6 – *pass.* 100,15 (colera nigra humor niger) 100,15 *item* 82,13 84,23 102,17

nominatio 100,16

non* 54,11. 20 56,9bis. 12. 14. 15 58,1. 16 non tamen 92,3 et non 106,26 112,22 non ... nec 80,16 non ... neque ... neque 120,1 non ... nisi 56,22 64,16 68,14 non ..., sed 56,1 78,9 80,7 82,13 non solum ..., sed 96,7 98,6 118,24

nos 54,20 58,8 78,14 82,6. 9 84,6 92,24 98,11. 19. 21 116,8 118,2. 4. 9. 19 → *ind. nom.* Galienus

noster 64,16 68,16 70,11 90,13. 22 102,16 110, 10 116,1

notitia 56,9 114,11. 21. 25 120,24 (firma) 104, 9 (uera) 114,24 116,6 (secundum modum sufficientie) 114,12

nouem (modi complexionum) 66,21

nullus -a scientia 58,3 *item* 68,2 80,5 82,2 86,4

numquam 100,7 n. ... nisi 100,8

nutrimentum 62,6 88,9 (*sc.* animalium) 102,10

nutrire *pass.* 88,24. [25] 102,4. 6

nutritio (membri) 86,21

ob 68,14

obliuio (domina) 60,9

obscuritas (ignorantie) 122,8 ([Arist.])

occasio 110,13 (modica) 100,19 (operatiua) 110,14 (motus et sensus) 60,2 -ne apostematum 76,8. 15 *item* 76,18 – *pl.* (certe) 110,12

octo VIII primi libri 122,13 ([Arist.])

oculus 78,4 – *pl.* (animalium) 124,1 ([Arist.])

oleum fex in -o 100,18

omittere 82,17. 18 *c. inf.* 82,11

omnipotens (deus) 94,15

omnis* 56,17 60,2 64,9 66,25. 26 68,1. 6 80,3 104,16 – *subst.* -es 106,22 114,28 -ia 62,1

operari 78,15 112,4. 5. 21bis 114,5 120,8 (proprias operationes) <78,20> *item* 110,7

operatio (motus pulsus) 60,18 (uirtutis) 62, 7 per -nem 82,11 – *pl.* 56,22 110,7. 11. 15. 19 (naturales) 78,15 86,15 (proprie *sc.* anime) 78,20 (*sc.* deitatum) 58,5 (dei) 58,7 (*sc.* uirtutum) 56,21

operatiuus occasio -a istarum operationum 110,14 *item* 114,2

opinari → oppinari

opium 86,10

oportere -et 120,11 *(f. l.)* (quod) 68,24 72,4 78,15 82,6 *c. inf.* 82,7 100,3. 4 *c. acc. c. inf.* 82,9

oppinari 78,11 102,8 116,13 (de alqa re) 90, 19 (quod) 64,13 74,5 76,18 90,24 102,4. 7 – *pass.* (quod) 70,11 90,14 104,3

opponere *pass.* 74,5 *(f. l.)*

opus (medicine) 100,1 (speculatio medicine) 98,18 (pratice) 120,11 ad -us discipulorum 106,7 *item* 104,22 106,6

oriri 62,8

os 92,14

papauer (lac) 86,9

paratus (ad alqam rem) 80,14

pars (nerui subtilis ad modum capilli) 74,24 (nerui corporis) 74,2 (dicti) 108,25 (libri) 80,7 (partium) 80,5bis (philosophie) 84,4 108,20 (naturalis philosophie) 108,23 p. regitiua -tium anime 72,11 82,16 in -te 108, 27 – *pl.* 72,21bis (minute) 80,4 (similes) 112,13 p. -tium 80,5 p. regitiua -tium anime 72,11 82,16 p. -tium membri radicalis 80,5

participare *pass.* 104,1 *(f. l.)*

particula 120,6 – *pl.* (minime) 116,15

particularis receptio p. corporis 72,18

paruus (dolor) 76,16 (quantitas) 62,1 86,6 – *comp. adv.* magis minus 66,10 – *sup.* (particule) 116,14 – *adv.* 76,20

pati 58,12 (alqa re) 96,21. 23 98,2bis

paucitas (caloris) 102,22 (doloris) 76,14

paulatiuus (probatio) 106,16

paulus *subst.* -o ante 80,9 108,15

pectus 92,17

per* 54,7 72,13 80,3. 6 scio per operationes 58,4 *item* 58,13 80,15 96,11 apparuerunt per uirtutem suam 58,9 operationes naturales diuiduntur per unam qualitatem uel per duas qualitates 86,16sq. tria principia per motus tres 82,7 oppinatur per equiuocationem nostram 70,11 per contrarium 98,1 per operationem 82,10 per se 78,9 112,19

perceptibilis sensus doloris p. 76,10

perceptio (sensibilium) 60,17

percipere (quod) 92,2 – *pass.* 60,15. 17 70, 14 104,1 106,9

perfectus (etas) 92,1
permanere 88,22 100,14
perscrutari 72,5 76,21 82,7 84,3 (quot) 120,16
pertinere 114,5 *c. inf.* 112,21
peruenire (ad alqem) 54,6 *item* 92,6 (ad alqam rem) 78,19 92,1 122,14 ([Arist.])
philosophia 122,12 ([Arist.]) (moralis) 114, 26 (pars moralis) 108,21 (pratice) 82,18 (pars pratice) 84,4 (scientie) 82,17 (ars) 54,20 (pars naturalis) 108,24
philosophus *subst.* ph. (de secta reubach) 84,5 Plato ph. 62,13 -i 68,5. 15 80,14 (antiqui) 104,5
phleb- → fleub-
phlegm- → fleum-
placere -et *c. inf.* 120,6
planta 104,7 (radix) 88,11 – *pl.* 62,1 *(f. l.).* 3. 5. 13 86,25bis 90,20 102,15 104,2. 19 108,5. 13 122,3 (corpora) 68,17 (radix) 102,21
pluries 96,9
pluuia *pl.* 70,6 (Hipp.)
pluuiosus (constitutio anni) 70,8 (Hipp.)
ponere 64,1 82,4 106,29 120,10 – *pass.* 60, 18 92,14
popularis (medici) 62,17
populus 60,1
portanarius (uena) 102,3
portare *pass.* 102,21
posse *c. inf.* 56,2. 23 64,14 70,14 74,1 78,20 80,7 102,17. 18 112,10. 11. 12
possibilis est -e 102,6 (quod) 78,14 90,13 100,13 *c. inf.* 114,27 *c. acc. c. inf.* 76,26
post 76,10 80,19 – *c. acc.* 82,16 p. hoc 70,8 78,21 96,9
postea 92,15. 16 96,8
postmodum 94,1
postquam *c. ind.* 62,8 80,19 90,16 *c. coni.* 72,4 124,2 ([Arist.])
potatio (medicinarum) 118,22 *(v. l.)*
potens (ad intelligendum) 104,22 *item* 110,17
potentia (actiua) 110,18 (constipatiua) 110, 22 (laxatiua) 110,21 (mensura) 110,25
potio (medicinarum) 118,22
potus *pl.* 100,20
prae- → pre-
praticus (philosophia) 84,4 – *subst.* -a (opus) 120,11 (philosophia) 82,18
precedere (alqam rem) 90,25
precipere 58,19. 20
predicare 58,18
predicere *pass.* 74,9 92,1 *(f. l.)*
preparare *pass.* (ad recipiendum) 118,10
prestare (iuuamen) 82,19
primus 56,4 62,19 64,10 66,16 (dictio) 78,17 (genera) 66,15 (instrumentum anime rationalis) 80,12 (membrum sensibilium) 72,8 VIII -i libri 122,13 ([Arist.]) – *subst.* -a (compositio) 112,8 in -is 92,9. 14
principium (caloris) 102,20 (dictionis) 70,5 (motuum) 60,11. 18 82,9 (motus et sensus) 108,5 (motus et uirtutis regitiue) 62,3 facere -um 116,3 – *pl.* 82,7 84,6 90,13. 14. 15. 17
prior 92,23 – *subst.* secundum -us 98,23 – *adv.* 92,20 94,1. 5
probare 74,1 84,4 (quod) 56,7. 8 60,18 62,4 80,15 84,7 96,15 *c. inf.* 84,5
probatio 80,18 96,2 100,6 (paulatiua) 106, 15 (uera) 114,19 (*sc.* sententiarum) 106,11 (de alqa re) 64,1 – *pl.* 82,4 100,6 *(f. l.)*
procedere 60,17 64,16 96,2 114,3
prodesse 86,10. 11 -est (multum scire) 84,7 (medicis scire) 84,6
prohibere (alqem de alqa re) 82,5
proicere *pass.* 94,10
promittere *c. inf.* 116,2
propinquus *c. inf.* 58,12 – *comp.* -ius est *c. inf.* 94,14
proponere 60,14
proportionatus (alcui rei) 102,11
propositio *pl.* -nes sillogismi 100,6 sillogismi -num 82,5
proprietas (corporis) 112,19 (totalitatis) 84,21 86,14
proprius (loca) 106,13 108,9 (natura) 112,5 (operationes) 78,20 (sanguis) 96,16 (substantia) 64,15
propter* 54,19 56,2 72,19 74,3bis. 7 p. hoc 76,2 102,14 104,1. 3
prouidere 100,8ter
prout 54,5 62,14 78,21. 24bis 80,1. 4. 8 82,18 94,7 108,26 110,5 114,16
puer 62,8 – *pl.* 66,4. 7
pulsatilis (uene) 90,2 92,11. 12. 13. 15. 21 94,6
pulsus (adiutorium uenarum) 90,8 (operatio) 60,19 – *pl.* (iuuamentum) 90,11 *(tit.)*
punctura (carnis) 74,3 (nerui) 74,4
pungere 74,2. 16 – *pass.* 74,13. 15
purgare medicine -antes 100,23 *(tit.)*
purgatiuus (medicamentum) 102,5 (medicine) 96,10 *(tit.).* 11. 12. 20 98,2
purus (nigrum) 100,19
putredo (humorum) 66,18

putrefacere *pass.* 106,20

quaerere → querere
qualitas 64,22 86,12. 17 qu. -atum 84,9 – *pl.* 78,11 84,9. 17 86,17 116,23 (contrarii) 64,6 (*sc.* elementorum) 64,1 (*sc.* substantiarum) 116,18 qu. -atum actiuarum 84,9
quam in aliis locis quam in propriis 106,12 *item* 96,3 *apud comp.* †58,9 64,14 66,5. 7. 8 72,3. 27 74,3 94,7 108,9 120,13 quam <si> 76,19
quamuis 56,3 qu. ..., tamen 78,13
quando 68,16 74,12 118,13. 16. 17. 18
quantitas (magna) 98,3 (parua) 62,1 86,6 (magna humiditatis) 96,22 – *pl.* 78,11 *(f. l.)*
quantus -o magis 60,5 tantum ... -um 76,22 -o magis minus ..., tanto deterior 66,9
quatuor (complexiones) 66,21bis (compositiones) 94,21 (elementa) 68,1 78,7 98,23 112,7 116,9. 10 118,6 (humores) 98,21 (uirtutes) 62,10
querere (de alqa re) 100,5
qui* 54,15 56,3. 4. 21. 22 58,10. 11 uirtute naturali, in qua uirtute 86,24 occasio que est motus 60,2 *item* 60,17 duos gramaticos ..., unus quorum 54,8 *item* 82,15 qui cum noluisset 54,13 *item* 80,12 118,12 secundum quod 54,9. 11. 17 58,23 hoc quod 56,8 62,21 hec in quibus 106,27 108,6 110,1 iudicium suum hoc quod 108,1 ille qui 54,11 56,4 58,12 62,22 70,12 illud quod 56,7. 9 58,19 62,6 illius rei que percipitur 106,9 is qui 60,15 80,15 112,21 iste res que 56,11. 18 quidam sunt qui 100,7
quia* 54,20 62,16. 18 64,15. 20 66,11. 22 – manifestauimus quia fluit 72,12 *item* 54,5 84,13 90,22 intelligatur quia illa est complexio 68,13 differentia (*sc.* est), quia Berthenis indiguit 56,5 *item* 86,3 intelligas quia materia aliquo modo sit materia 78,10
quicumque 74,1 – *relat.* 98,19
quidam 84,5 – *subst.* 86,18 94,22 96,5. 6 100,7 quidam ... quidam 94,8/11 110,25/112,3 medicinarum quedam ... quedam 84,14/16 86,11/13 aliqui ... quidam ... quidam alii 112,16/17 aliqui ... quidam ... quidam ... quidam 112,10–12
quidem 118,2
quis *interrog. subst.* 68,9 80,8 106,24 108,12 120,2. 16 – *adi.* 56,19 76,25 90,18. 19 – *indef. subst.* si quis 76,20
quod* hoc est quod 68,11 78,13 86,9. 22 96,3 id est quod nos dicamus 98,21 dicitur quod accidit 54,5 *item* 54,6 56,7. 8. 9. 12 58,3. 4 ego uideo quod ego debeam 56,10 58,18 *item* 56,15 58,16 60,14. 18 62,20 manifestum est quod elchadir est egritudo 76,5 *item* 54,19 90,14 manifestum est quod non habeam 56,16 *item* 68,24 72,4 78,8. 14. 16 timeo quod ymaginatio mea sit infecta 54,16 – *caus. c. ind.* 60,19 eo quod 76,17 92,24 100,18 106,8 110,6 *c. coni.* 58,9 – *consecut.* non sunt sic exercitati quod uenirent 56,1 *item* 60,17 80,5bis – *fin.* membra indigent ad hoc quod remaneant 88,7 *item* 90,6 uolens quod esset (*sc.* liber) defensio 60,9 *item* 68,10 70,12 96,12 – quod cum 70,2. 4
quoniam 58,5 64,19 68,20 70,18. 23 100,10
quot 64,17 120,15 *(e corr.)*. 17
quousque *c. ind.* 78,18 92,17 106,16 118,28 *c. coni.* 88,4 104,8 122,14 ([Arist.])

radicalis (membra) 70,19 80,3. 5
radix (*sc.* arboris) 88,12 (plante) 88,11 102,20 (brance) 88,15 (extremitas spine) 92,15
ramus *pl.* (in arbore) 74,11 *item* 88,14
rarefactio 76,12 *(f. l.)*
rarus *adv.* 100,8
ratio 62,14 *(f. l.)* 70,21 100,12 *(f. l.)* †114,1 (maneries) 60,15 – *pl.* 98,20
ratiocinari (quod) 102,9
rationalis (anima) 80,12
recedere (ab alqa re) 118,25. 27
receptio 72,18 (*sc.* anime) 118,12
recipere 54,13. 15 62,22 74,4 78,2 92,19. 21 ad -iendum 118,11 – *pass.* 106,9 *(f. l.)*
rectus (semita) 124,11 ([Arist.]) – *subst.* -um (uia) 124,6 ([Arist.])
recusare *c. acc. c. inf.* 62,18 -ando *c. acc. c. inf.* 58,2
redarguere 96,13
redire dispositio -eundi 110,8
referre non -fert (utrum) 78,22. 23
regere 62,4. 12 116,25 – *pass.* 78,2
regimen (animalium) 58,5 90,14. 16 (corporum) 90,13
regimentum 98,13 (sanitatis) 78,17 *(tit.)*
regitiuus (pars) 72,11 82,16 (uirtus) 62,3
remanere 88,7 90,6 (arbor intacta) 88,13
remotus (membra) 72,13
renouare 88,21
renunciare *c. inf.* 60,4
reperire *pass.* 56,21 100,10
replere *pass.* (alqa re) 118,18

reprobare 54,10 62,21 76,19 80,6. 17 82,2 84,5 100,6 (de alqa re) 64,11
reprobatio (sillogismi) 100,6
requiescere 122,20 ([Arist.])
res 60,13 62,14 *(f. l.)* 80,18 100,4. 12 102,7. 20 (contraria) 120,23 (conueniens) 120,22 (simplex) 64,5 (diffinitio) 106,9 (inuentio) 80,17 – *pl.* 62,21 64,1. 8 80,15 104,8 106,6 114,3. 18 (cause) 84,2 (creator) 56,18 (narratio) 56,11 (scientia) 56,16 116,19 (sensus diuersarum) 110,11
respicere 124,4 ([Arist.]) – *pass.* †114,1
respondere 54,13 122,10 ([Arist.])
restare -at *c. inf.* 120,16
retentiuus (uirtus) 62,7. 10 108,17
retinere 62,7
reuerti 92,17
reuoluere *pass.* 92,14
rubeus 100,15 *(f. l.)*

sanguis 64,15 92,5. 6. 9. 12. 19. 21 94,18. 23 96, 17bis. 18bis 98,6. 8. 9. 10. 26 *(f. l.)* 100,11 102,1. 8. 9. 10. 11 118,17 (niger) 102,3 (conturbatio) 100,17 (generatio) 86,20
sanitas 98,14 (corporis) 114,22 (conseruatio) 120,4 (regimentum) 78,17 *(tit.)*
sanus corpora -a uel non -a 94,22 – *subst.* -i 66,8
sapiens 122,12 ([Arist.])
satis longior s. 92,12
scamonea 110,20
schola → scola
scientia 56,10 108,23 *(f. l.)* 116,27 (naturalis) 82,13 104,21 108,1 110,23 (uirtuosa) 56,8 (loyce) 60,15 (metheororum) 84,3 (rerum) 56,15 116,19 *(e coni.)* (substantie anime) 76, 25 (de alqa re) 58,3 (finis) 108,3 (lux) 122,9 ([Arist.]) (philosophia) 82,18 habere -am (de alqa re) 56,17 62,19 (utrum) 56,12 – *pl.* 112,4 *(f. l.)*
scilicet 56,20 76,11 90,15 108,16 110,5
scire 56,17 *(v. l.)* 60,1. 4 78,12 82,19 84,4. 6. 7 114,15. 18. 28 (de alqa re) 58,2 (quod) 58,4 82,6. 9 90,16 116,5. 9 118,9 (de alqa re quod) 58,23 (utrum) 60,5 *item* 120,2 sc. de scientia uirtuosa 56,7 sc. secundum uiam sufficientie 56,8
scola *pl.* (locus) 54,8
scribere 96,9 (de alqa re) 62,12
secta s. reubach 84,5
secundum* 54,14 56,8 62,13. 14 64,2 *(tit.)*. 7 66,3 *(tit.)* s. hoc 102,17 s. quod 54,9. 11. 15. 17 58,23 66,7 68,10 70,1. 11 s. quod ..., ita 80,8
secundus 60,12 66,17 84,10 (dictio) 70,2. 5. 7
sed* 56,6 58,4. 7. 22 62,8. 12 66,23. 26 70,3 sed et 102,4. 7 non ... sed 56,2 58,2 64,22 78,9. 21 80,8 82,14 96,9 non solum ..., sed 96,7 98,6 118,26
sedes (anime) 122,17 ([Arist.])
semel 58,10
semita (recta) 124,11 ([Arist.])
semper 78,18 90,2
senectus 60,9 (tempora) 70,15
senex *pl.* (membra radicalia) 70,20
senium (finis) 78,19
sensibilis (complexio) 78,16 (corpus) 78,3. 8 80,9 (membrum) 72,17 (nerui) 74,6 76, 19. 20. 23 (partes) 72,21 (substantie) 112,2 – *subst.* -ia 60,18 (primum membrum) 72,9 (perceptio) 60,17
sensibilitas 76,21. 22 (nerui) 76,17
sensitiuus (uirtus) 72,14 120,25
sensus 72,2. 26 88,17 104,1 (calidus) 102,21 (manifestus) 104,13 (perceptibilis) 76,10 (doloris) 74,4 (rerum) 110,10 (genus) 122,4 (occasio) 60,3 (principium) 108,6 – *pl.* 106,10 *(e coni.)*
sententia 54,14 64,4 82,2 (uerisimilis) 96,1 (antiquorum) 72,9 (expositionis) 54,12 (Platonis) 108,23 (uersuum) 54,8. 12 (Ypocratis) 64,2 *(tit.)* 66,3 *(tit.)* 94,20 *(tit.)* 96,2 (de alqa re) 94,19 – *pl.* 82,4 96,3 106,8 114,6. 8 (false) 80,19 (Ypocratis et Platonis) 60,8 *(tit.)* 80,10 *(tit.)*
sentire 74,19. 21 [102,22] 110,5 114,20 (de alqa re) 110,5 114,9 (quod) 110,11 *c. inf.* 114, 17
septimus (dictio) 80,10
sequi 58,18 76,2 90,23 98,25
sermo 106,22. 25 (meus) 56,5 (Berthenis) 56, 5 (sillogismus) 106,17 – *pl.* 106,11 (Aristotilis et Theopha) 106,3 (*sc.* Platonis) 104,27
si* *c. ind.* 76,20 78,6 88,12. 20 98,27 100,8. 14 *c. coni.* 58,17 68,22 74,19 96,21. 23 98,2 ac si 74,27 et si 82,2 quam si <76,19> *ellipt.* 98, 1 *i. q.* num [Arist.] 122,18. 19. 20. 21 → etsi
sic sic ... quod 56,1
siccitas 66,25 68,23 70,1 78,18 84,10. 16. 19 (ultimitas) 78,20
siccus (complexio) 68,11 70,17. 20 100,15 (elementum) 66,23 – *subst.* -um (dominium) 66,24
sicut 58,1 60,10 72,24 74,11 86,19. 26 88,18

100,11. 12. 17 102,8. 19 120,10 uerbi gratia s. 84,22 s. . . ., ita etiam 78,22
significare 58,1 64,5. 7bis 68,9 100,16 (quod) 76,14 s. significatione manifesta 58,14
significatio 64,19 100,20 (manifesta) 58,14 (colere) 100,12 (corporis) 80,9 (humoris) 100,11
signum (dispositio) 84,1 – *pl.* 58,13
sillogismus 100,7. 10 (sermonis) 106,17 (propositiones) 100,7 (reprobatio) 100,6 – *pl.* (inuentio propositionum) 82,5
similis 96,16 102,11 (partes) 112,13 *c. dat.* 76,7 88,1. 9 94,23 96,5. 18 98,3. 10 102,5. 7. 20 112,14 – *subst.* -e *c. gen.* 54,19 -ia 106,15 *c. dat.* 62,7 – *adv.* 62,21 64,8 90,1 94,6
similitudo 98,10
simplex (complexiones) 66,21. 22 (medicina) 84,13 *(tit.)* (res) 64,5
simul 66,24 84,18. 19
sine 70,8 (Hipp.) 76,10 78,11. 12 92,5 102,9. 10 106,15 110,13
sinister (uenter cordis) 92,18 – *subst.* ad -tram 124,8 ([Arist.])
siue 54,16 124,7 ([Arist.]) s. . . . s. 120,7
socius *pl.* (Platonis) 62,13
sol 80,16 84,1
solus *adv.* 96,17 98,9 non -um . . ., sed 96,7 98,6 118,24
sompnium *pl.* 58,7
spatula *pl.* 92,17
species (doloris) 76,7 secundum -em 78,9. 10 – *pl.* 82,11. 12. 14
speculatio 98,18
sperma 64,15 94,10. 11. 14
spina (longitudo) 92,16 (extremitas radicis, cauda) 92,15
spiritus 80,1 92,11bis. 19. 21 112,17 (animalis) 80,10 (anime) 80,2. 11
splen 98,28 102,2. 4
spleneticus *subst.* -i 98,27
stare 118,15 *(f. l.)*
stillea 96,21 → listilia
stomachus 86,20
studere -entes (defectus) 54,19
studium 100,9
stultitia (tenebre) 122,9 ([Arist.])
subiectum 86,26 *(f. l.)*
substantia 62,12 64,23 90,19 92,18. 19 *(f. l.)* 116,19 *(f. l.)* 118,1 (incorporea) 112,16 (operatiua) 114,2 (magis subtilis) 62,11 (anime) 60,3 78,9. 13. 23 80,1. 8 120,2 (scientia anime) 76,25 (propria caloris) 64,15 (deitatis) 58,17 *item* 58,3 (membrorum) 90,4 (complexio membri) 90,7 (*sc.* plantarum) 86,26 (uirtutis) 62,9bis 110,4 (totalitas actiue) 84,11 (totalitas *sc.* medicinarum) 84,22 86, 14 (totalitas *sc.* operationum naturalium) 86,19 – *pl.* 112,4 (corporee) 116,15. 26 (sensibiles) 112,1
subtilis (pars nerui ad modum capilli) 74, 25 (substantia) 62,11
sufficere (alcui) 104,14 -it *c. inf.* 104,12 (alcui) *c. inf.* 82,14 98,11
sufficiens (dictum) 108,27 110,2
sufficientia 108,3 scire secundum uiam -e 56,8 *item* 114,13
sui* 58,2 62,5. 7 88,21 102,5 in se 76,19 in seipsa 68,22 per se 78,9 112,19 118,1 secum 96,12 108,25
sumere 116,22 – *pass.* 62,13. 14 86,7
super *c. acc.* 62,18 92,14. 16 commentum s. librum Ypocratis 94,19 *item* 106,28 sunt exercitati s. libros 56,4 *sim.* 74,1 80,18 82, 4 – *c. abl.* locutus sum s. hiis 96,9
superare 68,2. 9. 24 100,14
superhabundantia (colerarum et fleumatis) 98,11
superhabundare 64,7 70,23 98,16 (ab alqa re) 60,19 (in alqa re) 64,14. 23
supracelestis (corpora) 62,18 *(v. l.)*
surgere 122,21 ([Arist.]) -endi 110,9
suscitare *pass.* 122,21 ([Arist.])
suus* 56,6 58,9 70,2. 5 78,20 82,13 *i. q.* eius, earum 54,6bis. 8. 12. 15 56,10 88,5 92, 12
syllogismus → sillogismus

tactus 102,22
tamen 62,1 78,14 non t. 92,3 etsi . . ., t. 78,2
tamquam 88,11
tantus -um . . . quantum 76,22 quanto magis minus . . ., -o deterior 66,11 – *adv.* 84,4 92,11. 19 94,23 96,6 116,18
temperamentum 68,2. 14 (complexionis) 90,6 (ignis terre aque et aeris) 62,20
temperantia (prima) 64,10 (caloris) 64,9
temperatus complexio inuenietur -a inter caliditatem et frigiditatem 68,23
tempus 116,1 (longum) 80,19 – *pl.* (anni) 68,20 70,13 (senectutis) 70,15
tenebre (stultitie) 122,8 ([Arist.])
terra 54,7 62,18 80,16 (motus) 84,1 temperamentum ignis -e aque et aeris 62,20

tertius 60,12 66,17 82,10. 15 (dictio) 70,3
testa *pl.* 106,19
testimonium conuocare in -um 56,6. 7 *item* 54,17
timere 108,9 (de alqa re) 74,17 (quod) 54,16 *c. inf.* 108,8
tonitrus dispositio -ui 82,19
totalitas (*sc.* commixtionis) 116,12 (substantie) 84,11 86,18 (proprietas substantie) 84,21 86,14
totus 70,4. 7 (Hipp.) 74,15 80,16 100,23 102,21 104,26 106,17
trahere 122,7 ([Arist.])
transire 54,7 92,13. 16
transmittere *pass.* 90,2
tres (dictiones) 62,4 64,3 (genera prima febrium) 66,16 (loca) 82,14 (motus) 60,11 82, 7. 9 (principia) 82,7 84,6 90,13. 17 (species) 82,11. 12. 14
tribuere 100,23
tristiuus †108,18
tu 72,4 74,1 102,17 110,19
tunc cum ..., t. 78,20 124,5 ([Arist.])
turbatio 100,17 (*f. l.*)
turpis -e est *c. inf.* 94,3
turpitudo 82,1. 2

uadere 60,16
ubi 122,16 ([Arist.])
uehemens (alteratio) 118,14
uel 56,3. 14 74,2 84,9 86,12. 17 88,14 94,22 96, 6 98,10 106,20 118,15 uel ... uel 80,19/82,1 84,18/19 92,19 98,27/28 uel ... uel ... uel ... uel 84,15sq. → aut, utrum
uelle 54,11 78,24bis 80,4 98,20 114,28 120,10 (quod) 60,8 68,10 70,12 96,12 *c. inf.* 76,21 82,17 84,4 90,14 104,11 122,11 ([Arist.]). 12 ([Arist.])
uena 74,26 92,24 102,2. 3 (pulsatilis) 92,15 – *pl.* 90,3 92,7. 10 96,8. 20 100,14. 23 102,6 (non pulsatiles) 92,12 (pulsatiles) 90,1 92, 11. 13. 20 94,6 (congregatio) 92,25 (pulsus) 90,8
uenenum *pl.* 86,2
uenire 88,16 92,9. 11. 13. 26 (ad complementum) 56,1
uenter (sinister *sc.* cordis) 92,17 – *pl.* (cordis) 92,18
uentriculus *pl.* (cerebri) 80,12. 13
uentus *pl.* 70,8 (Hipp.)
uer 68,20 (complexio) 68,22 70,13
ueraciter 62,21 90,12 92,20 114,18
uerbum -i gratia 84,22 96,21 – *pl.* (*sc.* Berthenis) 54,15
uerisimilis (dictum) 92,3 (sententia) 96,1 est -e (quod) 92,22 98,9
ueritas 80,19 (amator) 80,16 (uia) 124,10 ([Arist.]) in -te 80,16
uero 54,10 62,18 64,1 88,21
uersificator Berthenis u. 54,6. 9. 14
uersus *pl.* 54,9. 14 (*sc.* Berthenis) 54,6 (sententia *sc.* Berthenis) 54,8. 12
uerum 76,1 96,2
uerumptamen 66,25 68,1. 7. 22 72,26 76,21 80,17 90,5 102,11 104,20 110,13 114,2. 17 118,1
uerus 62,15 (*f. l.*) 100,3 108,8 (dicta) 104,23 (notitia) 114,24 116,6 (probatio) 114,19 – *subst.* -um 70,20 – *comp.* (sententia) 96,2
uesica *i. q.* uesica urinaria 92,14
uia (recti) 124,6 ([Arist.]) (*sc.* uenarum pulsatilium) 92,12 (ueritatis) 124,10 ([Arist.]) secundum -am sufficientie 56,8
uidere* 58,13 78,4 110,6 (quod) 56,10 58,16. 17. 22 60,1 92,8 94,21. 22 96,6 108,19 *c. acc. c. part.* 92,24 *c. acc. c. inf.* 54,20 – *pass.* 58,11 (*e corr.*) (michi conuenibile) 78,2 -tur (quod) 54,19 (michi quod) 108,7 (michi) *c. inf.* 76,26
uincere 68,11
uinum fex in -o 100,18
uiolentia (magna) 98,4
uir *pl.* 82,3
uirtuosus scire de scientia -a 56,8
uirtus 62,5bis. 8 72,15. 23 80,16 (*f. l.*) 86,24 88,12 90,1. 18. 20 96,11 102,18 108,15. 18 (appetitiua) 62,10 (appetitiua, expulsiua, retentiua et digestiua) 108,16 (attractiua) 120,17 (digestiua) 62,6. 10 (operatio digestiue) 62,7 (expulsiua) 62,11 (mirabilis) 58,15 (motiua uoluntaria) 72,14 (naturalis) 86,24 102,17. 18 (natura naturalis) 90,4 (principium regitiue) 62,3 (retentiua) 62,7. 10 (sensitiua) 72,14 120,25 (deitatis) 56,20 (*sc.* deorum) 58,9 (alteratio) 72,20 (dispositio) 88,16. 19 (natura) 88,19 – *pl.* 56,21 62,15 80,16 (*f. l.*) 90,18 114,4 (incorporee) 112,2 (naturales) 62,16 (*tit.*) 88,10 100,22 (*tit.*) 120,15 (substantia) 62,10 110,4
uita 78,21 (*sc.* Berthenis) 54,6 (dispositio) 118,9
uiuere 86,26
ultimitas (frigiditatis et siccitatis) 78,19 in -te 118,23

ultimus *subst.* in -o 56,3
uniuersalis *adv.* 60,1
unus* 66,21. 22 70,3 84,4. 9 86,12. 16 96,9 -um elementorum 64,6 *item* 64,10 68,12 96,2. 7 u., alter ..., tertius 82,10. 15 -um ..., secundum ..., tertium 60,12 *sim.* 84,9 – *subst.* -um ... aliud 78,8 u. ..., alter 54, 8 – *i. q.* aliqui 58,10 74,24
unusquisque 72,16 80,4 86,21 88,17 96,17 102,5. 12 110,18 unaqueque sententiarum 82,4 *item* 60,16 82,12 86,23 88,2. 4 96,4. 10. 19 102,6 112,3 – *subst.* u. 110,24 120,9 unumquodque 106,2
uocare *pass.* (uena portanaria) 102,3
uoluntarius (motus) 60,3. 16 108,14 (uirtus motiua) 72,15
uoluntas (amatoris ueritatis) 80,16
uomica 100,19 (*f. l.*)
uomicus (medicine) 96,4
uos 124,10 ([Arist.])
usque 92,16 u. ad 92,17 102,2
ut ut si 98,2 – contingit ut intelligatur 68,12 *sim.* 100,19 *fin.* 88,8 *i. q.* quotienscumque 74,1
uti (alqam rem) 86,9 -endo 98,14
utrum 56,13 60,5 u. ..., nec u. 116,24/27 u. ... aut 56,18 60,10. 11 76,26 78,23bis u. ... uel 56,13 62,9 116,15 u. ... uel ... uel 80,2

ymaginatio (*sc.* Berthenis) 54,16
ypostasma [100,17]
yris (dispositio) 84,1

zarolus *pl.* 110,21

E. Index nominum Hebraicorum

(גאלינוס) אני 56,15 58,1. 2. 3. 5. 16. 22 60,1. 5
פרטאגורס 58,2

F. Index verborum Hebraicorum

אבל 58,4 60,4
אדם בני אדם 58,17. 23 60,1
אות 58,14
אחר אחריו 56,14. 15 אחר שחשבו 58,13 מאחר שאני 56,15
אי אי אפשר 56,22
אי זה 56,19
אין אין אני אומר 58,1 item 58,16 אני איני יודע 58,2 אין דבר 56,14 אין לי ידיעה 56,12. 15. 17 58,4 60,5
אלא 56,22 58,3
אלהי הכחות האלהיים 56,20 58,18
אלהים 56,20
אמנם 56,20
אמר 56,12 58,2 אני אומר 56,15 58,1. 4
אניה pl. 58,12
אפשר אי אפשר 56,22

באר המבואר 56,16
בחירי התנועה הבחירית 60,3
בטח יבטחו 58,14
בן בני אדם 58,16. 23 60,1
בעל בעלי חיים 58,7 60,4
ברא הבורא 56,23
ברור ראיה ברורה 58,15

גִדֵּל לגדלם 58,19
גוף 56,18 זולתי גוף 56,19

דבר *res* 56,14 אין דבר 56,14 – pl. 56,16
דת 58,20

הוה מהווה 56,13
הִלֵּל להללם 58,19
הצלה 58,12
הרכבה הרכבת בעלי חיים 58,6
השגחה (sc. השם) 58,10

זולתי זולתי גוף 56,19 זולתי מקבלת המות 60,7

חוב יחייב 58,19
חוץ מחוץ 56,14
חיים בעלי חיים 58,7 60,4
חלום pl. 58,8
חשב 58,13

ידה אני מודה 60,5
ידיעה 56,12. 16. 17 58,4 60,5
ידע 58,17 imperf. 60,6 יודע 58,3. 5. 22. 23
יחס מיוחס 58,1
ים 58,12. 13

יצר היוצר 56,17 יצורים 58,10
ירד היורדים בו (sc. הים) באניות 58,12
ירה יורה 58,15 יורו על 58,9 מורים 56,23
יש 56,13 כל מה שיש בזה העולם 56,18 יש לנו 58,22
ישע ויושעו 58,15

כח 58,10. 15 – pl. 56,21 הכחות האלהיים 56,20
58,18
כי 60,1 זה כי 58,23
כל 56,17 58,3. 23 60,1. 5
כמו 56,16 58,2. 23
כן כל שכן 60,6 כמו כן 56,17 על כן 56,23 58,18
כפי 58,19

מות מקבלת המות 60,7
מחלה 58,11
מעשה מעשי השם 58,9
מצא נמצא 56,21 58,5
מקום 56,19 – pl. 56,19
מת 60,6

נזק יזיק 58,16
ניחוש 58,7
נפלא 58,16
נפש 58,22 60,4bis
נשג ישיגו 60,3

סבה 60,2

עולם 56,13. 18. 22
עונן עוננות 58,8
עיקר כל עיקר 58,3
ענין 58,3
עצם עצם הנפש 60,4 item 58,17 בעצמם 58,4

פֹּעַל pl. 56,21 58,6bis

צד מצד 56,22

קִבֵּל מקבלת המות 60,7
קרא קוראים לסבה . . . נפש 60,1

ראה 58,18 – imperf. 58,7. 11. 14 אני רואה 58,16
60,1
ראיה ראיה ברורה 58,15 ראיית החלומות 58,8
רגש ההרגש 60,3
רפא 58,10

שבר השבר (בים) 58,13
שם השם ית׳ וית׳ 58,9
שקוע ש. בים 58,13

תנועה התנועה הבחירית 60,2

G. Voces Arabicae Latinis litteris scriptae

(al-)istisqā' listilia, stillea
al-khadir, al-khadr elchadir
al-khaṭir, al-khaṭar elchatir
riwāq reuac, reubach *(ind. nom.)*
al-wāfida elguefete
yaraqān iarcan

Bei Fragen zur Produktsicherheit wenden Sie sich bitte an:
If you have any questions regarding product safety,
please contact:

Walter de Gruyter GmbH
Genthiner Straße 13
10785 Berlin
productsafety@degruyterbrill.com